FETAL SECTIONAL ANATOMY
and ULTRASONOGRAPHY

FETAL SECTIONAL ANATOMY and ULTRASONOGRAPHY

LEWIS H. NELSON III, M.D.
Professor of Obstetrics and Gynecology
Associate in Radiology

WALTER J. BO, Ph.D.
Professor of Anatomy

GEORGE C. LYNCH
Professor of Medical Illustration

The Bowman Gray School of Medicine
Wake Forest University Medical Center
Winston-Salem, North Carolina

Cover Design by George C. Lynch

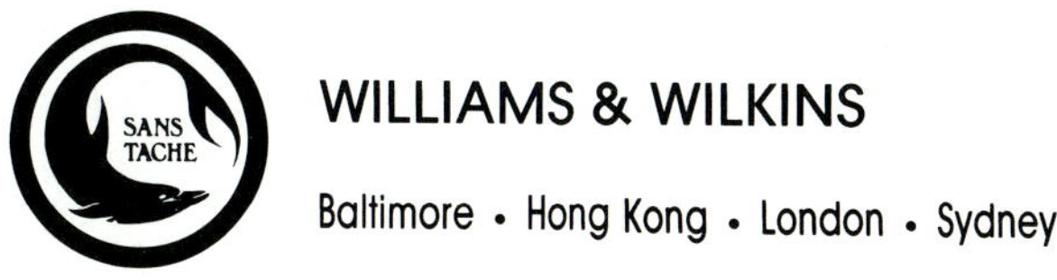

WILLIAMS & WILKINS
Baltimore · Hong Kong · London · Sydney

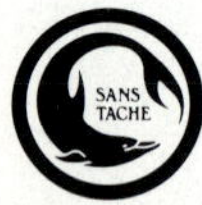

Editor: Carol-Lynn Brown
Associate Editor: Victoria M. Vaughn
Copy Editor: Stephen Siegforth
Design: JoAnne Janowiak
Illustration Planning: Wayne Hubbel
Production: Anne G. Seitz

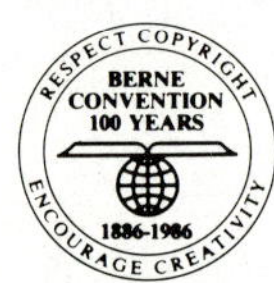

Printed in the United States of America

Nelson, Lewis H.
    Fetal sectional anatomy and ultrasonography / Lewis H. Nelson III
Walter J. Bo, George C. Lynch
    p. cm.
    Includes index.
    ISBN 0-683-06400-2
    1. Fetus—Anatomy. 2. Fetus—Ultrasonic imaging. I. Bo, Walter
J. II. Lynch, George C. III. Title.
    [DNLM: 1. Fetus—anatomy & histology—atlases. 2. Ultrasonic
Diagnosis—atlases. WQ 17 N427F]
RG605.N45 1988
611'.013—dc19
DNLM/DLC
for Library of Congress

88 89 90 91 92
1 2 3 4 5 6 7 8 9 10

To Kenneth R. Gottesfeld, M.D. (1938–1984) and Charles W. Hohler, M.D. (1945–1986) who by their example inspired excellence in learning, teaching, and research in obstetrical ultrasonography.

To Zachary (10/3/86–12/12/86) whose many ultrasound images help make this atlas possible.

To our students and teachers.

Preface

*There are more things in heaven and earth, Horatio,
Than are dreamt of in your philosophy.*
(HAMLET, 1.5.166–67)

With the advent of ultrasonography, magnetic resonance imaging, and computed tomography, knowledge of sectional anatomy has assumed great clinical significance. During the years that ultrasound has been available, operator expertise and technology have increased as partners—advancement in one leading to new discoveries in the other. Improvements in resolution and imaging techniques enable us to see more than we have "dreamt of" in the past. A thorough knowledge of fetal anatomy remains the foundation upon which is constructed the framework of basic ultrasound.

It is not always possible to extrapolate adult or neonatal anatomy to the fetus, especially in early pregnancy. For example, the fetal brain is less developed with few gyri; the fetal liver occupies a considerable portion of the abdomen; and the umbilical vessels, remnants in the neonate, are prominent landmarks in the fetus. Adding further to the difference is the fact that the active fetus is less cooperative than the adult patient, who generally remains in one standard position for imaging studies. Cross sections of this enthusiastic, young patient are composed of fleeting glimpses of oblique sections in which familiar landmarks are often distorted. The purpose of this atlas is to help novice and experienced imagers correlate sectional anatomy with other forms of imaging by using xeroradiography and ultrasound as guides. We accept that imaging techniques will change but submit that anatomy, at least for a relatively long time in human evolution, will remain constant.

Cross sections and sagittal views of fetuses at approximately midpregnancy are used as the basis for the atlas. Since the major changes in growth near term are more in the longitudinal axis, sagittal sections of an anencephalic fetus at 36 weeks gestation are presented. The sagittal sections should facilitate grasping contiguous cross-sectional relationships.

Accompanying many of the anatomical sections are xeroradiographs and ultrasound images. Xeroradiographs have been included to portray the ultimate in the detection of differences in absorption coefficients of tissue and the ultimate in "edge enhancement" of the junction of tissues with different absorption coefficients. Xeroradiography is not presented as a clinical tool in this instance; rather, we offer it as a learning tool. The ultrasound images are similar to the anatomical sections and are from fetuses in utero.

For ease of interpretation, labeling of the anatomical sections has been restricted to main structures, and commentary has been omitted since this is primarily a visual atlas. The gross section appears on the left page with the xeroradiograph and ultrasound on the right page to facilitate comparisons and learning.

Acknowledgments

Few books are ever written without the support of many. The authors wish to express sincere appreciation to: Robert K. Bowden, Anatomy Specialist, for preparing the gross sections; Robert O. Karraker, RBP, for his photography; Charles E. McCreight, Ph.D., Professor Emeritus in Anatomy, and J. Keith Sutton for assistance in labeling the sections; Joan Lincoln, Senior Staff Technician, and Diana Pulliam, RTR, for the xeroradiographs; Jack Dent and the staff of the Audiovisual Department of Bowman Gray School of Medicine; Mary F. Penry, BSRN, RDMS, for ultrasound sections; and ADR Ultrasound/Advanced Technology Laboratories for equipment. Preparation of the atlas was supported by a grant from the Center for Medical Ultrasound, the Bowman Gray School of Medicine.

A special thanks is due Nancy Hunter Nelson, MS, for her graphic arts skills, diligence in proofreading labels, preparing overlays, and tolerance of the senior author during preparation of this atlas.

A Note for Using this Atlas

A suggested study method for the inexperienced sonographer is to look at the atlas while scanning the patient who, also, may enjoy correlating the real thing with the atlas images. The arrow on the line drawing indicates the direction from which the section is viewed. Studying from a picture will not be quite as effective as studying from the ultrasound scan in "real time." Small movements of the transducer help fine tune the scan image to correlate better with the anatomical section in the atlas. If you get lost, return to a known anatomical section and work to the area of special interest, scanning slowly. Frequently the novice scans too fast, missing important features before the brain is able to register their presence.

The experienced sonographer will hopefully be able to find more information in the images than previously recognized.

Enjoy!

Contents

1

CROSS SECTIONS

22-week fetus

Occipital lobe
Dura mater
Superior sagittal sinus
Frontal lobe

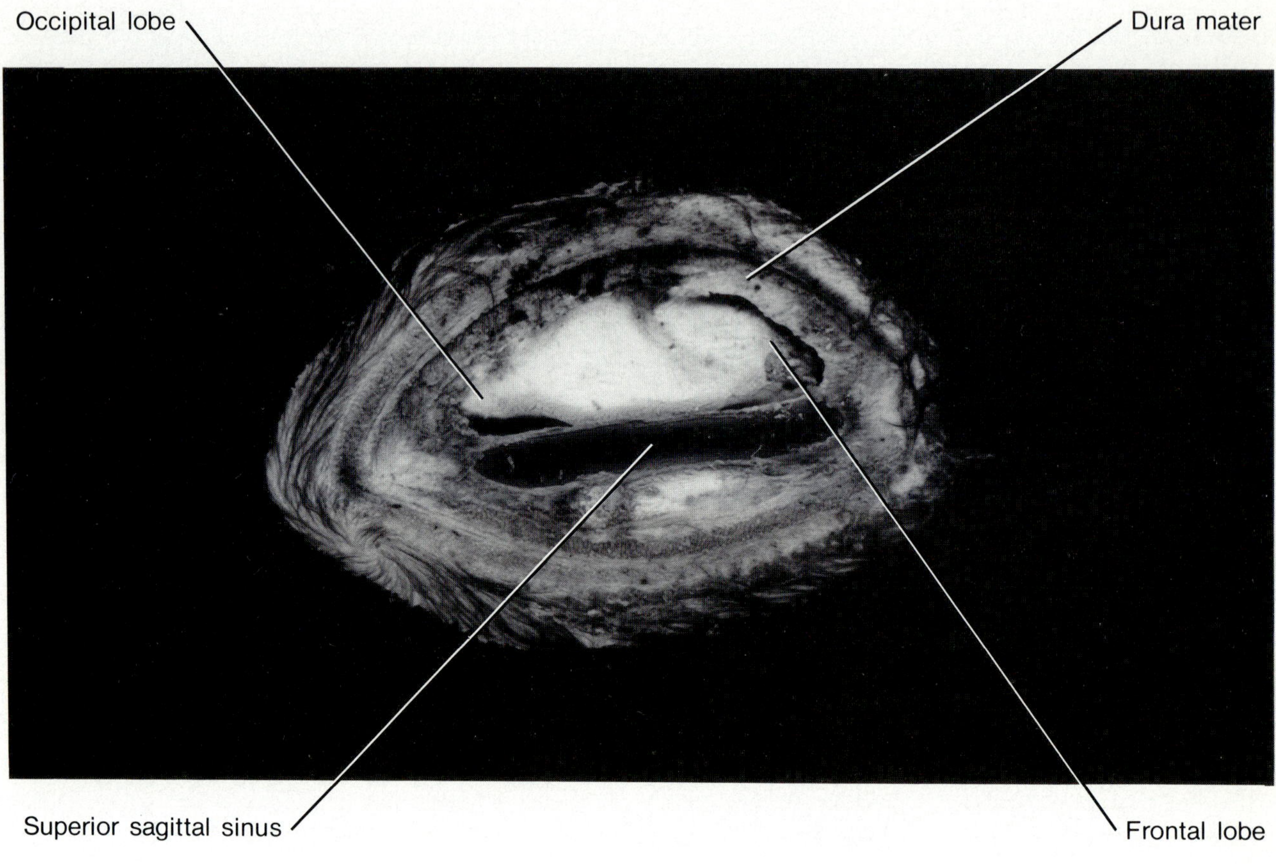

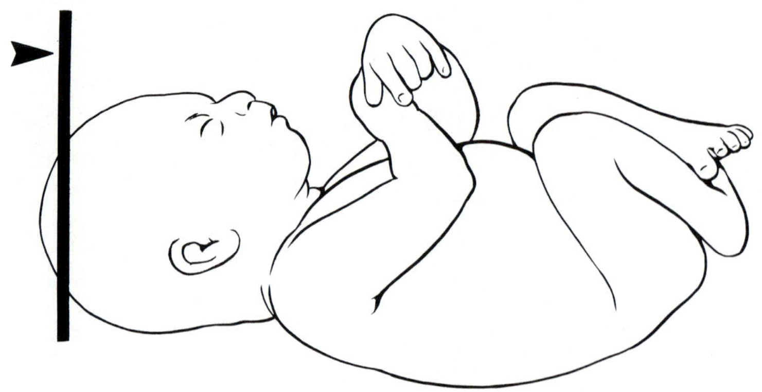

Figure 1.1

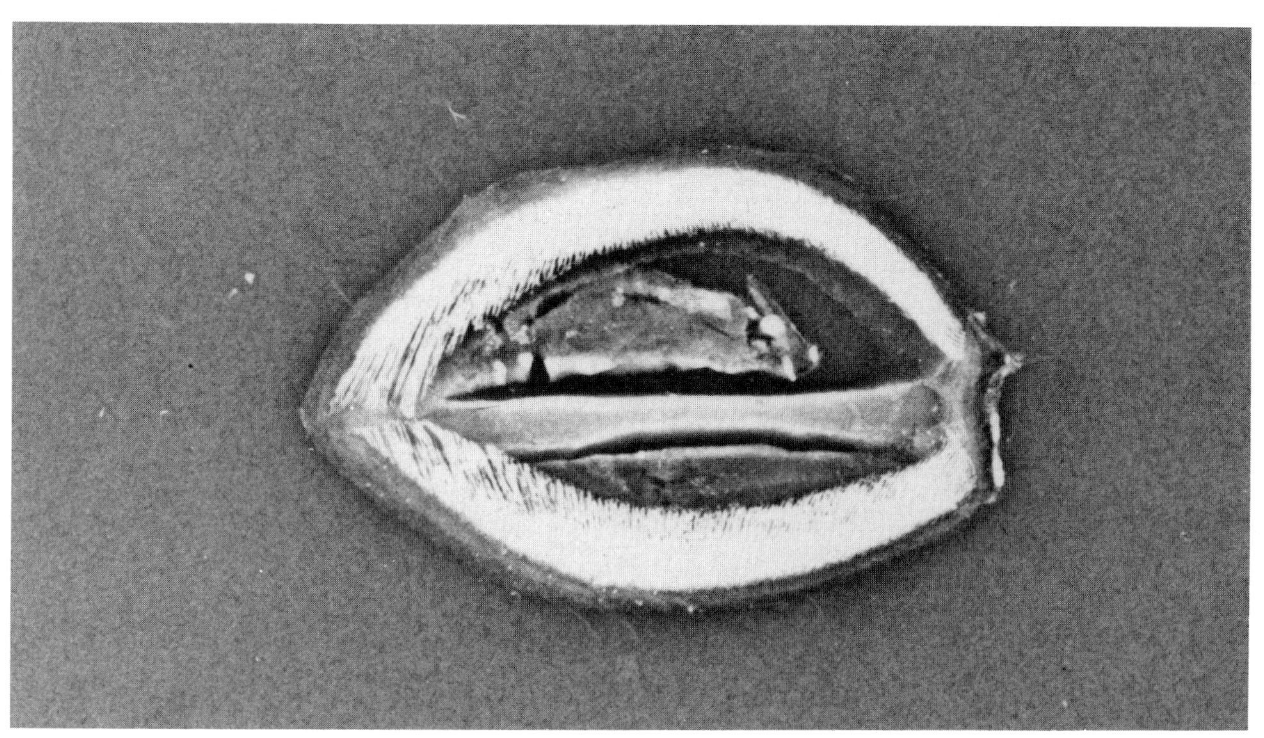

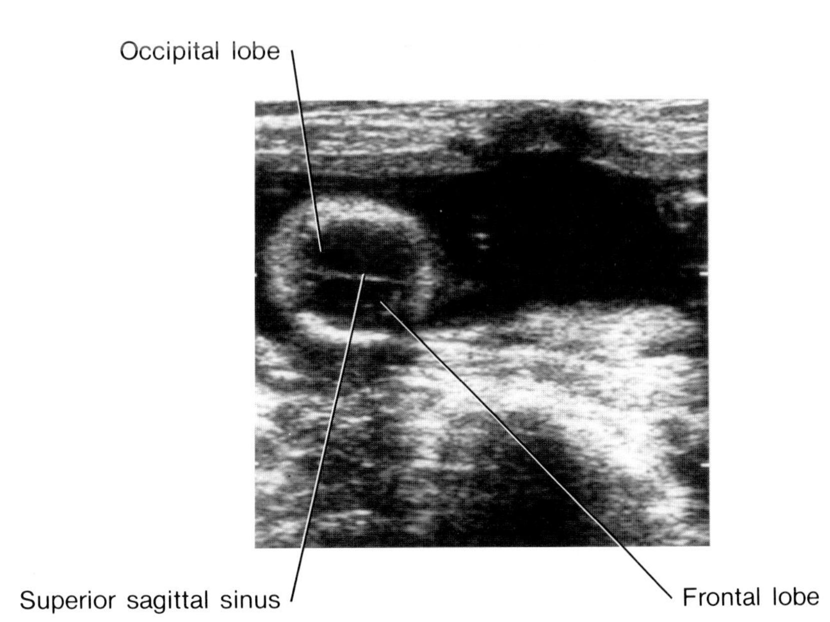

Occipital lobe
Superior sagittal sinus
Frontal lobe

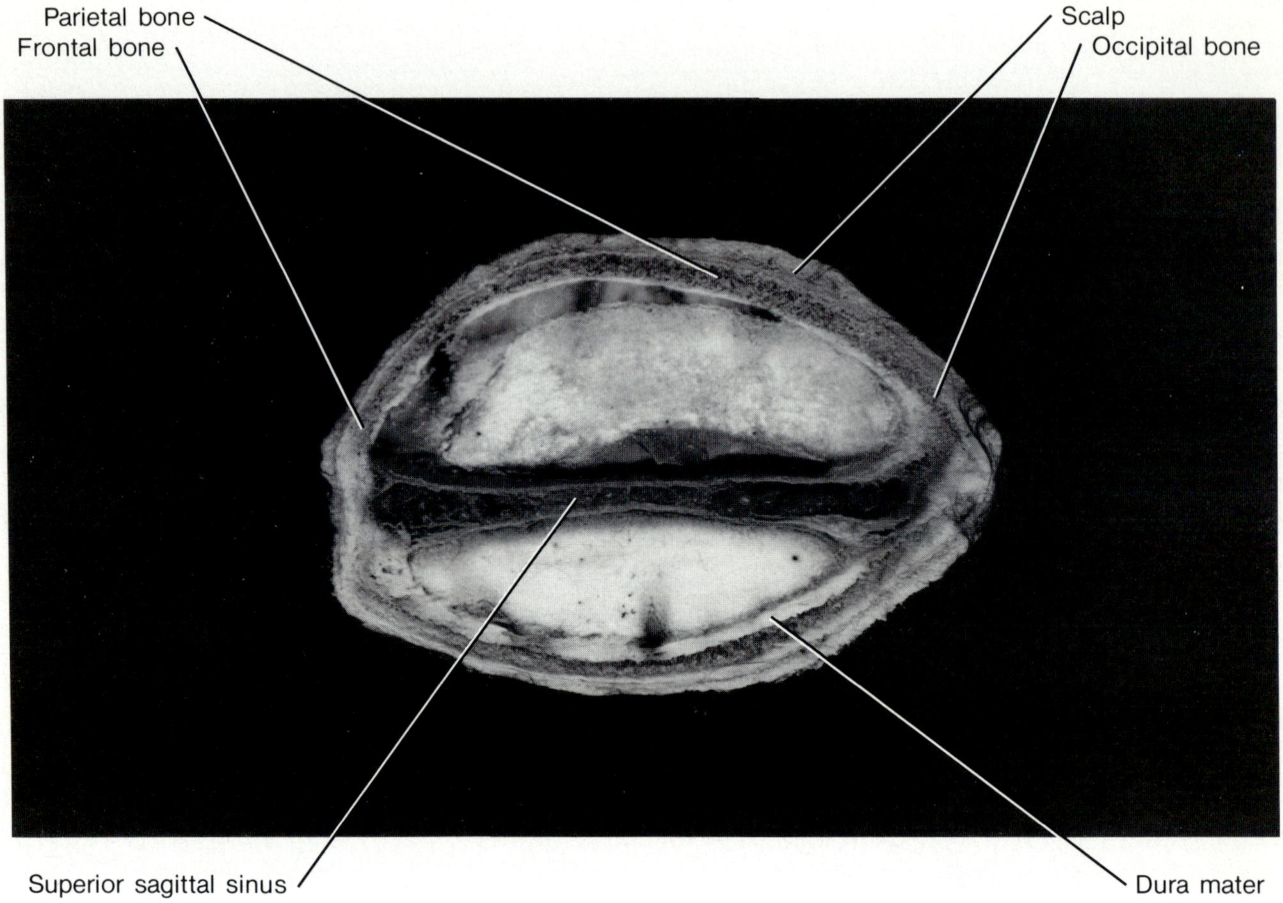

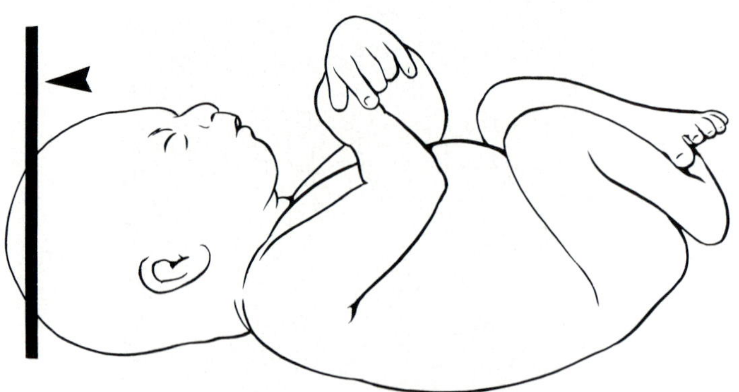

Figure 1.2

    FETAL SECTIONAL ANATOMY AND ULTRASONOGRAPHY

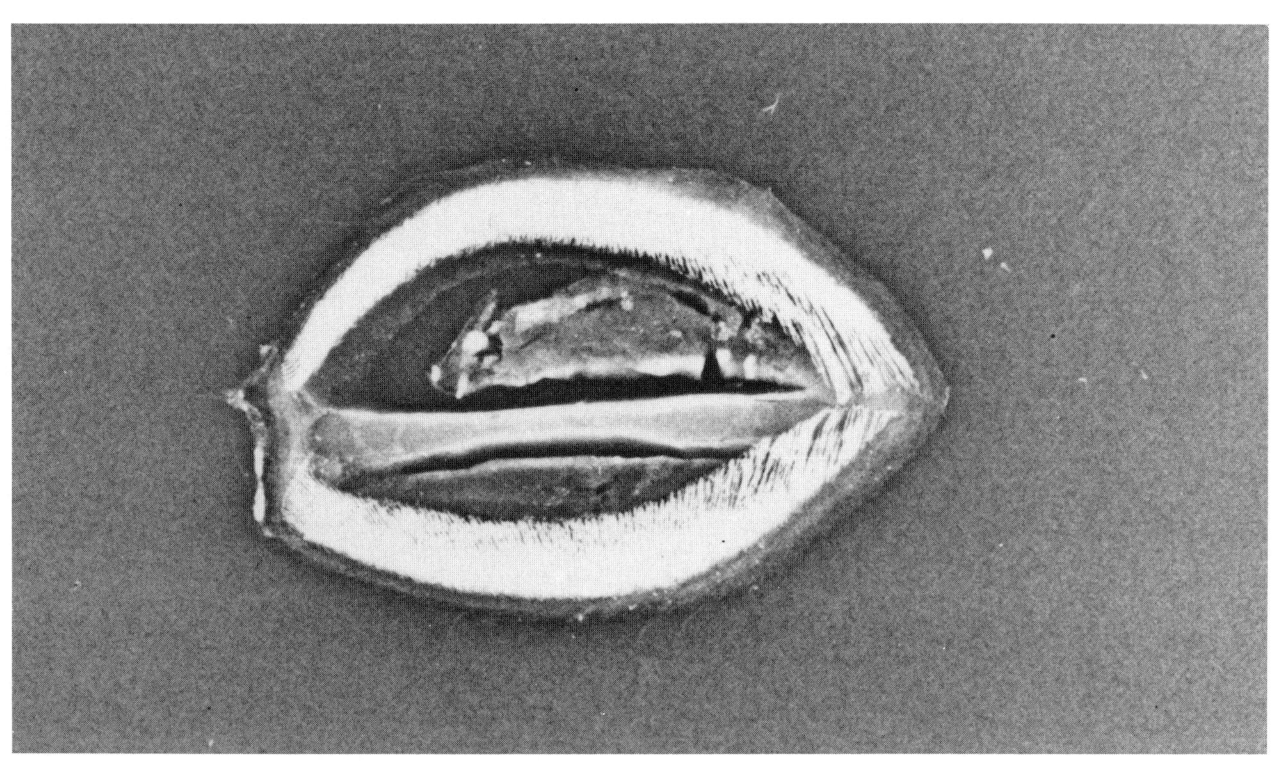

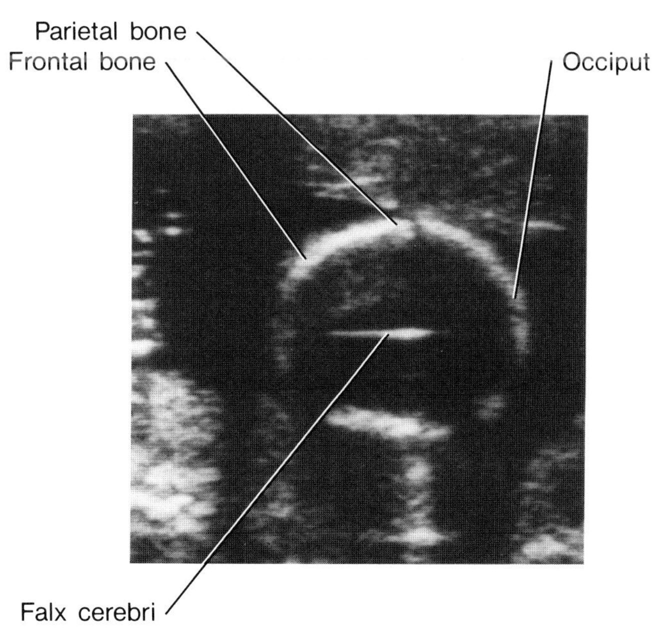

Parietal bone
Frontal bone
Occiput
Falx cerebri

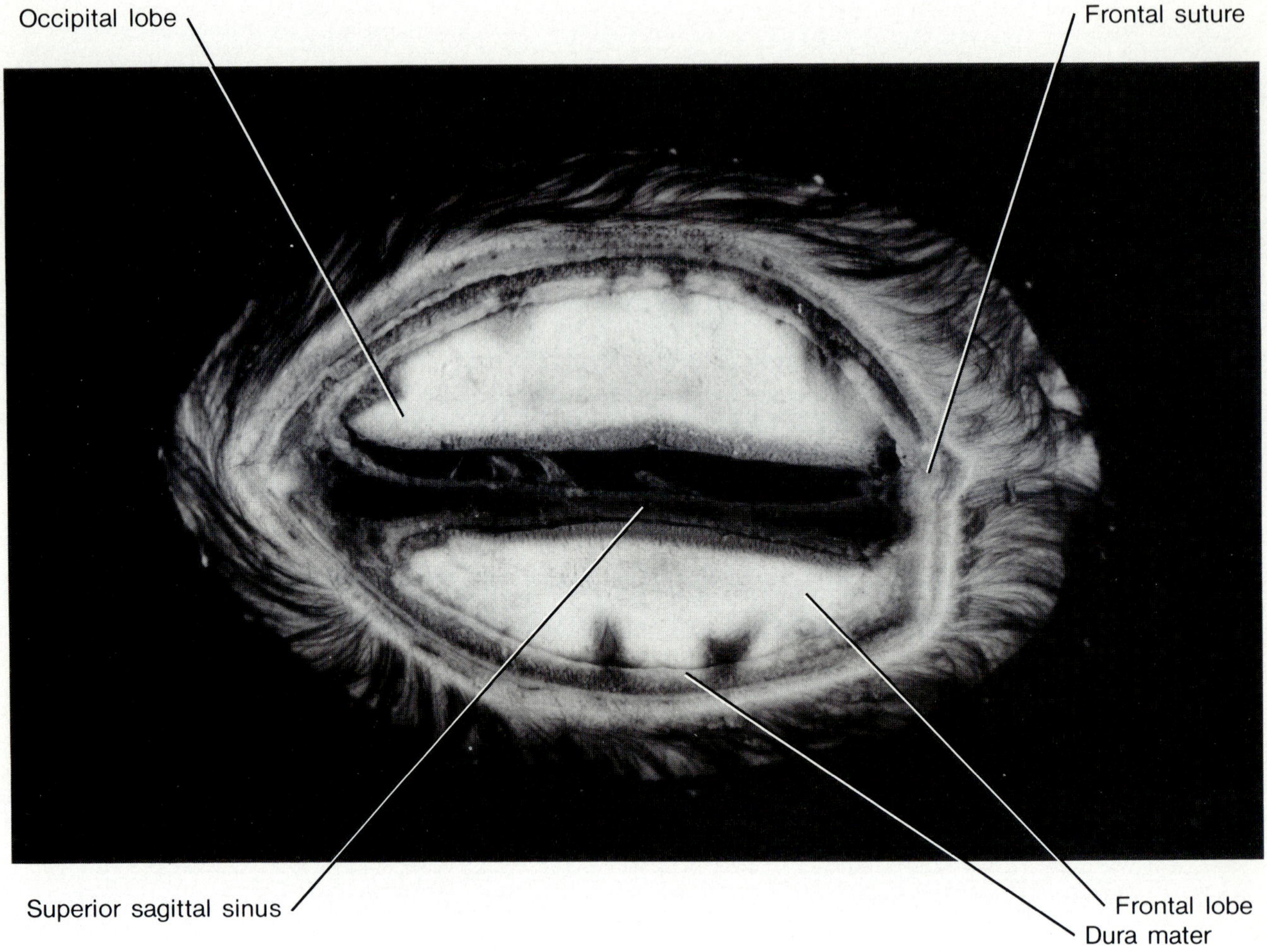
Occipital lobe
Frontal suture
Superior sagittal sinus
Frontal lobe
Dura mater

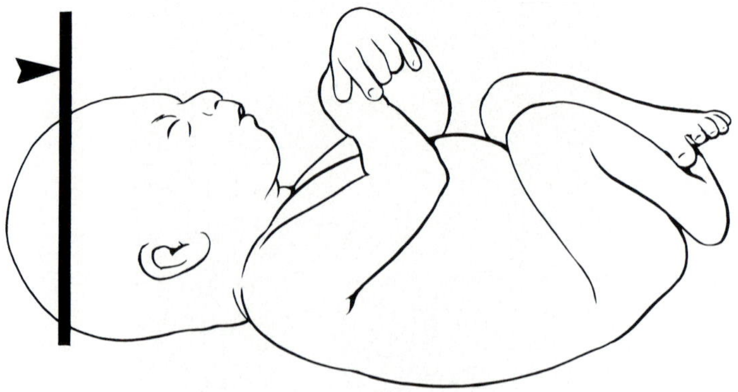

Figure 1.3

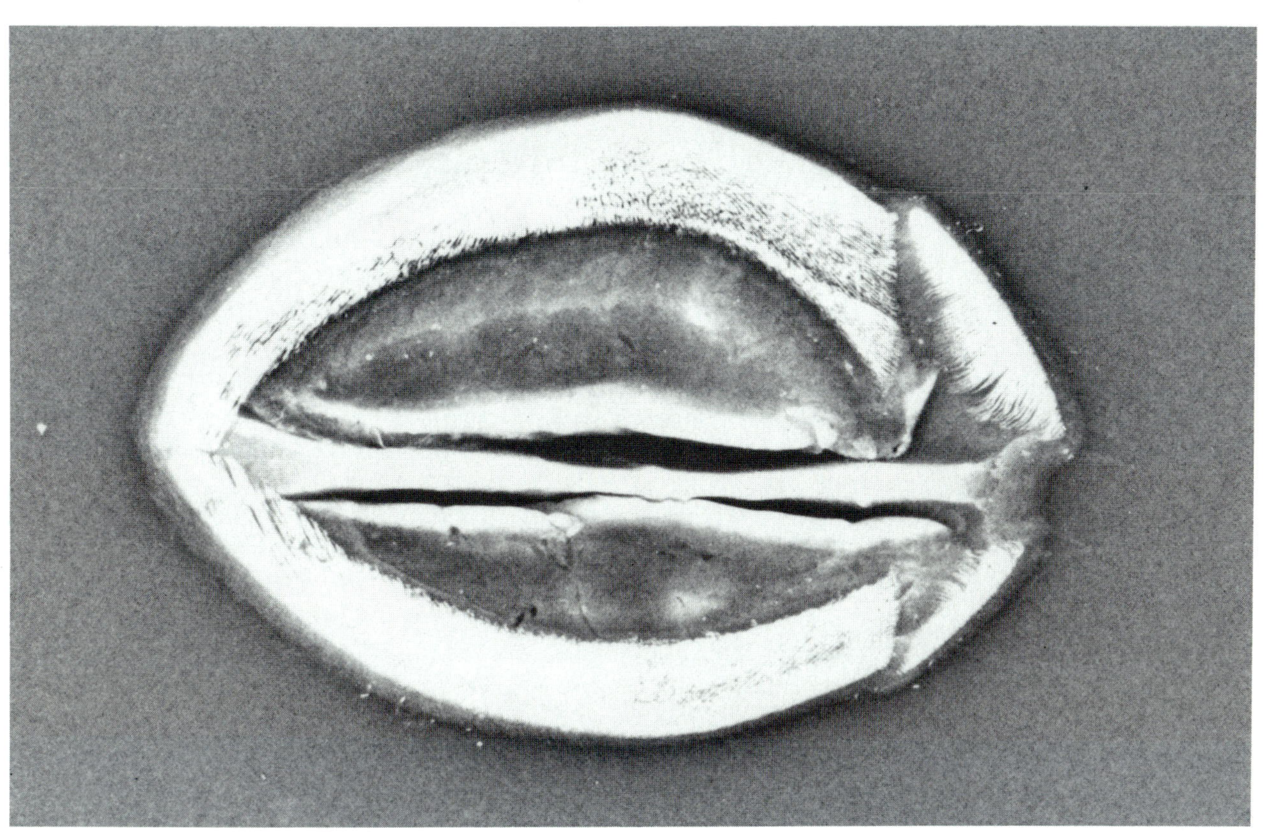

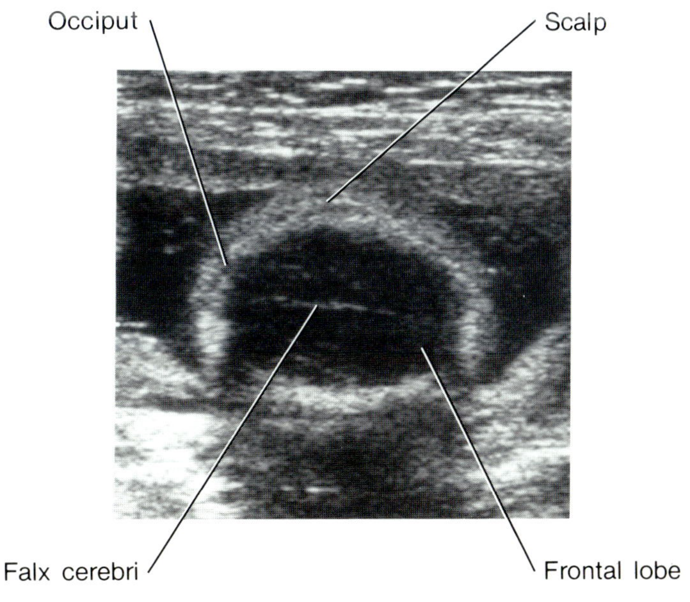

Occiput
Scalp
Falx cerebri
Frontal lobe

Falx cerebri
Arachnoid membrane
Superior sagittal sinus
External occipital
protuberance
Coronal suture
Frontal lobe
Parietal lobe
Central sulcus

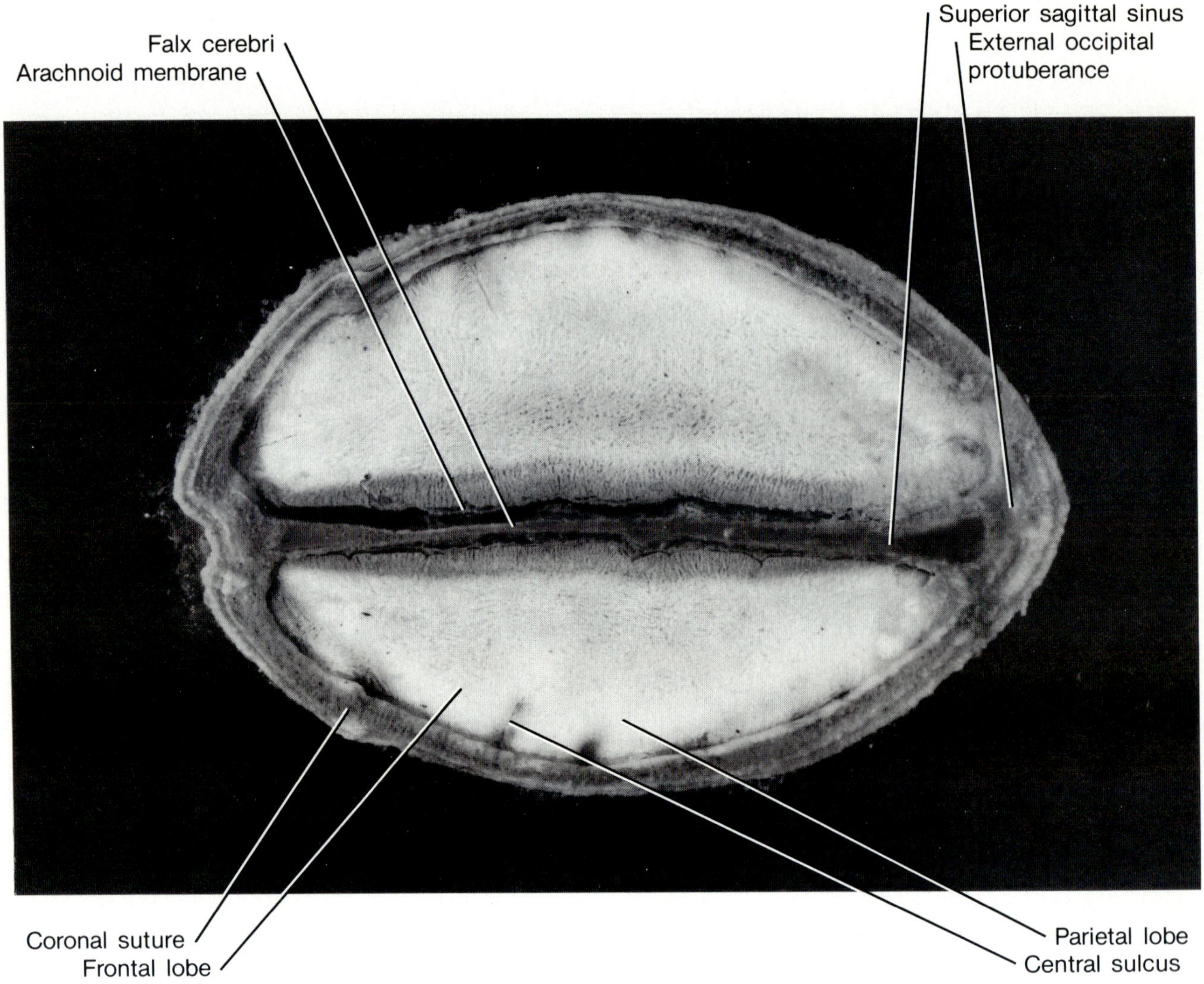

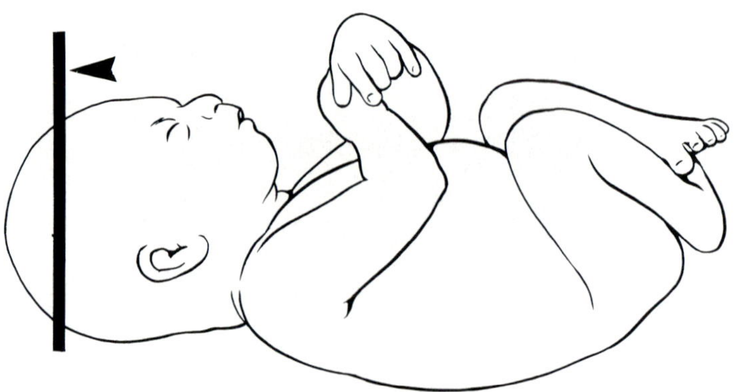

Figure 1.4

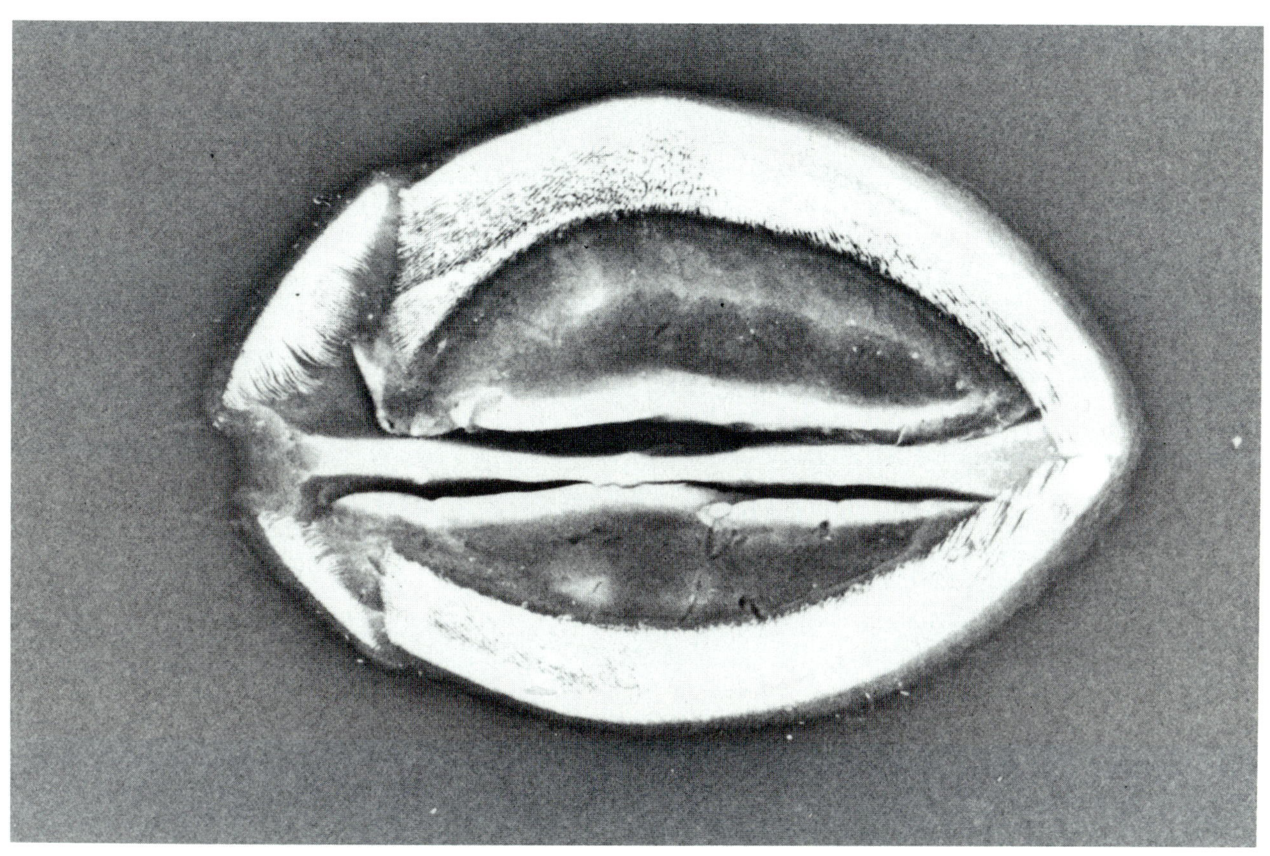

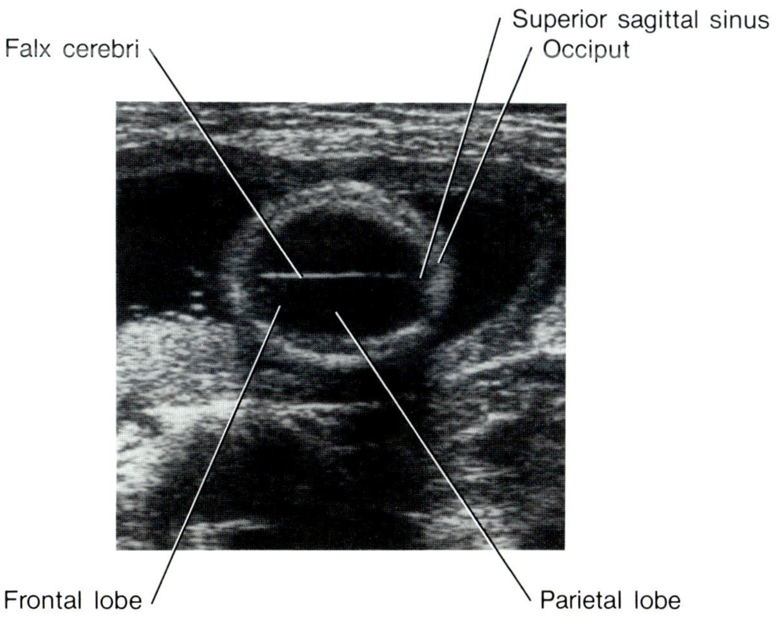

Falx cerebri
Superior sagittal sinus
Occiput
Frontal lobe
Parietal lobe

External occipital
protuberance
Central sulcus
Falx cerebri
Superior
sagittal sinus
Coronal suture
Frontal lobe

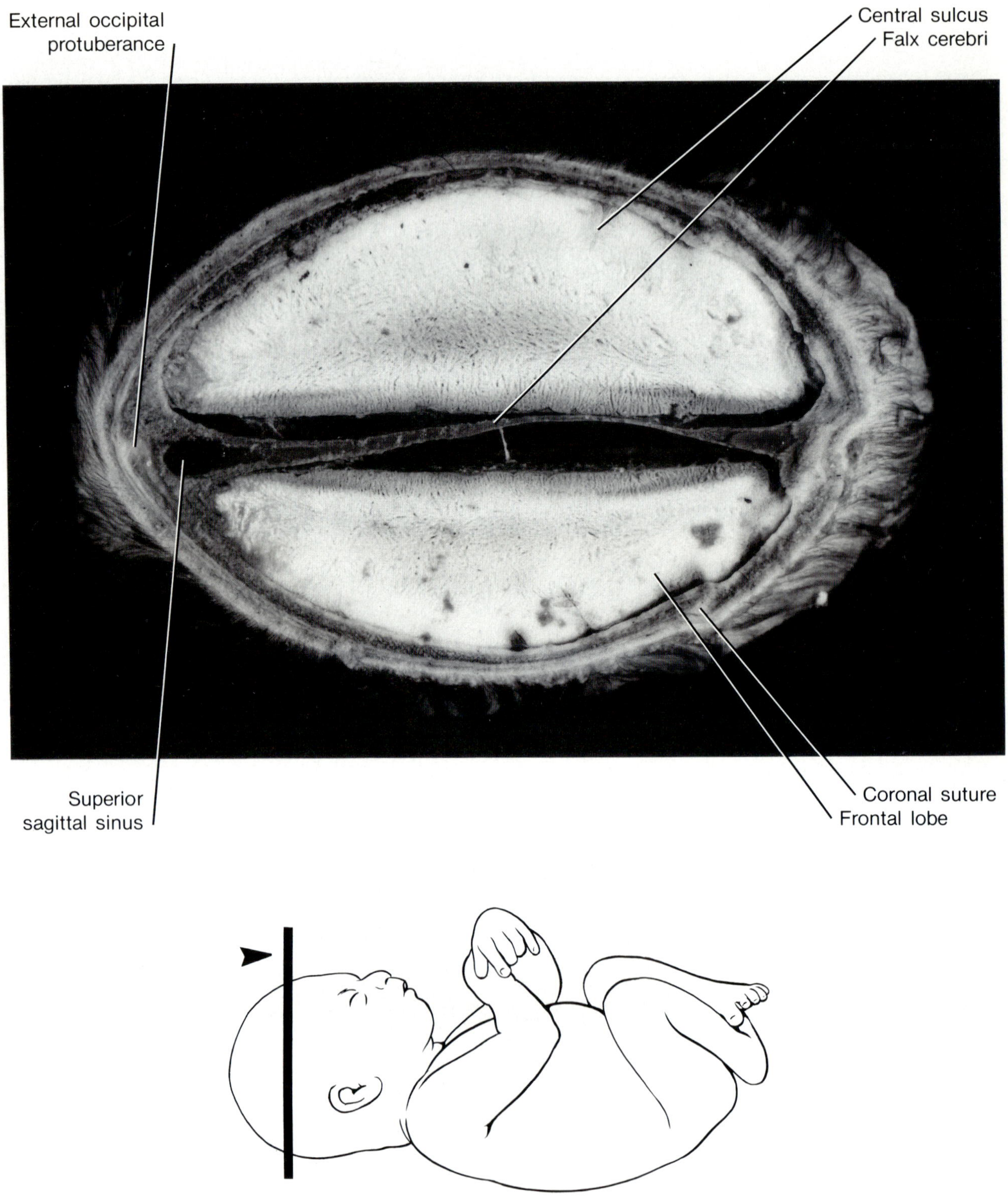

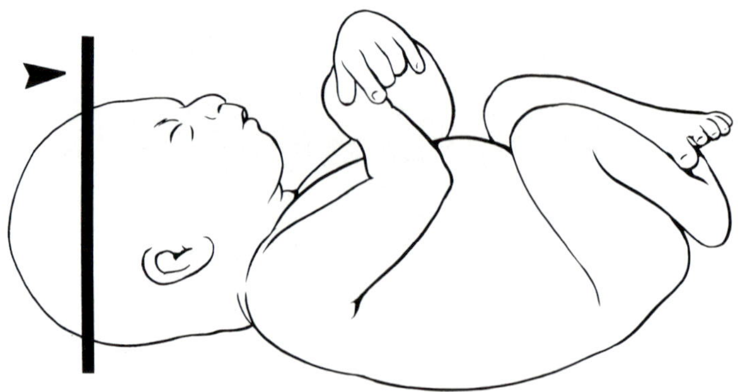

Figure 1.5

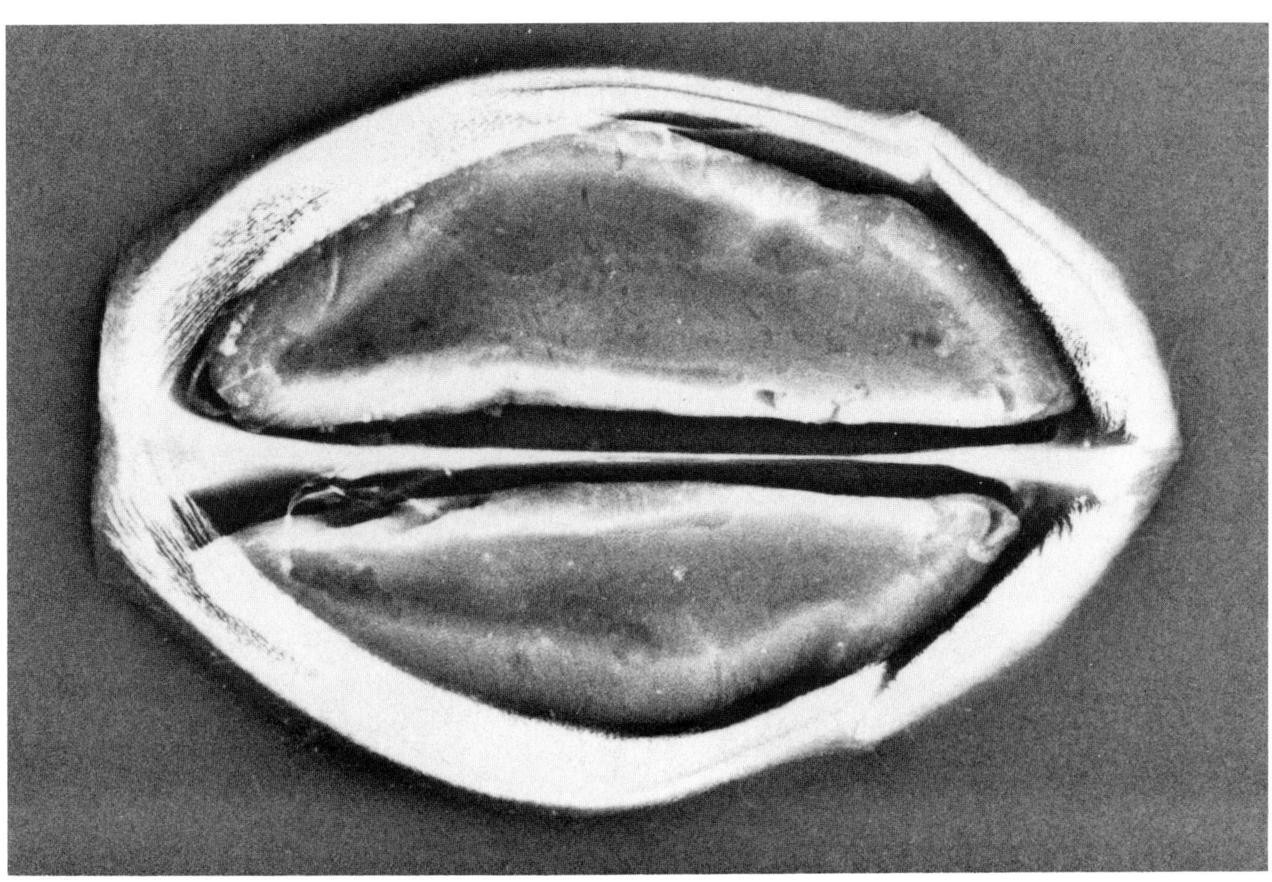

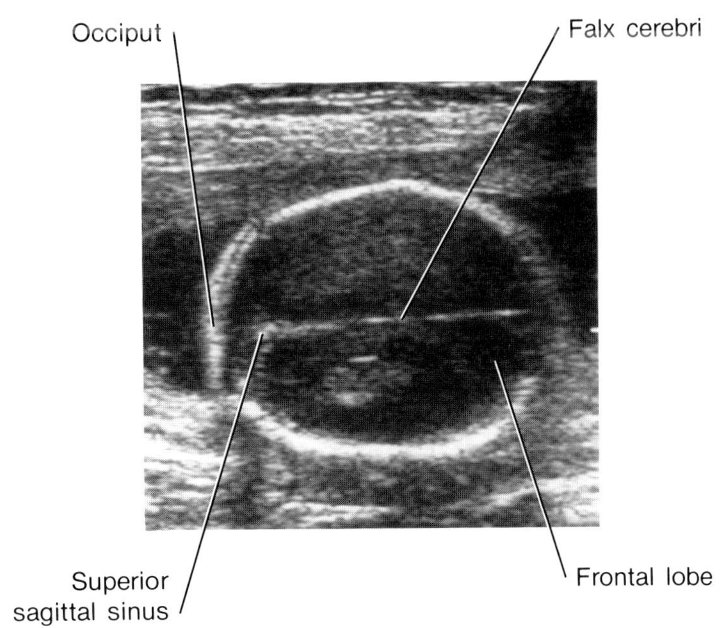

Occiput
Falx cerebri
Superior
sagittal sinus
Frontal lobe

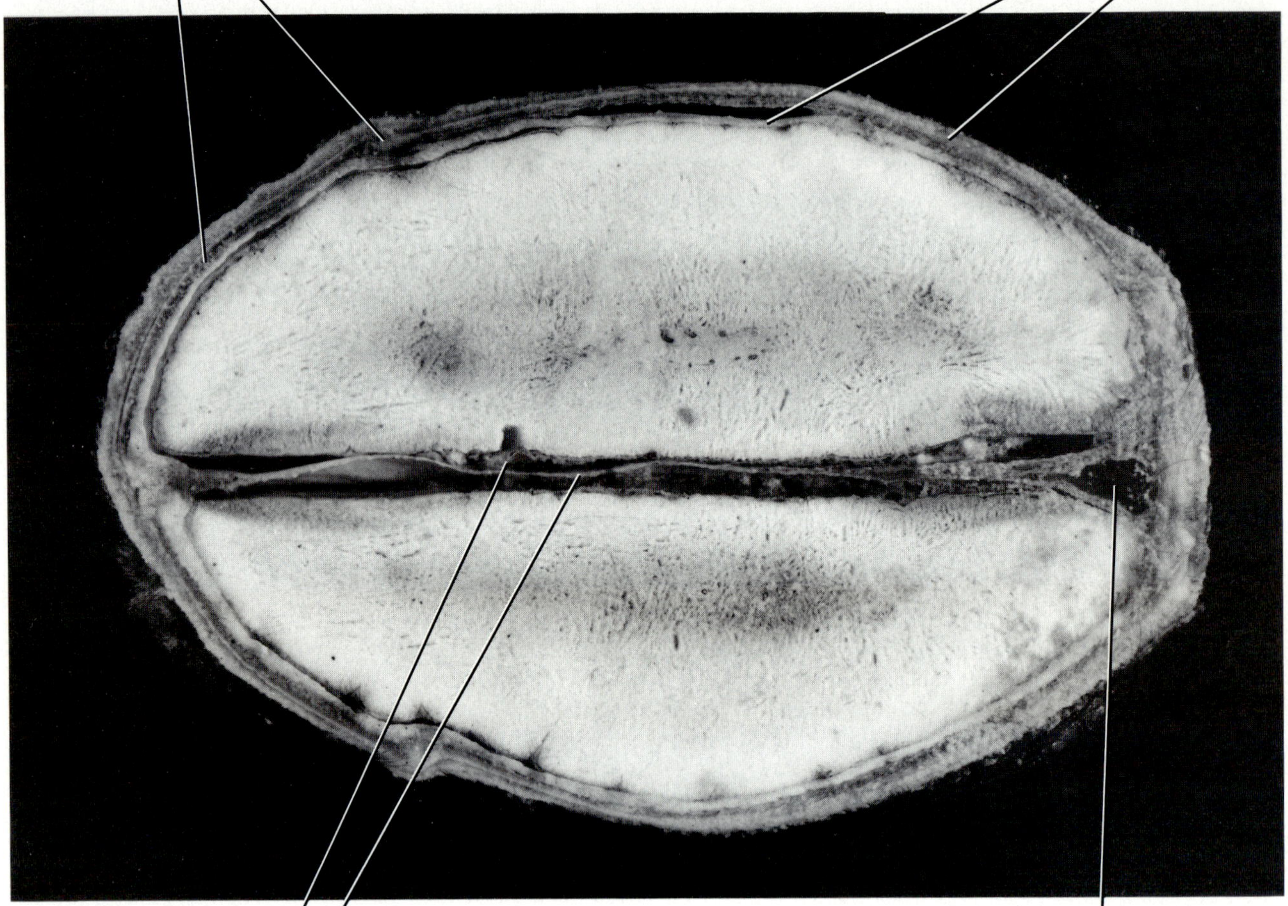
Coronal suture
Frontal bone
Dura mater
Scalp
Arachnoid membrane
Falx cerebri
Superior
sagittal sinus

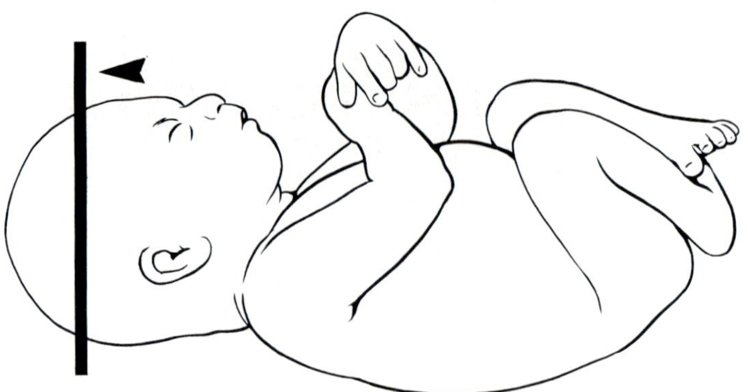

Figure 1.6

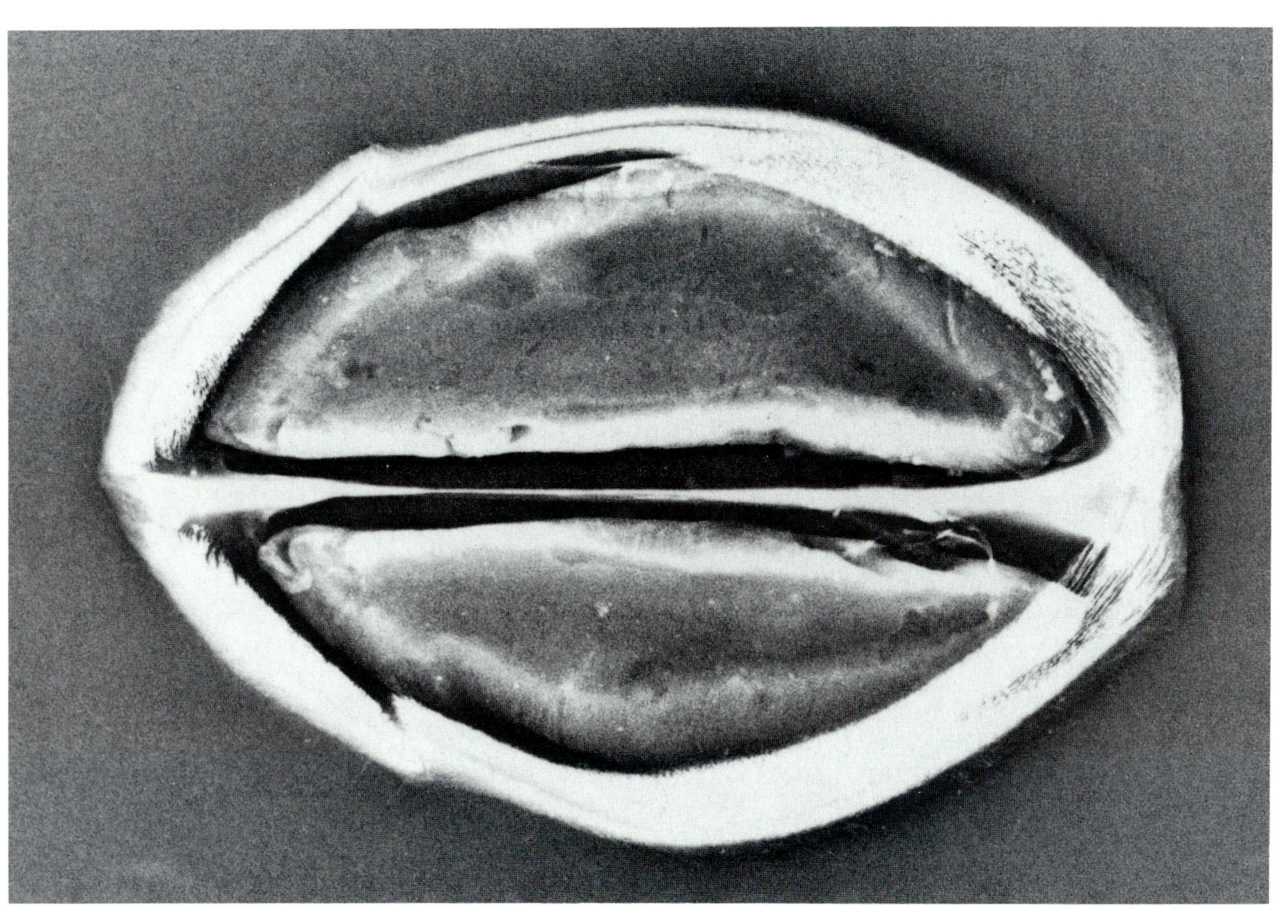

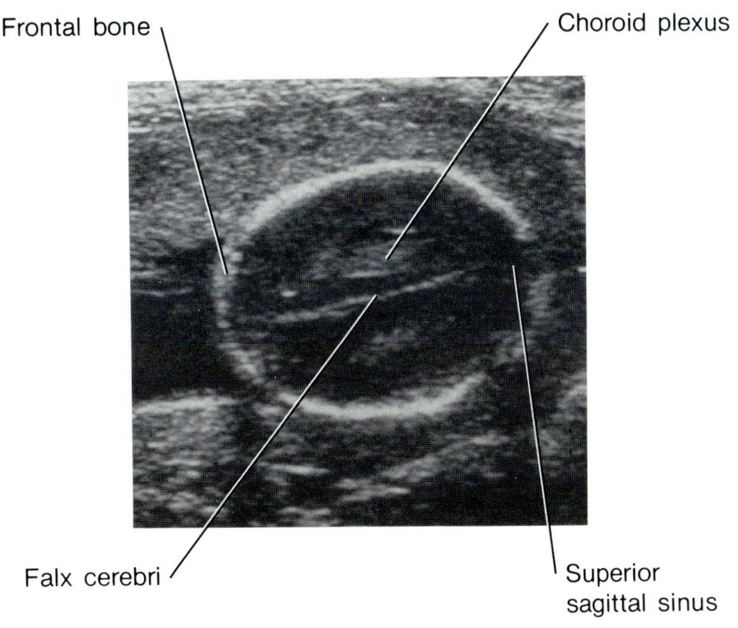

Frontal bone
Choroid plexus
Falx cerebri
Superior
sagittal sinus

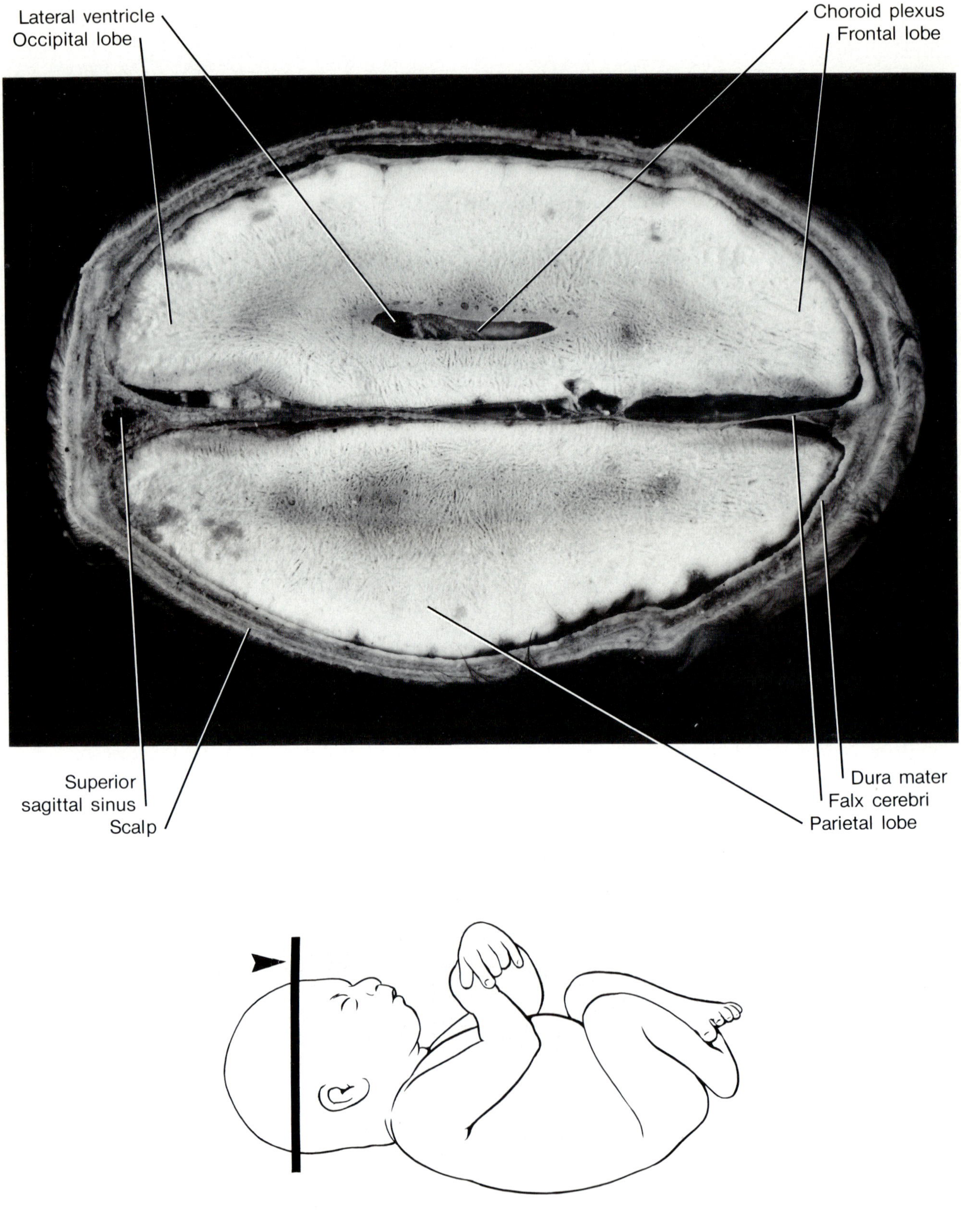

Lateral ventricle
Occipital lobe
Choroid plexus
Frontal lobe
Superior sagittal sinus
Scalp
Dura mater
Falx cerebri
Parietal lobe

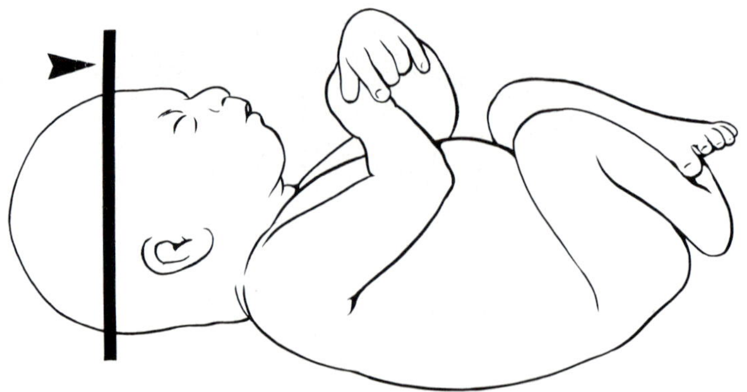

Figure 1.7

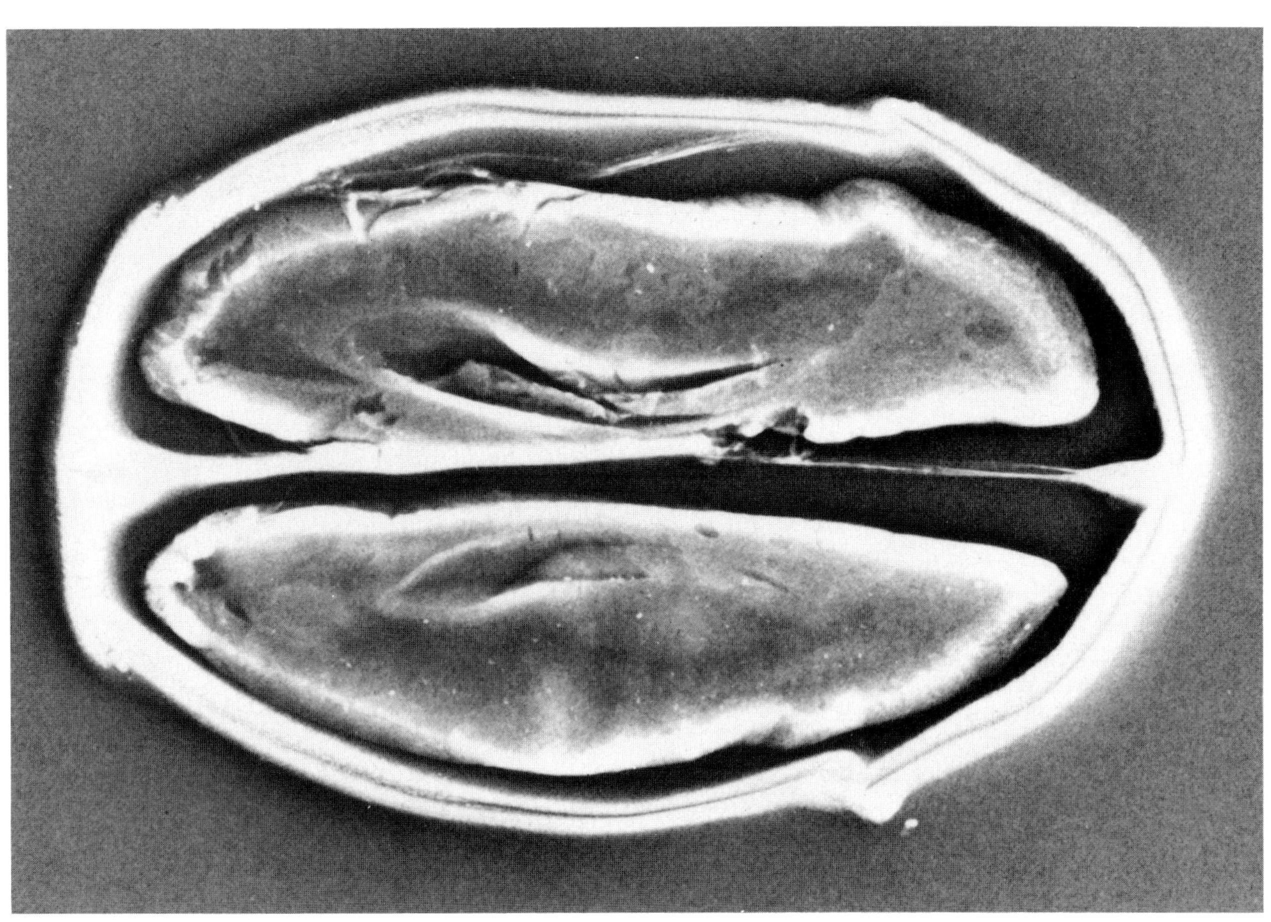

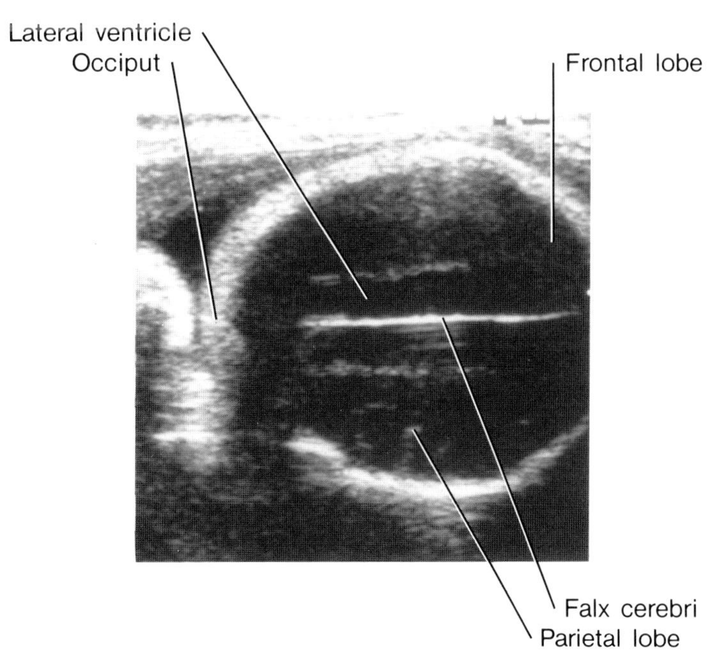

Lateral ventricle
Occiput
Frontal lobe
Falx cerebri
Parietal lobe

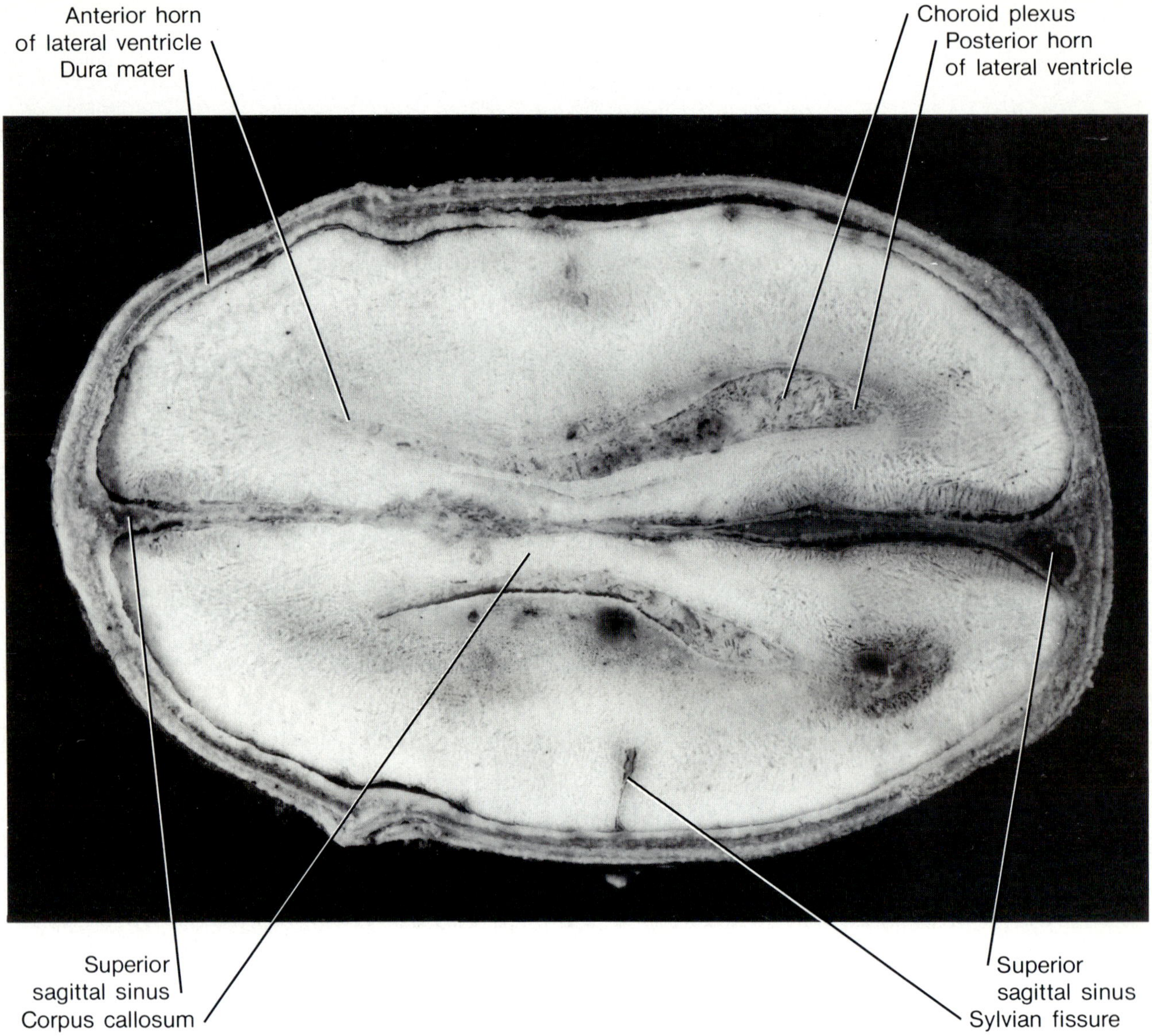

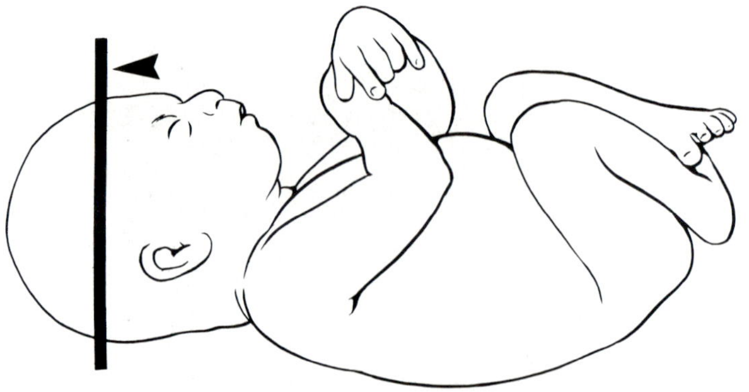

Figure 1.8

     FETAL SECTIONAL ANATOMY AND ULTRASONOGRAPHY

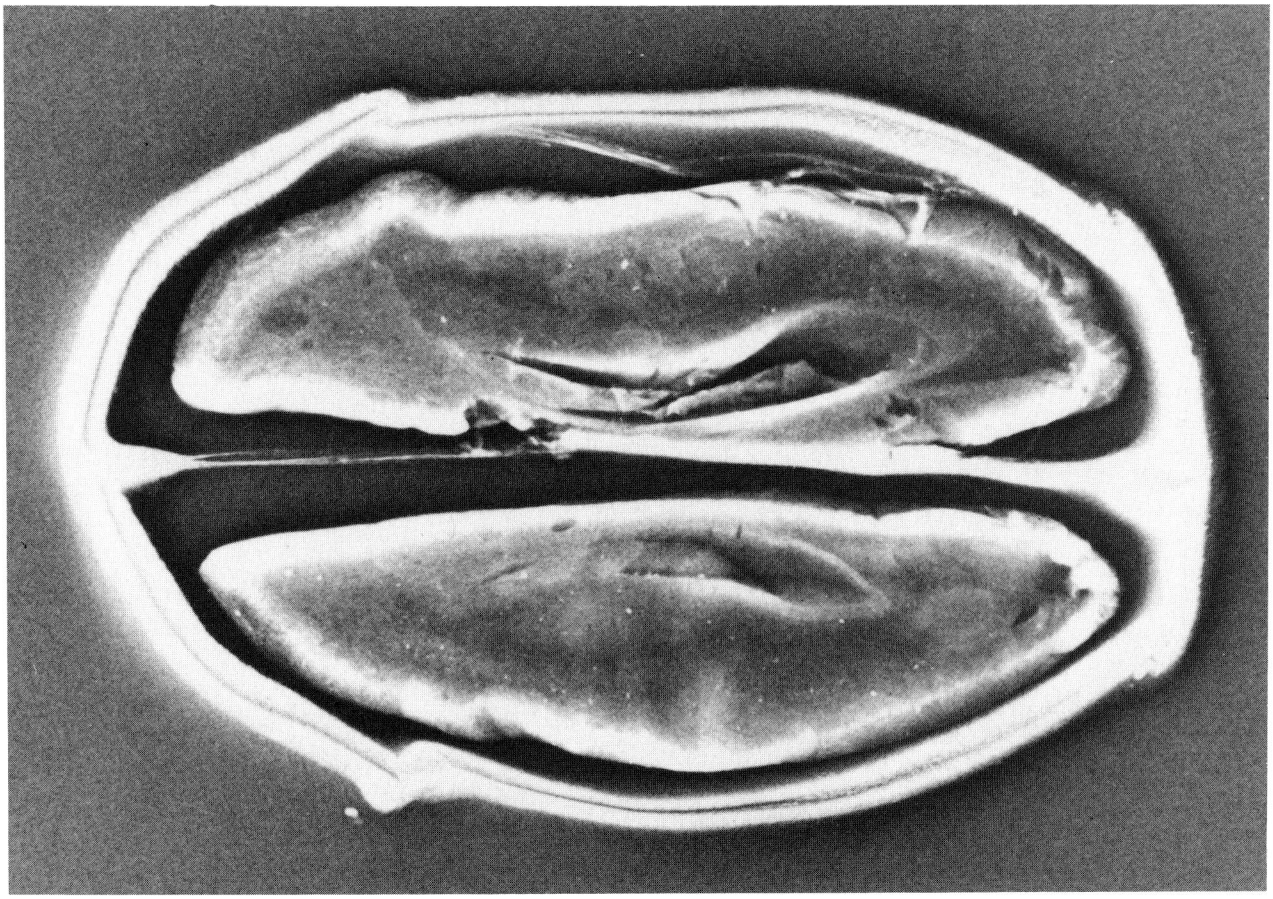

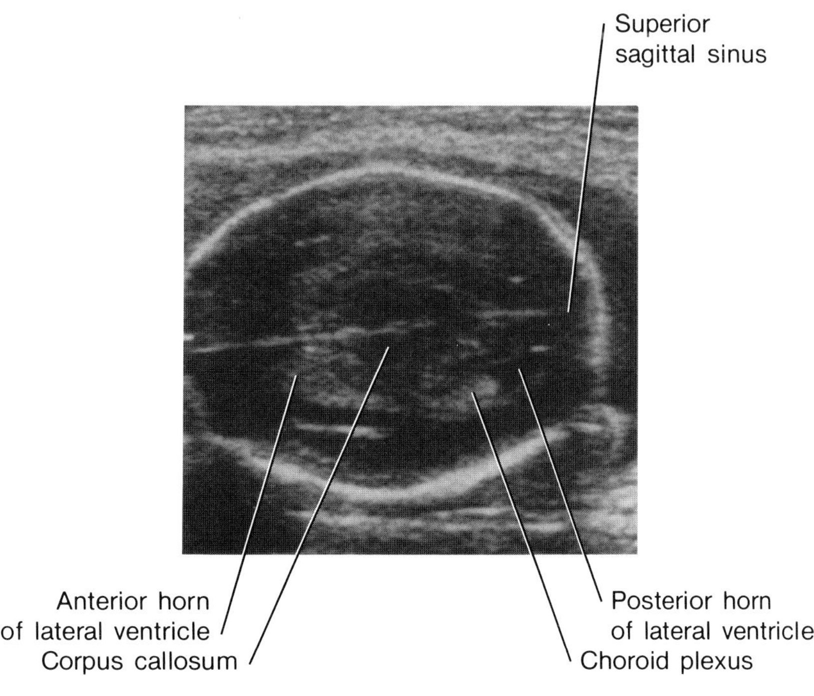

Superior
sagittal sinus
Anterior horn
of lateral ventricle
Corpus callosum
Posterior horn
of lateral ventricle
Choroid plexus

Insula
Dorsal thalamus
Choroid plexus
Posterior horn
of lateral ventricle
Body of fornix
Septum pellucidum
Anterior horn
of lateral ventricle
Superior
sagittal sinus
Falx cerebri
Sylvian fissure
Superior
sagittal sinus
Dura mater
Third ventricle

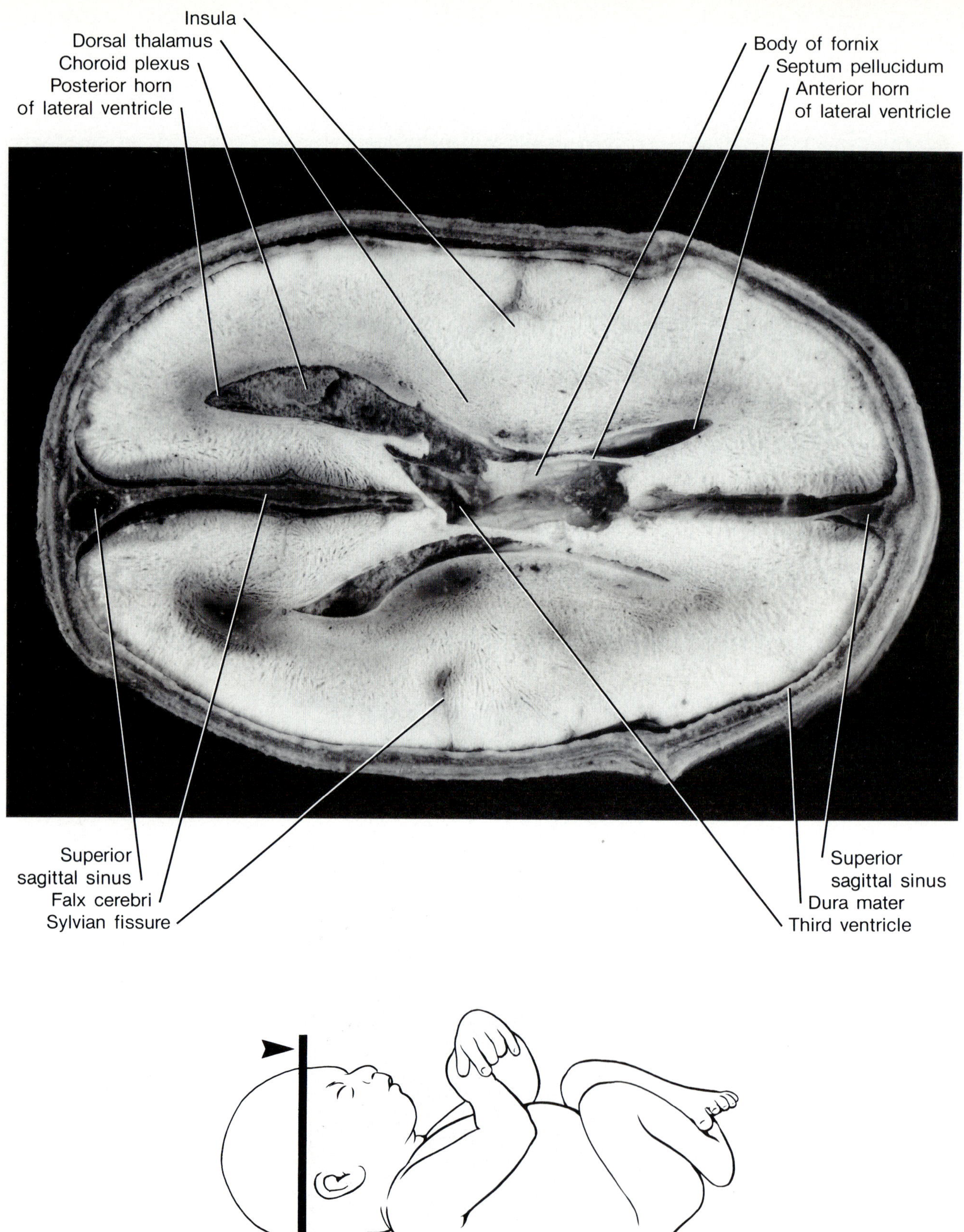

Figure 1.9

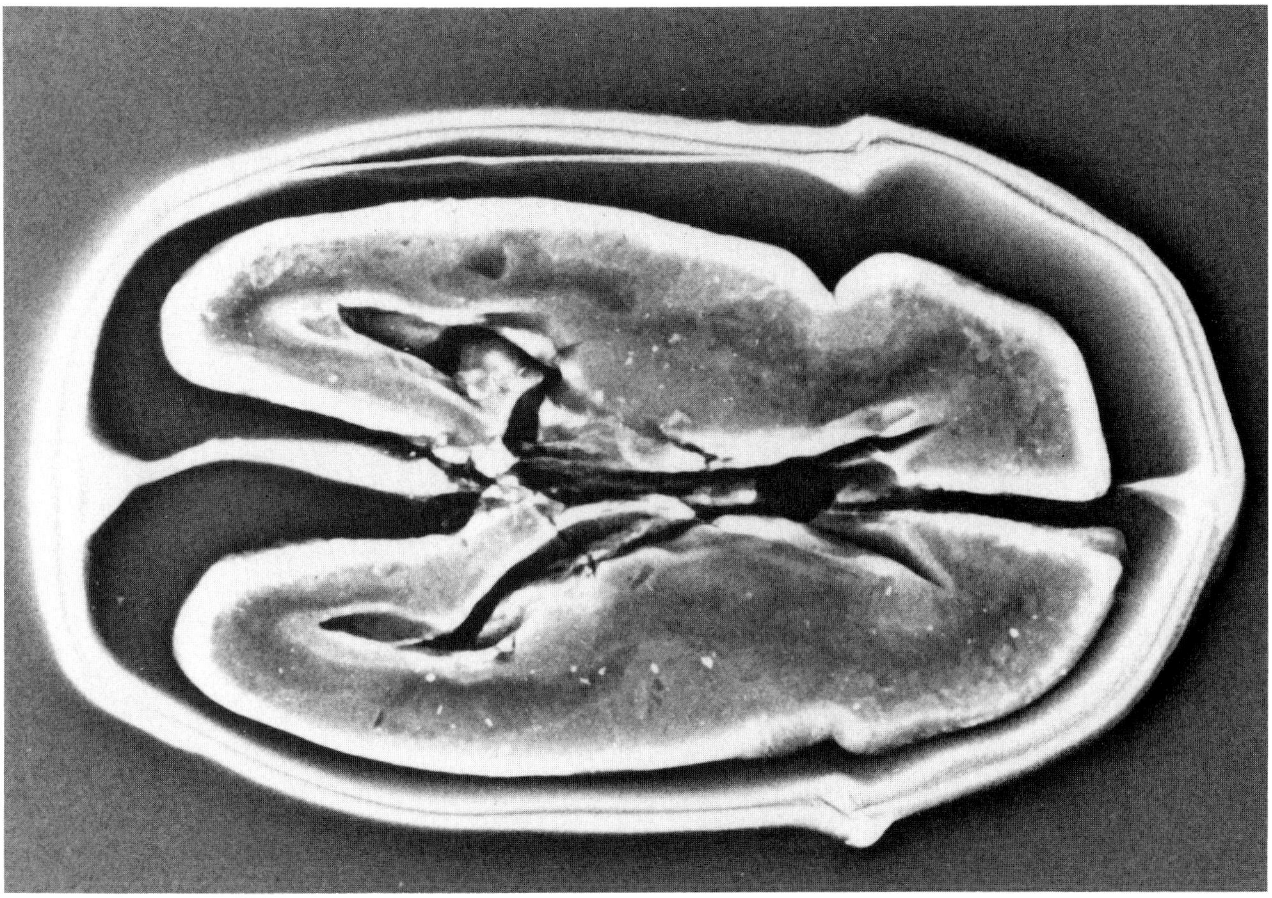

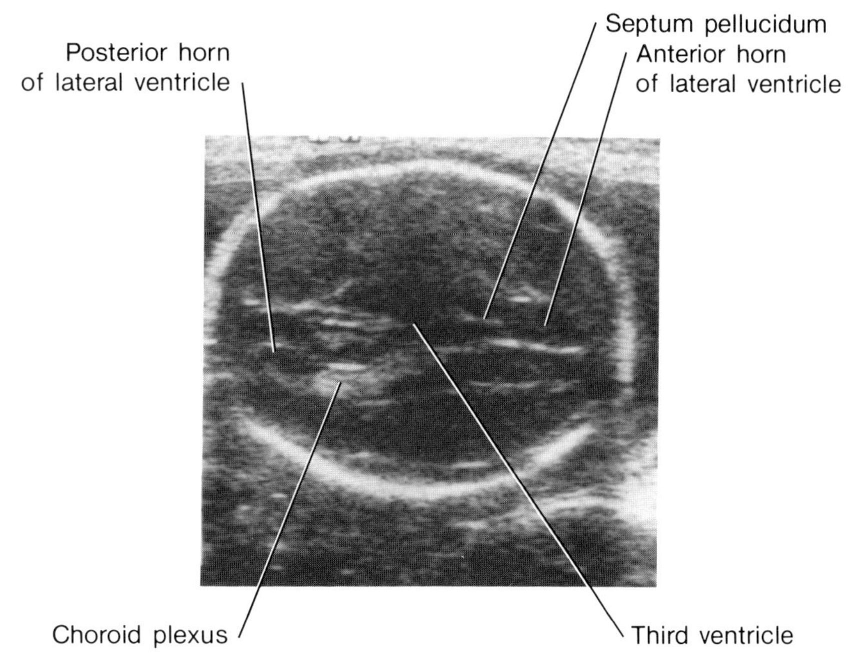

Posterior horn
of lateral ventricle
Septum pellucidum
Anterior horn
of lateral ventricle
Choroid plexus
Third ventricle

Head of caudate nucleus
Septum pellucidum
Anterior horn
of lateral ventricle
Genu of corpus callosum
Internal capsule
Dorsal thalamus
Hippocampus
Falx cerebri
Dura mater
Falx cerebri
Fornix
Sylvian fissure
Superior
sagittal sinus
Third ventricle
Insula

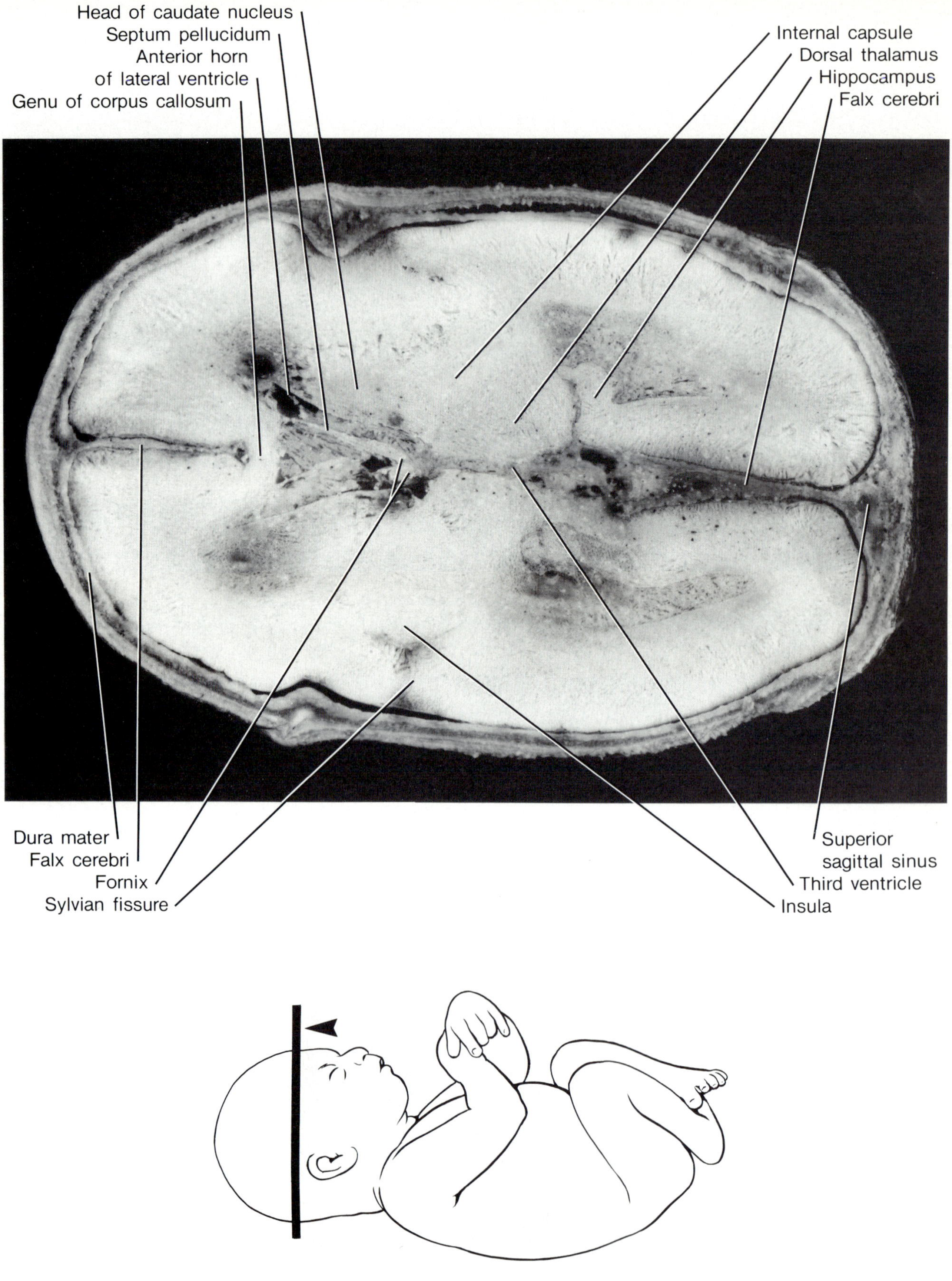

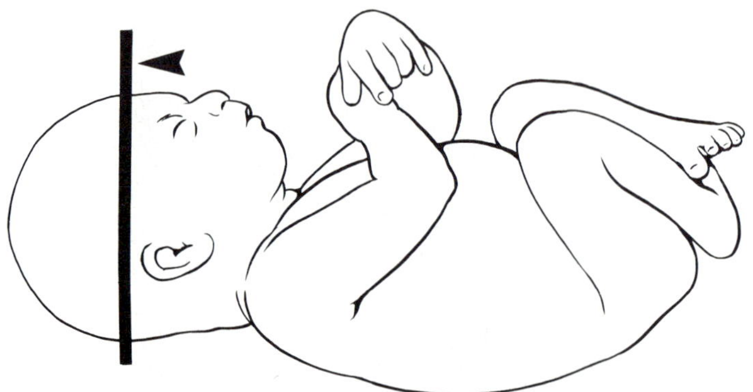

Figure 1.10

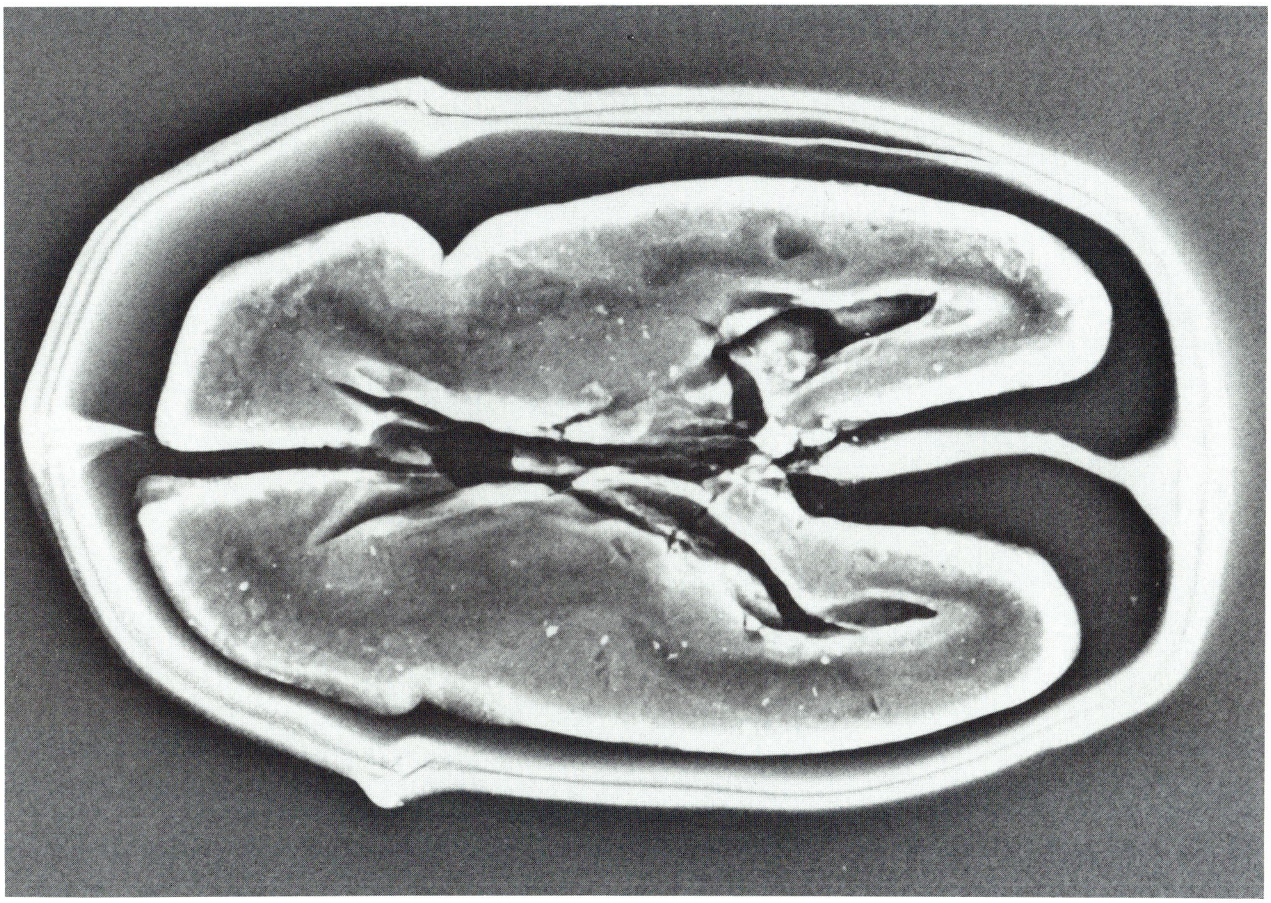

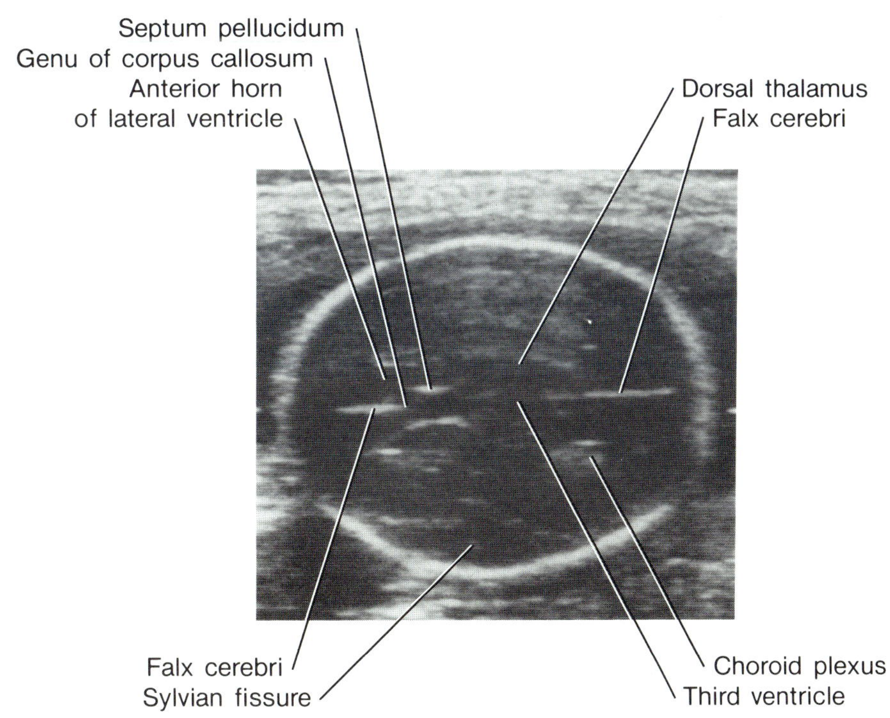

Septum pellucidum
Genu of corpus callosum
Anterior horn
of lateral ventricle
Dorsal thalamus
Falx cerebri
Falx cerebri
Sylvian fissure
Choroid plexus
Third ventricle

Fimbria of fornix
Hippocampus
Choroid plexus
Occipital lobe
Transverse sinus
Tail of caudate nucleus
Dorsal thalamus
Columns of fornix
Genu of corpus callosum
Falx cerebri
Posterior horn of lateral ventricle
Straight sinus
Tentorium cerebelli
Third ventricle
Internal capsule
Anterior horn of lateral ventricle
Cavum of septum pellucidum
Coronal suture
Septum pellucidum
Insula

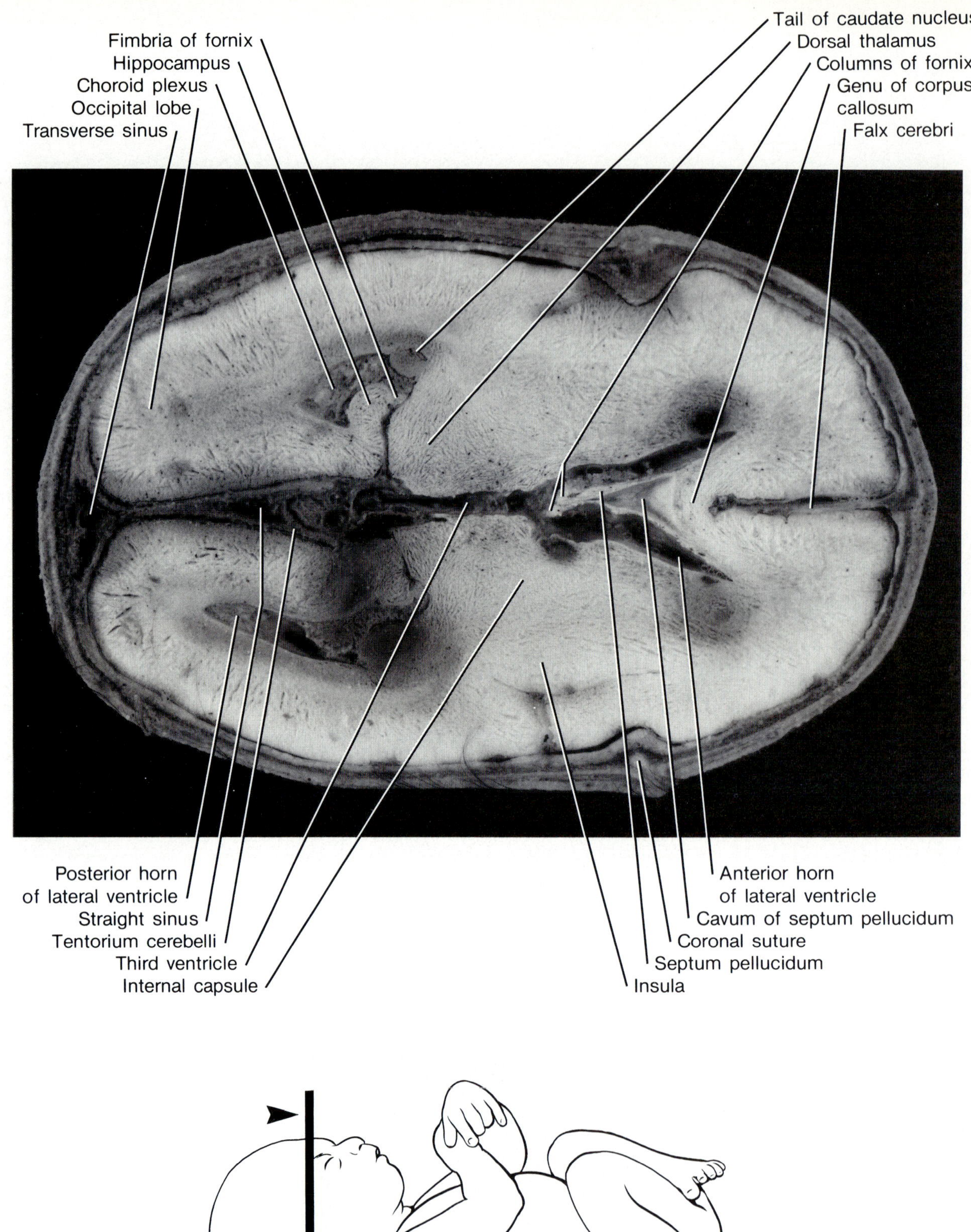

Figure 1.11

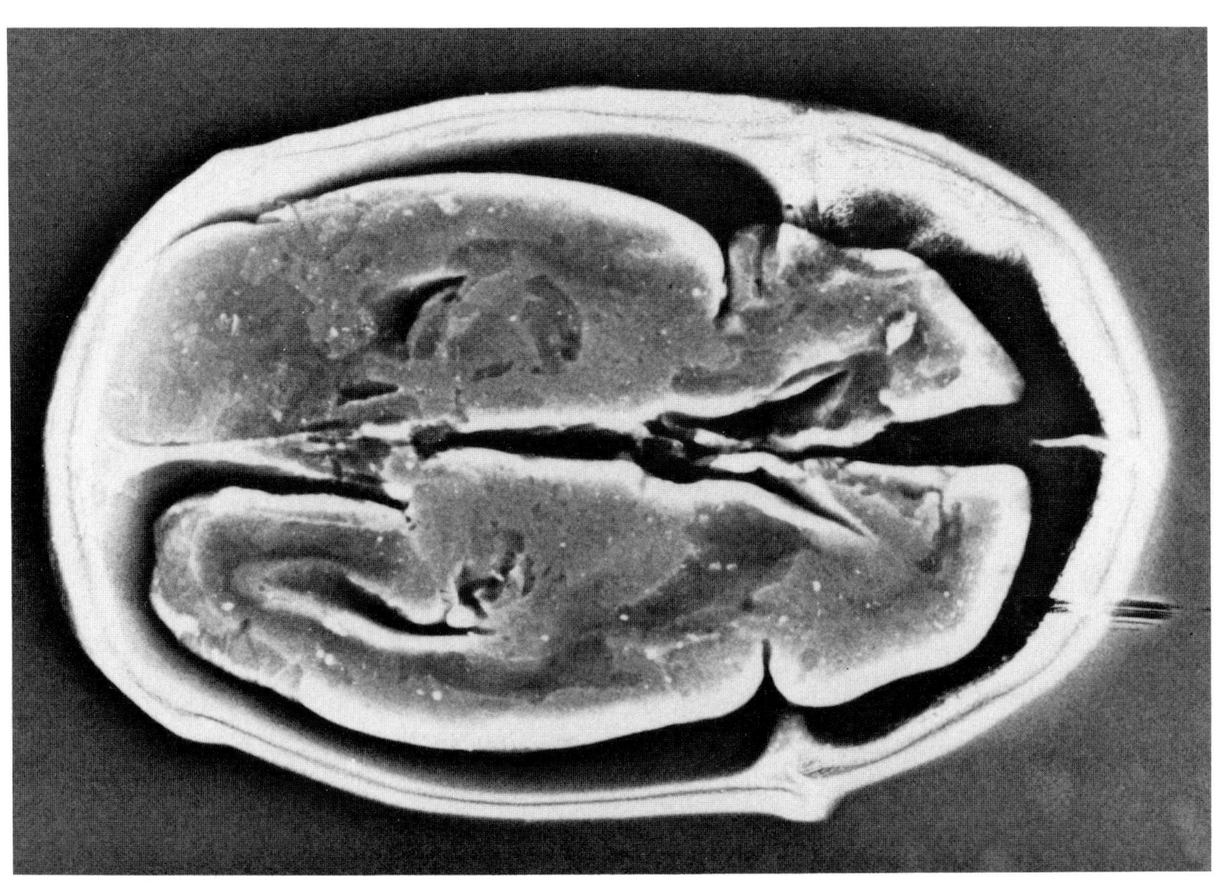

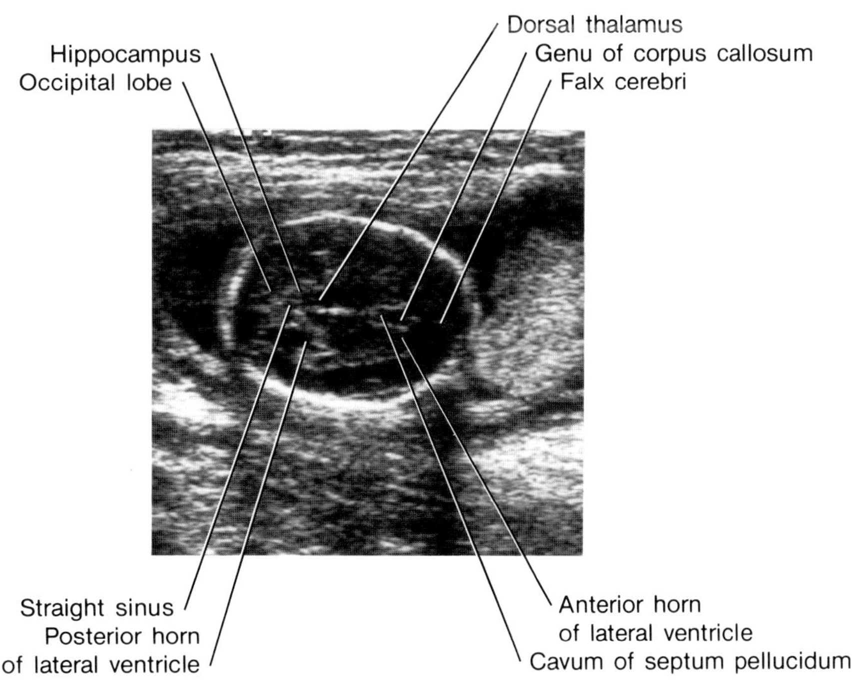

Hippocampus
Occipital lobe
Dorsal thalamus
Genu of corpus callosum
Falx cerebri
Straight sinus
Posterior horn
of lateral ventricle
Anterior horn
of lateral ventricle
Cavum of septum pellucidum

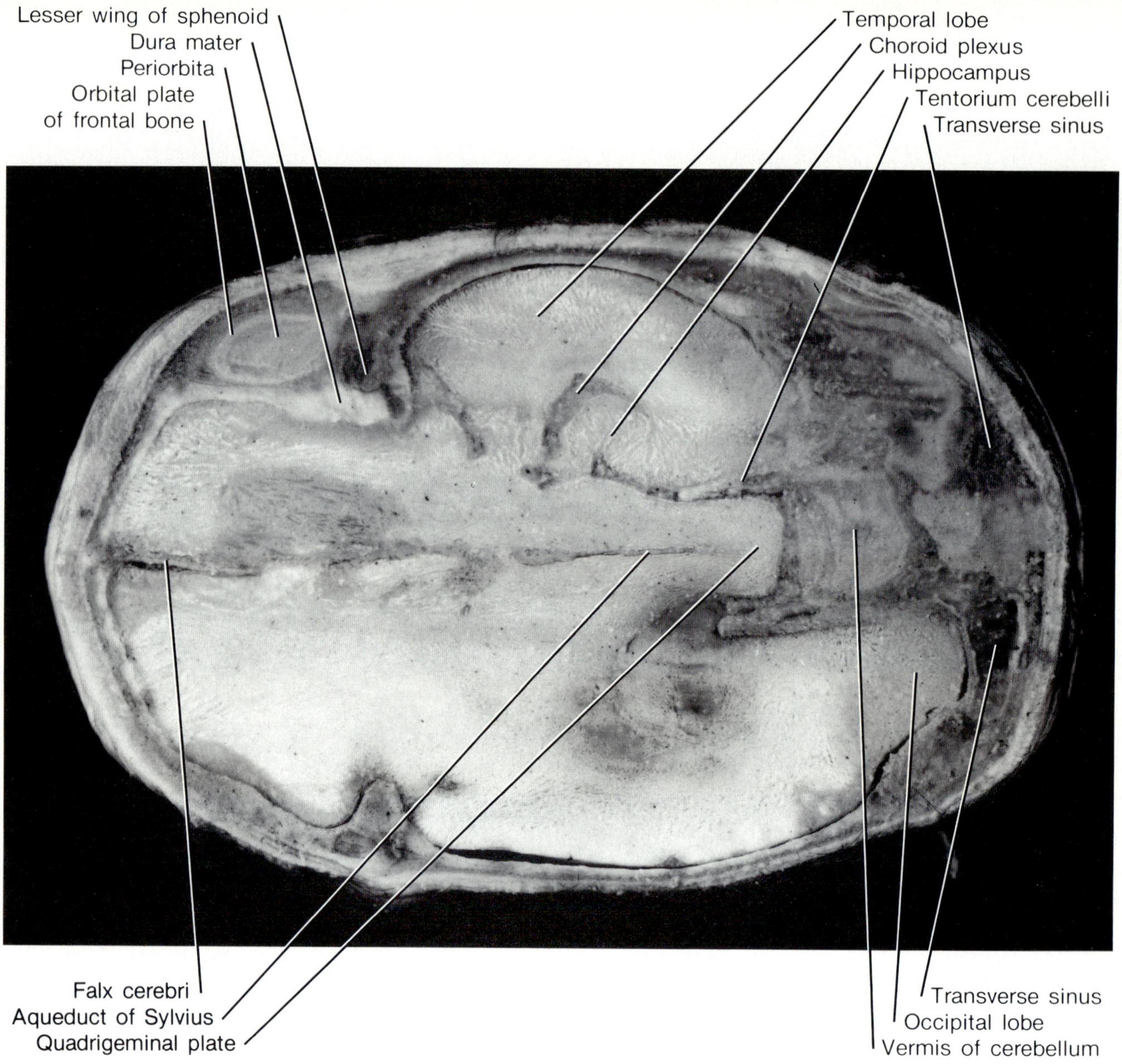

Lesser wing of sphenoid
Dura mater
Periorbita
Orbital plate
of frontal bone

Temporal lobe
Choroid plexus
Hippocampus
Tentorium cerebelli
Transverse sinus

Falx cerebri
Aqueduct of Sylvius
Quadrigeminal plate

Transverse sinus
Occipital lobe
Vermis of cerebellum

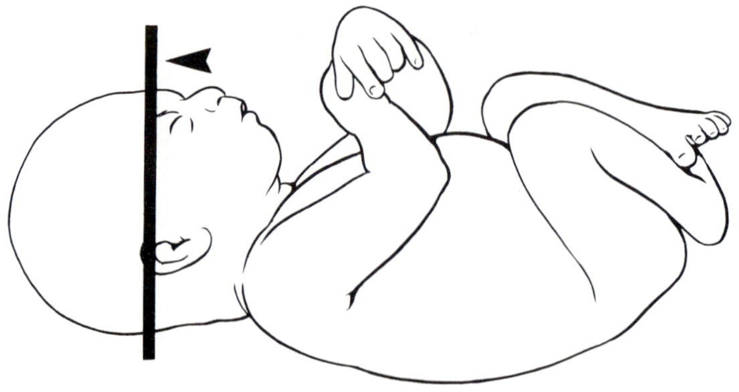

Figure 1.12

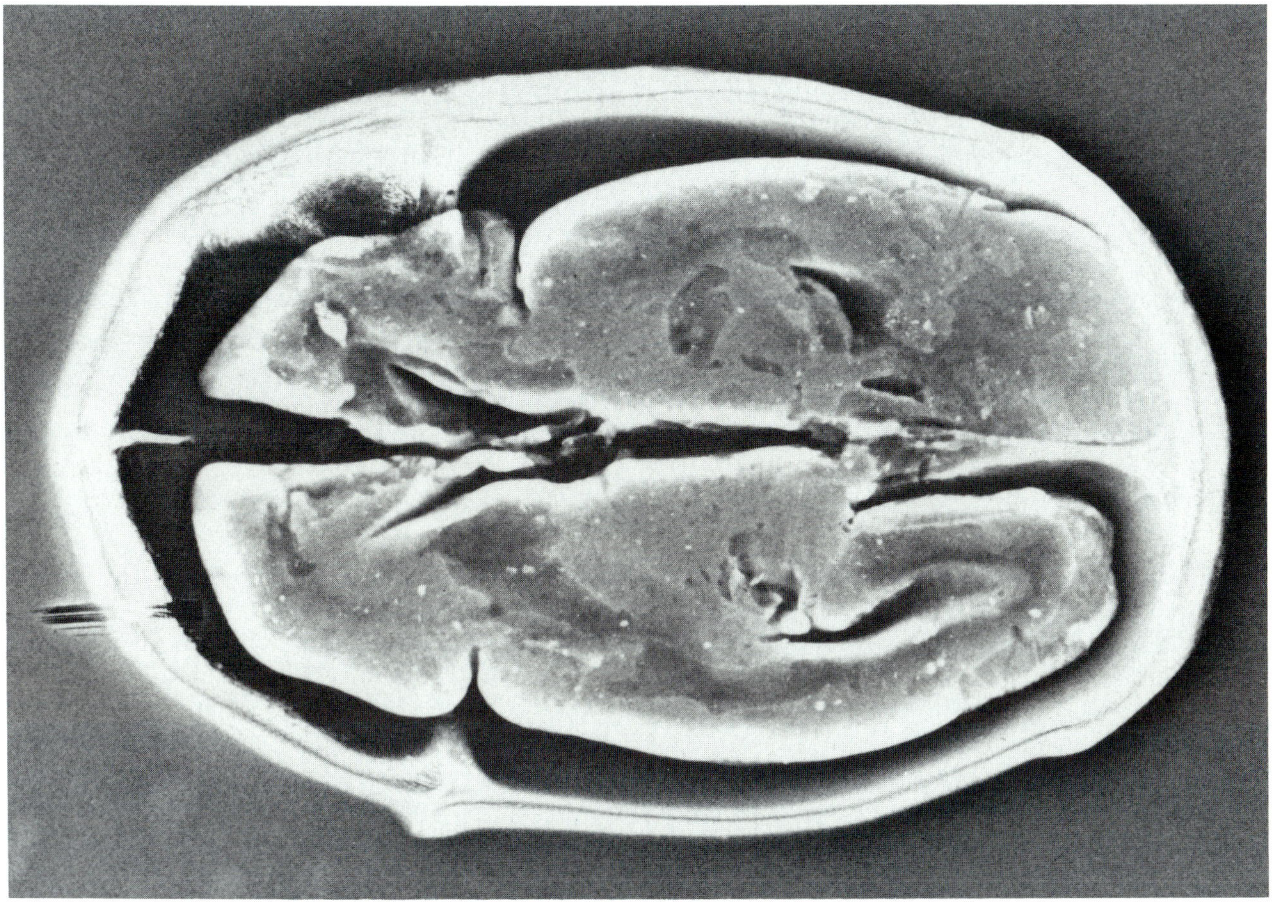

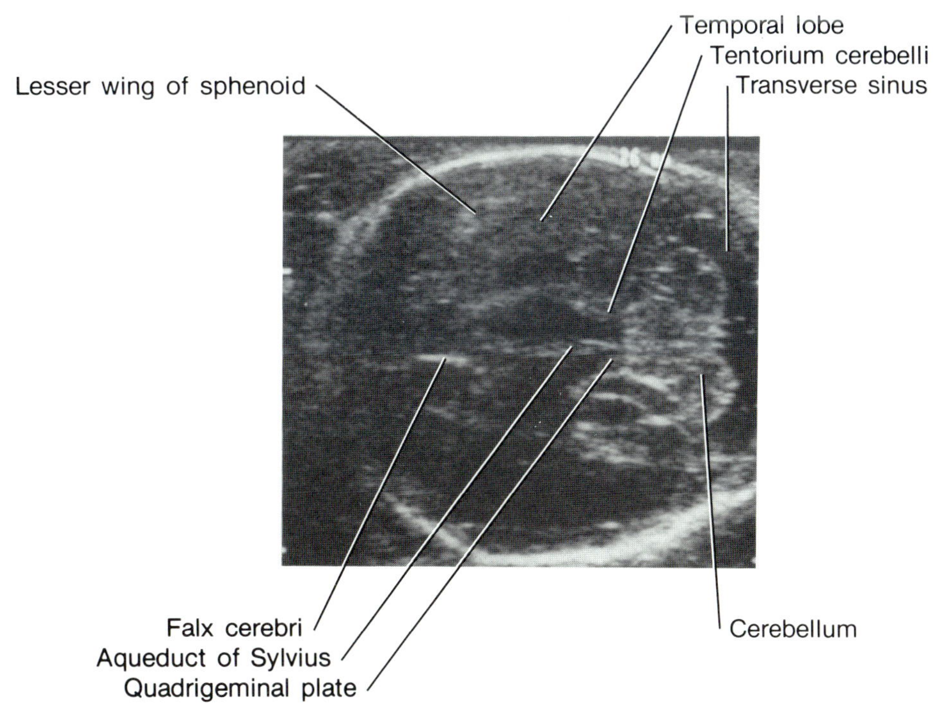

Temporal lobe
Tentorium cerebelli
Transverse sinus
Lesser wing of sphenoid
Falx cerebri
Aqueduct of Sylvius
Quadrigeminal plate
Cerebellum

Quadrigeminal plate
Tentorium cerebelli
Transverse sinus
Cerebellum
Temporal lobe
Temporal horn
of lateral ventricle
Lesser wing of sphenoid
Orbit
Internal occipital
protuberance
Transverse sinus
Tentorium cerebelli
Aqueduct of Sylvius
Dura mater
Falx cerebri
Third ventricle
Hippocampus

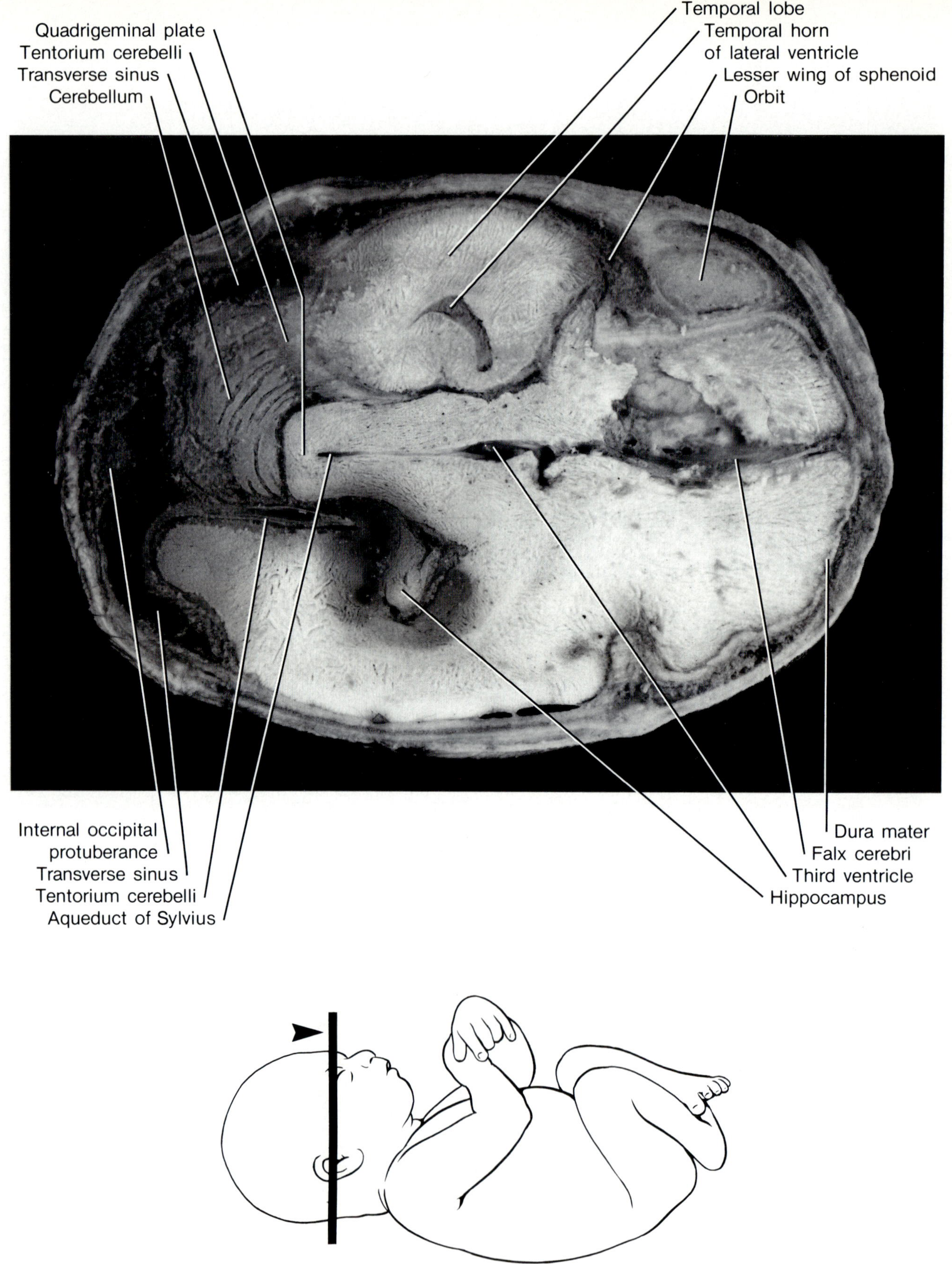

Figure 1.13

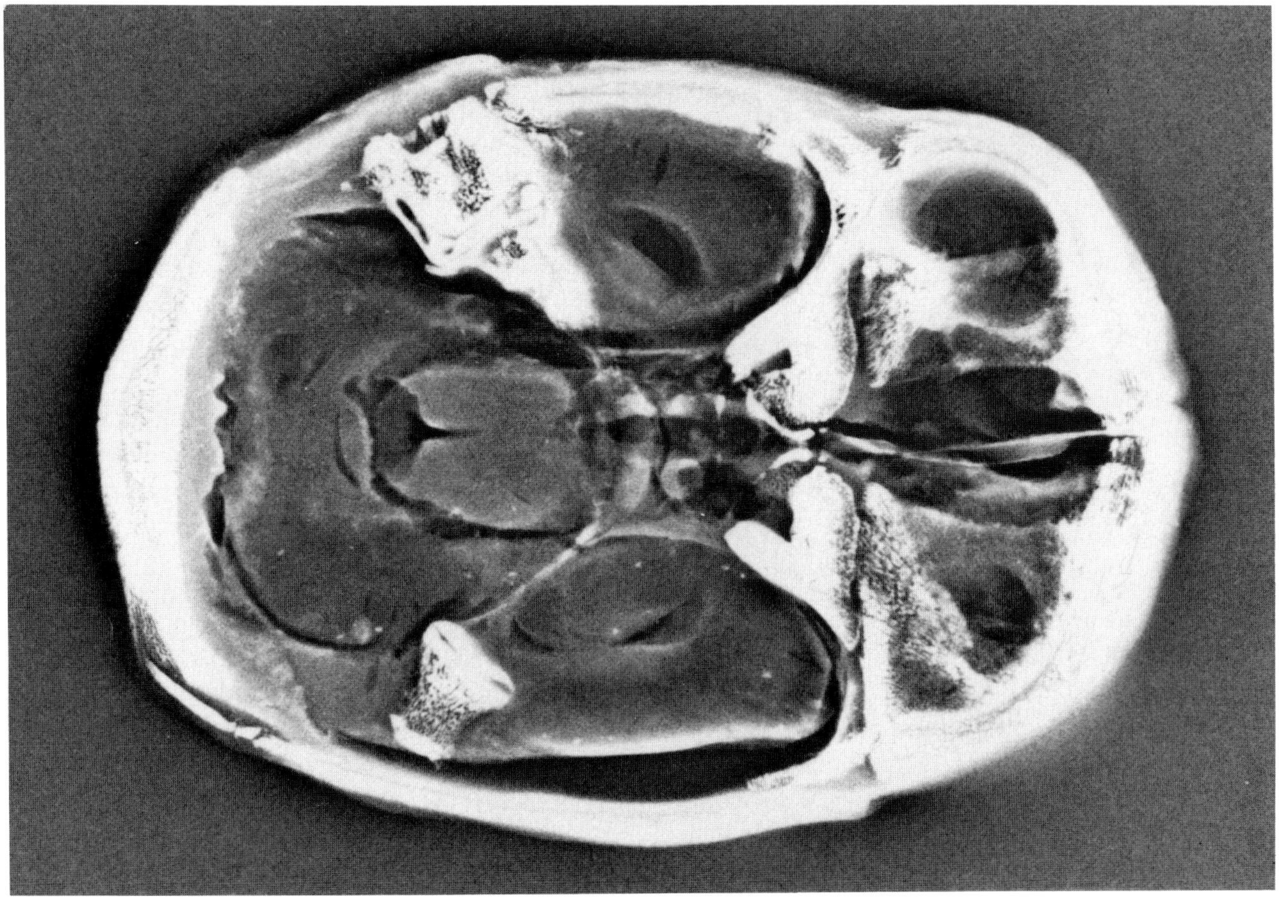

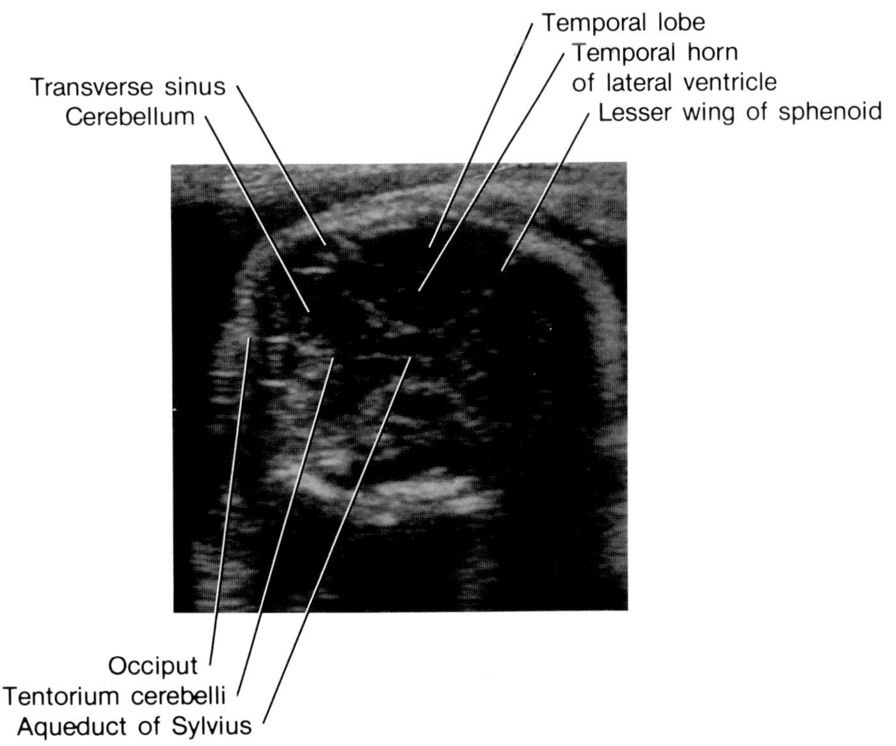

Temporal lobe
Temporal horn
of lateral ventricle
Lesser wing of sphenoid
Transverse sinus
Cerebellum
Occiput
Tentorium cerebelli
Aqueduct of Sylvius

Lateral rectus m.
Optic n.
Zygoma
Sclera
Pituitary
Dorsum sellae
Pons
Fourth ventricle
Transverse sinus
Christa galli
Ethmoid
Medial rectus m.
Body of sphenoid
Diaphragma sellae
Sigmoid sinus
Cerebellar peduncle
Petrous portion
of temporal bone
Internal carotid a.
Temporal lobe

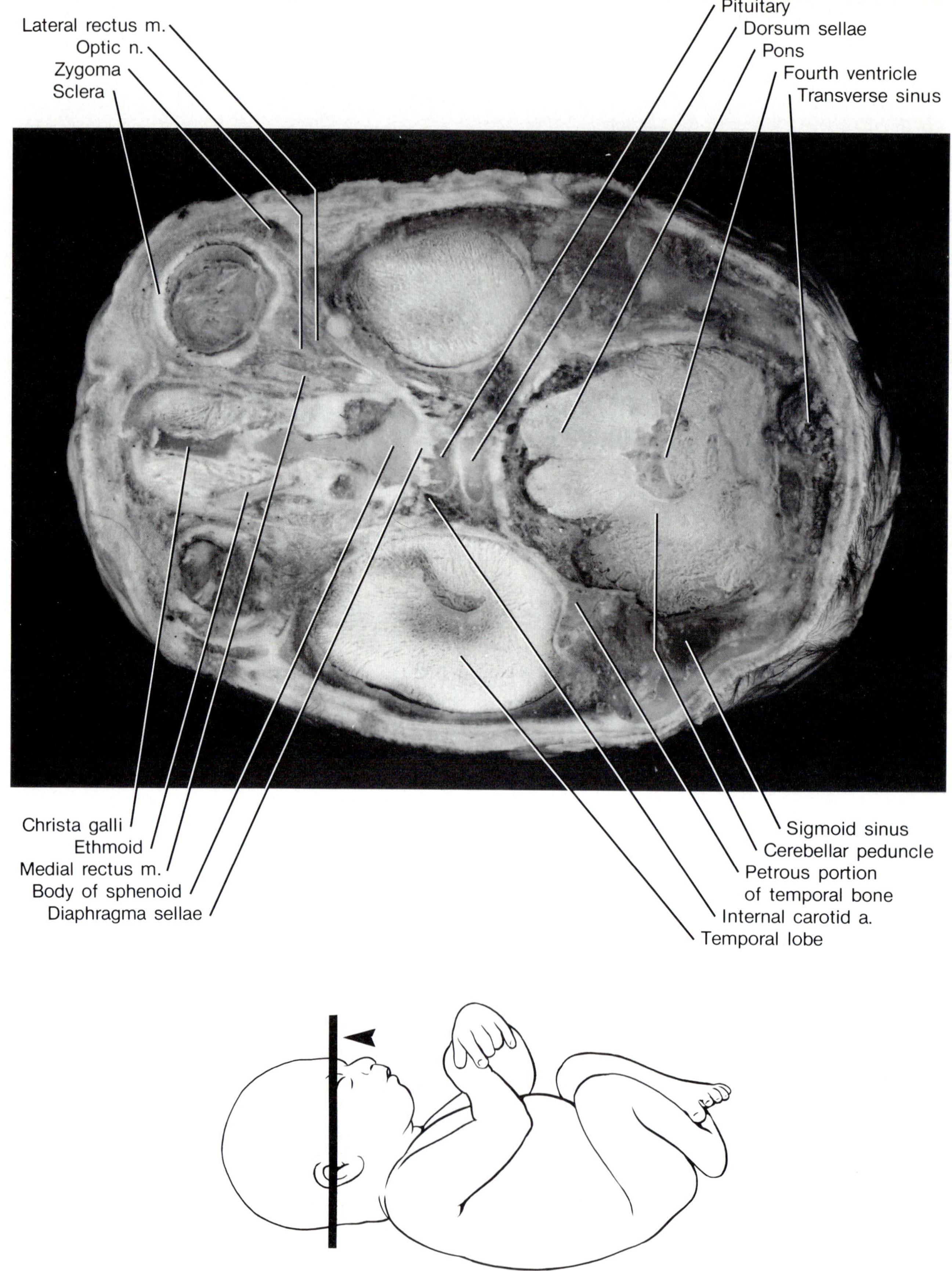

Figure 1.14

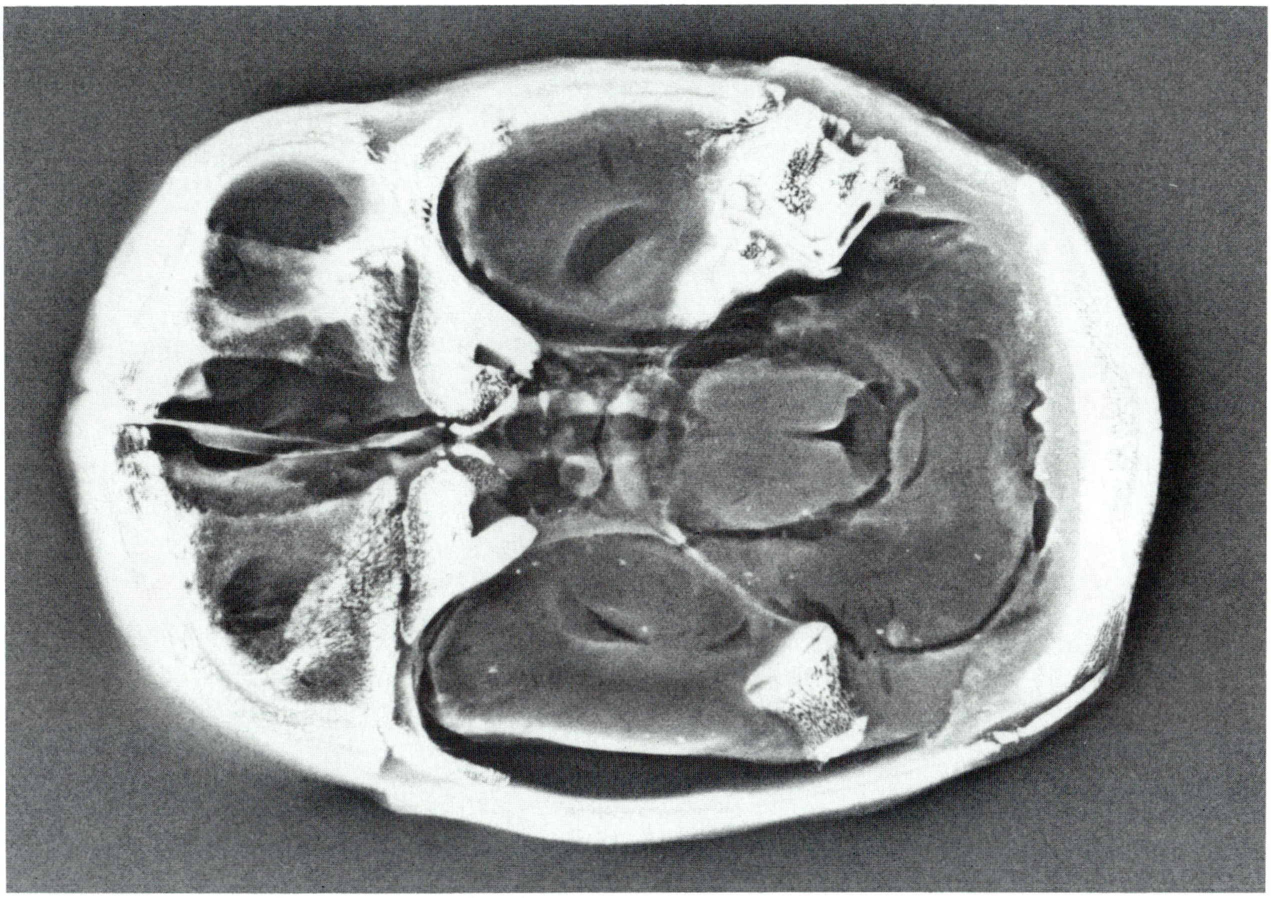

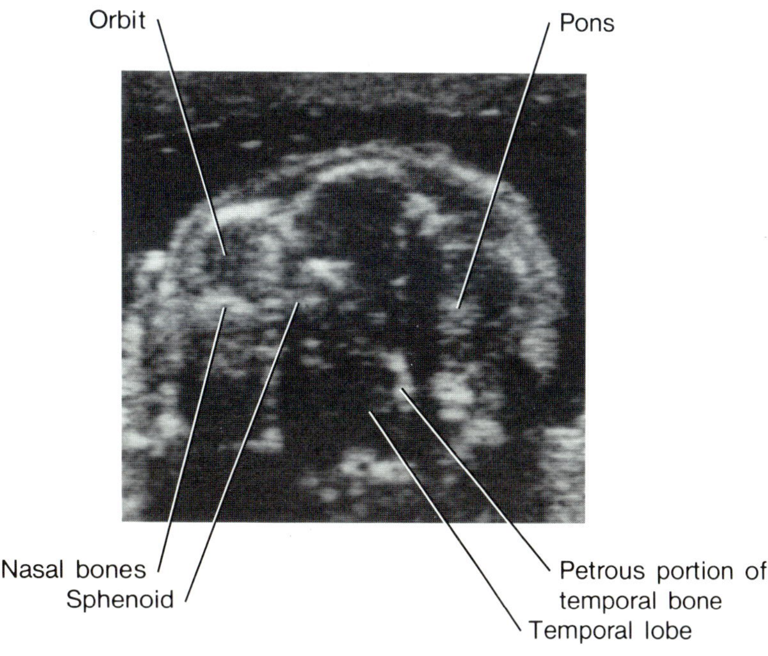

Orbit
Pons
Nasal bones
Sphenoid
Petrous portion of
temporal bone
Temporal lobe

Cranial nerves VII & VIII
at internal auditory meatus
Middle ear
Cerebellum
Transverse sinus
Occipital bone
Temporalis m.
Dorsum sellae
Zygoma
Lens
Sigmoid sinus
Fourth ventricle
Basilar a.
Cranial n. V
Internal carotid a.
Temporal lobe
Sclera
Nasal concha
Nasal septum
Optic nerve
Body of sphenoid
Sella turcica

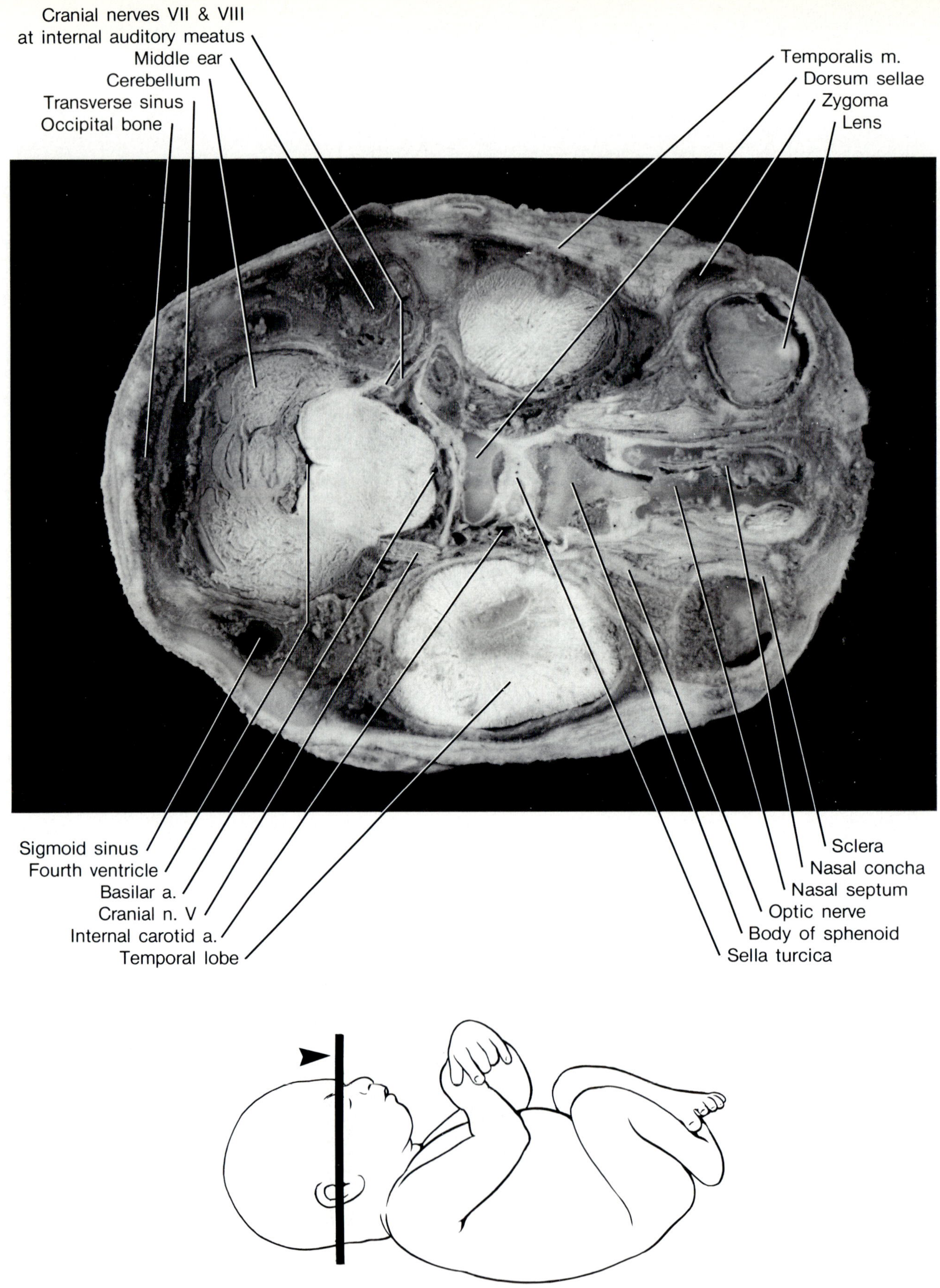

Figure 1.15

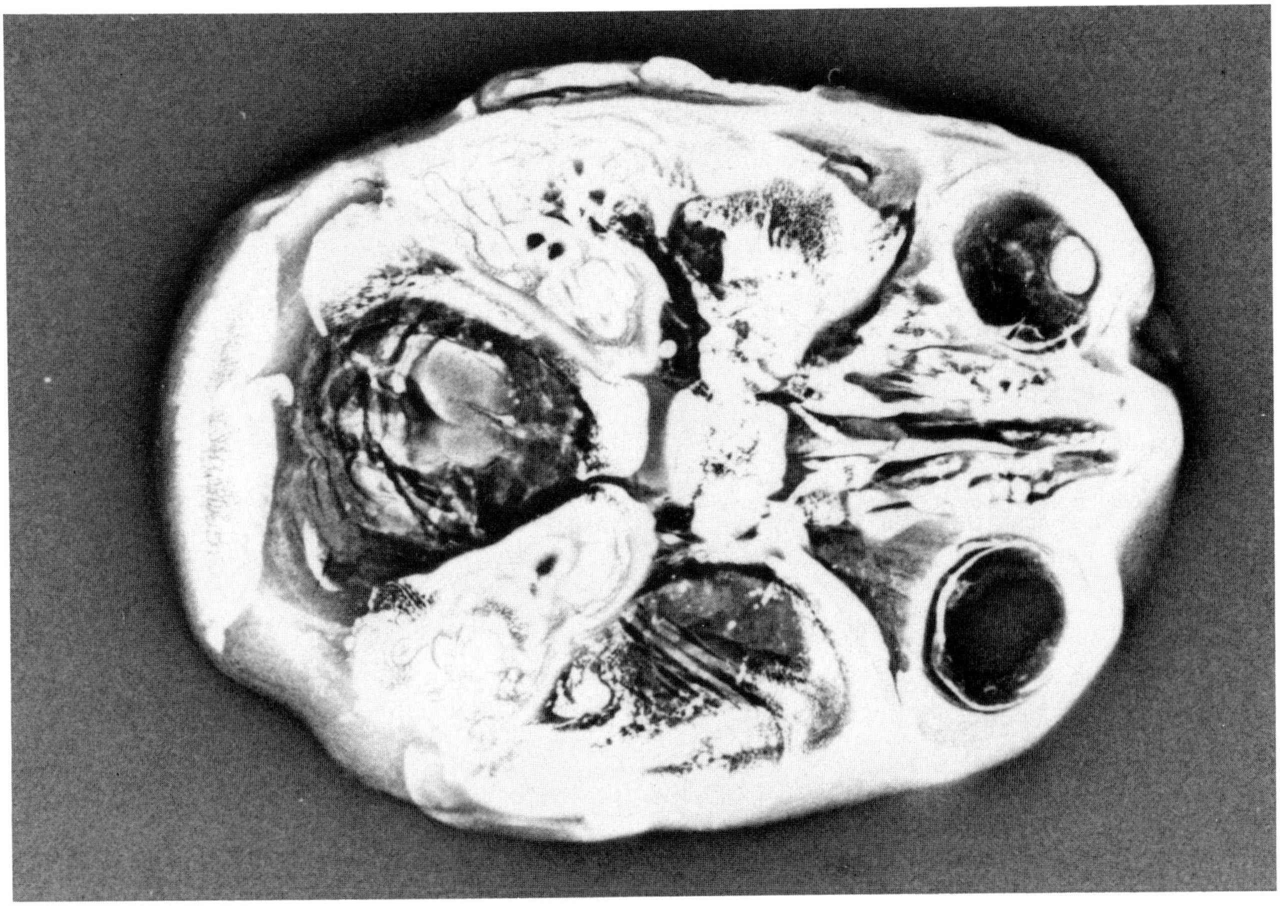

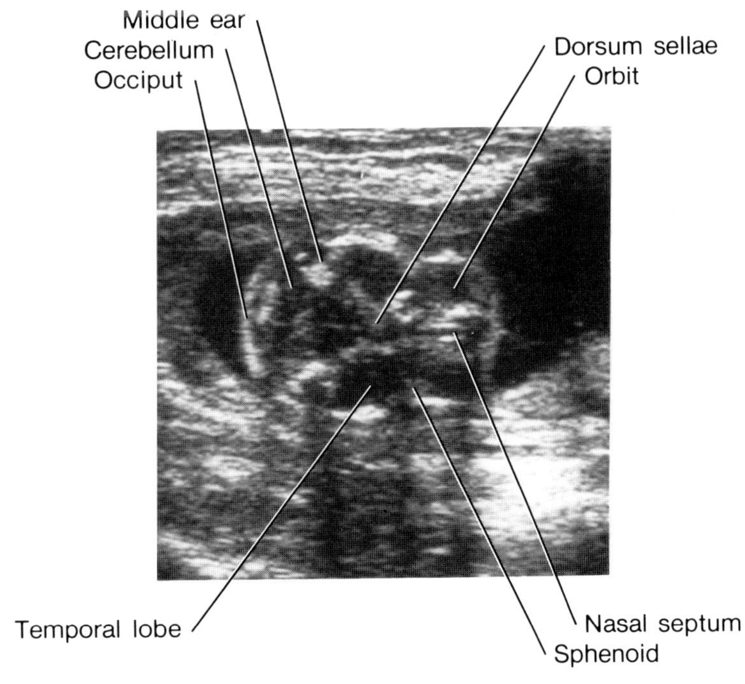

Middle ear
Cerebellum
Occiput
Dorsum sellae
Orbit
Temporal lobe
Nasal septum
Sphenoid

Middle ear
Inner ear
Sigmoid sinus
Lesser wing of sphenoid
Lateral rectus m.
Optic n.
Medial rectus m.
Sclera
External occipital protuberance
Medulla
Cranial n. VII-VIII
Basilar plexus of veins
Dura middle cranial fossa
Crista galli
Superior rectus m.
Temporalis m.
Cavernous sinus
Body of sphenoid

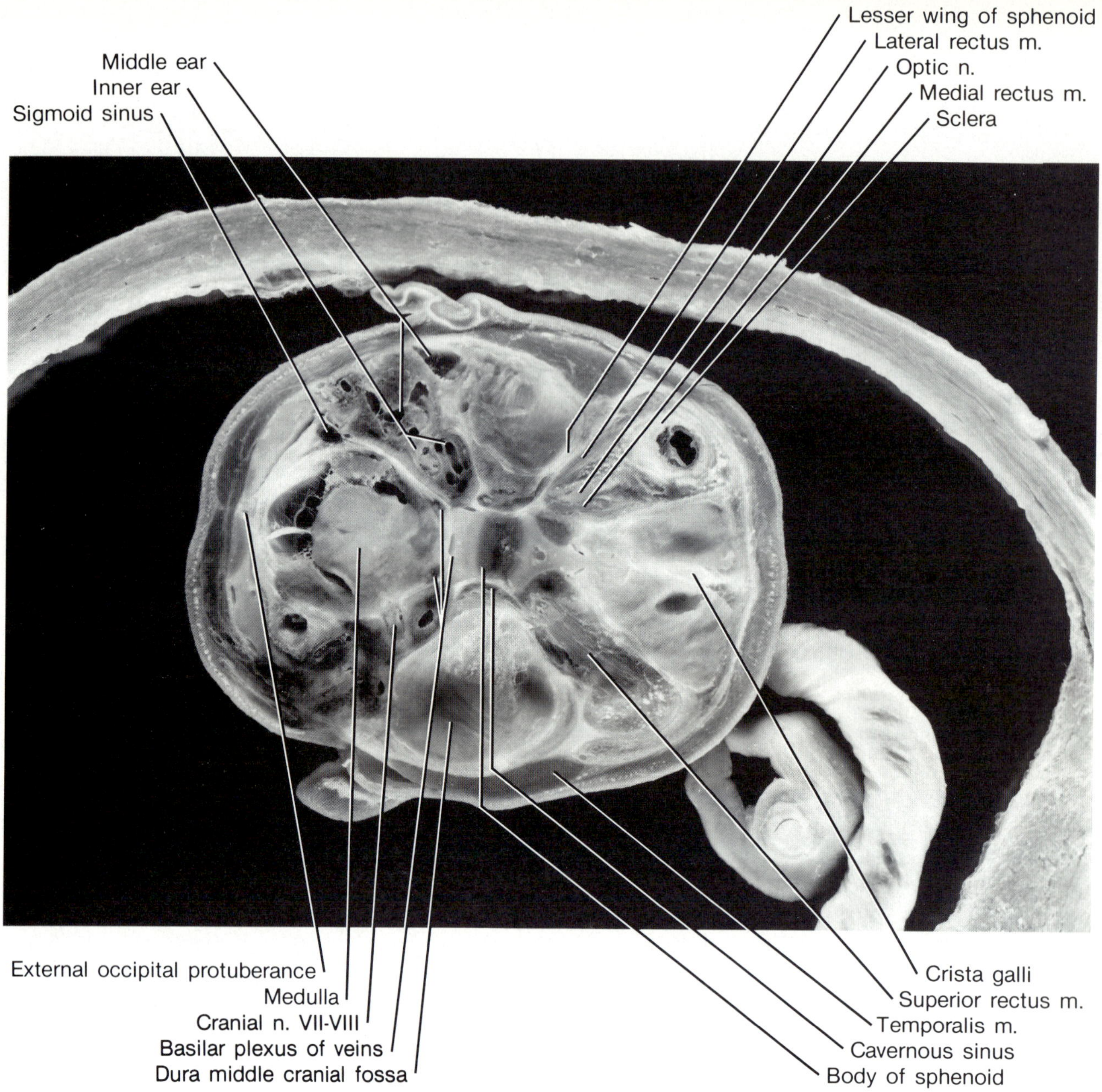

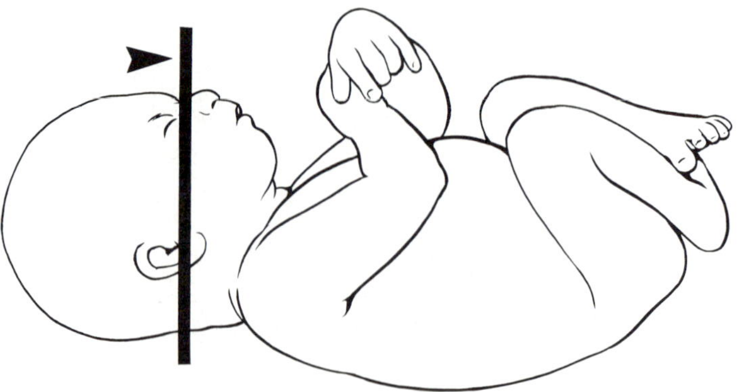

Figure 1.16

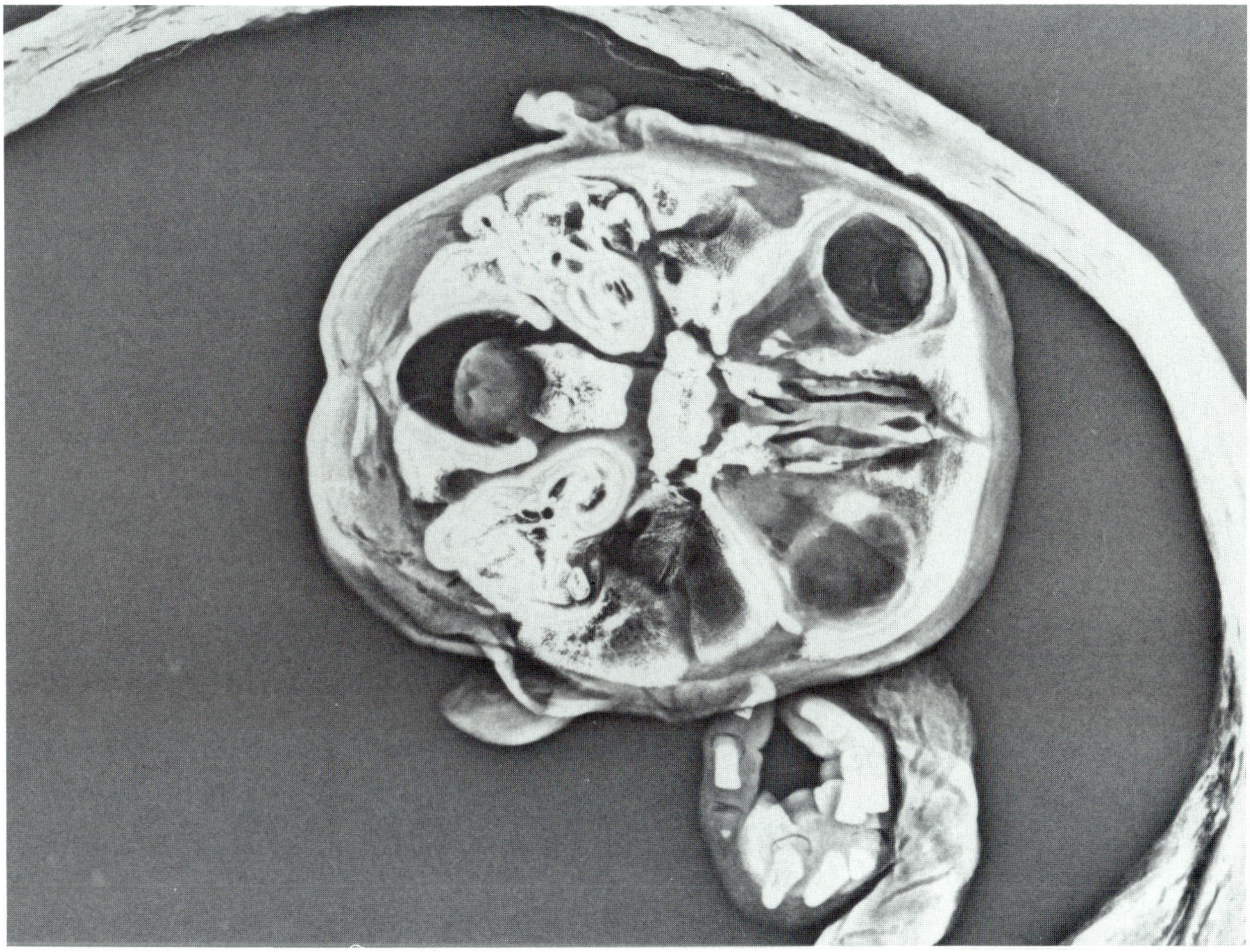

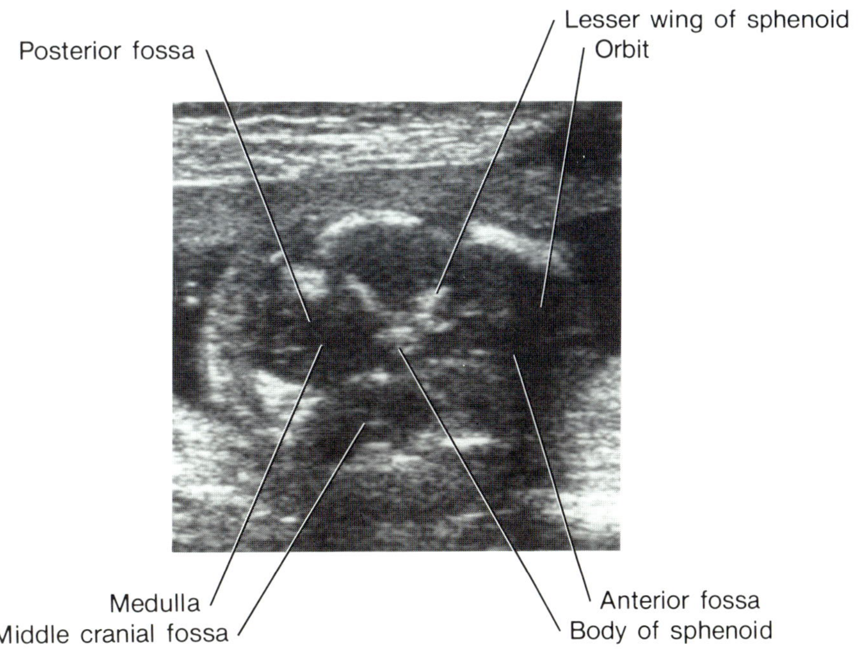

Posterior fossa
Lesser wing of sphenoid
Orbit
Medulla
Middle cranial fossa
Anterior fossa
Body of sphenoid

Temporalis m.
Vitreous
Lens
Cornea
Nasal septum
Lateral pterygoid m.
Condyle of mandible
Longus capitis m.
Sigmoid sinus
Foramen magnum
Inferior rectus m.
Lateral rectus m.
Body of sphenoid
Inner ear
Petrous portion of temporal bone
Middle ear

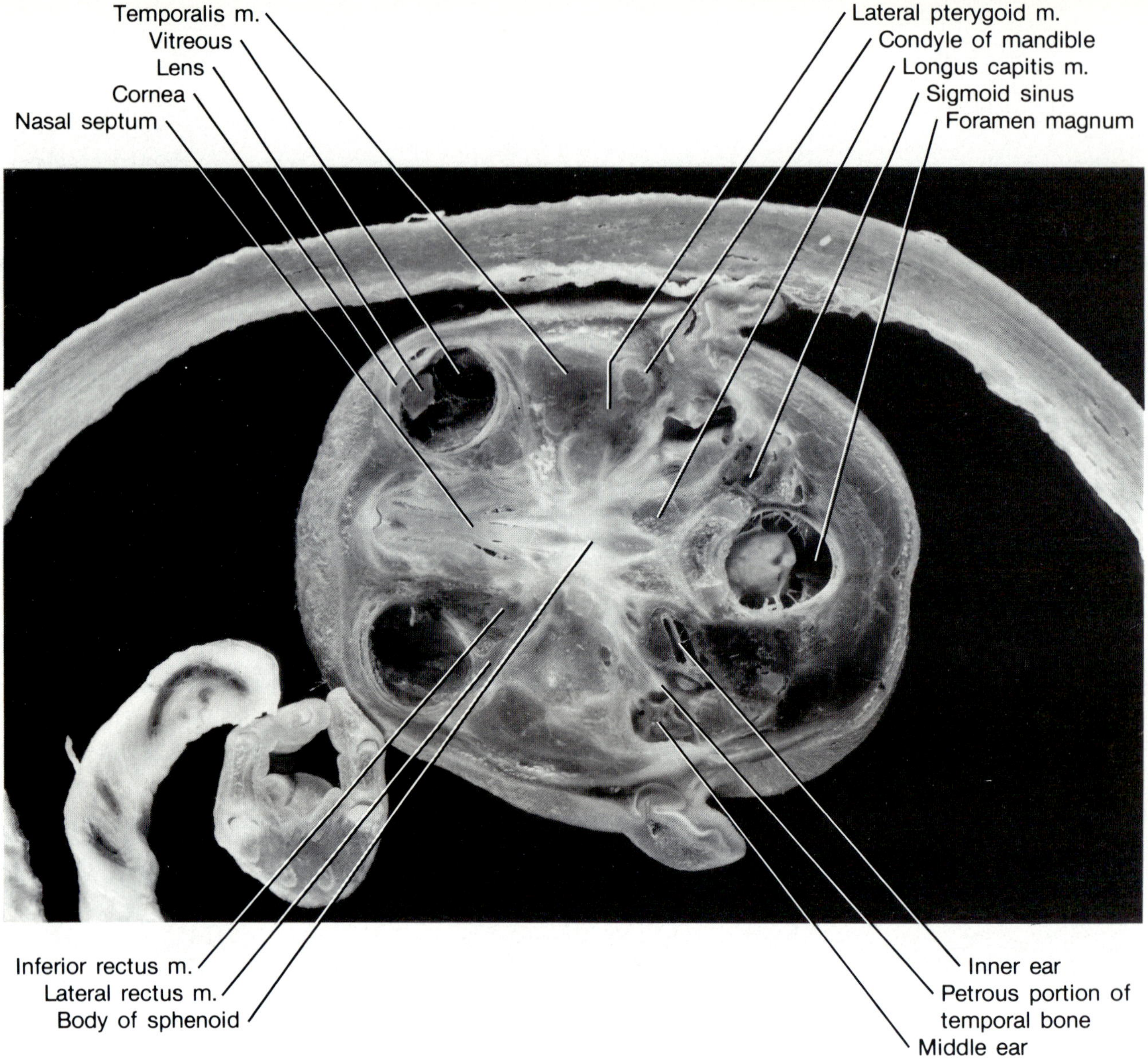

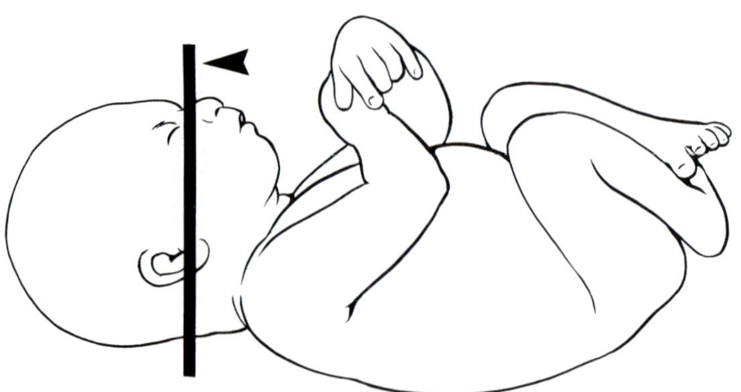

Figure 1.17

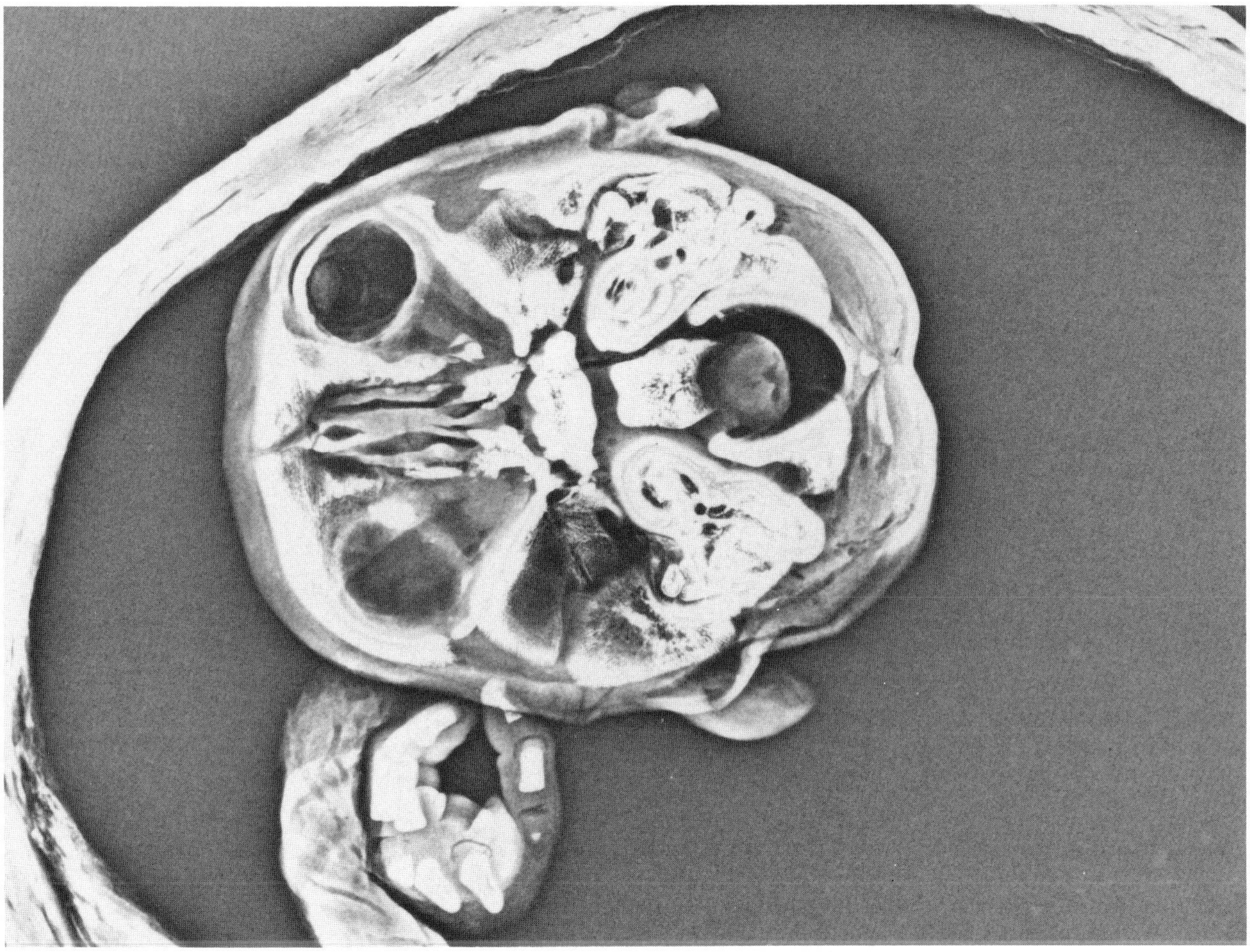

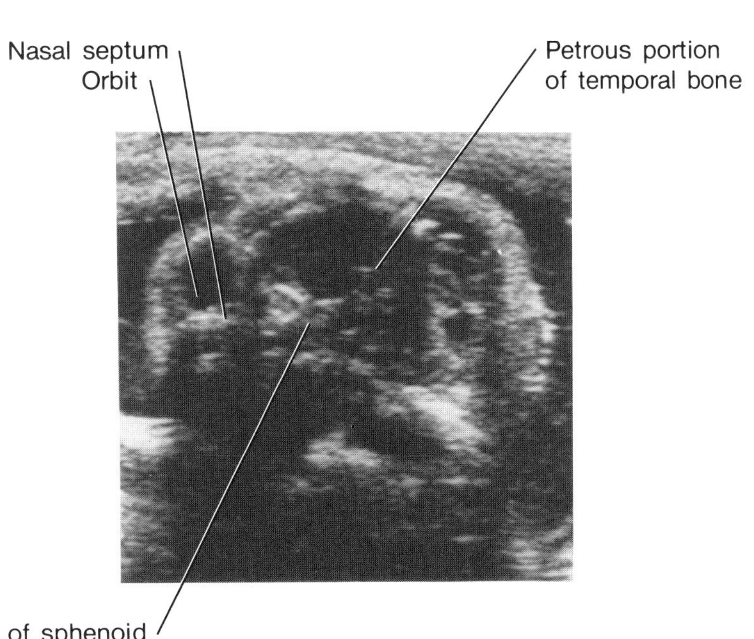

Nasal septum
Orbit
Petrous portion
of temporal bone
Body of sphenoid

Longus capitis m.
Parotid gland
Sternocleidomastoid m.
Occipital bone
Splenius capitis m.
Semispinalis capitis m.
Parotid gland
Head of mandible
Lateral pterygoid m.
Nasopharynx
Lens
Cornea
Tympanic membrane
Malleus
Head of mandible
Inferior rectus m.
Temporalis m.
Masseter m.
Nasal septum
Middle concha
Medial rectus m.
Sclera
Lateral rectus m.

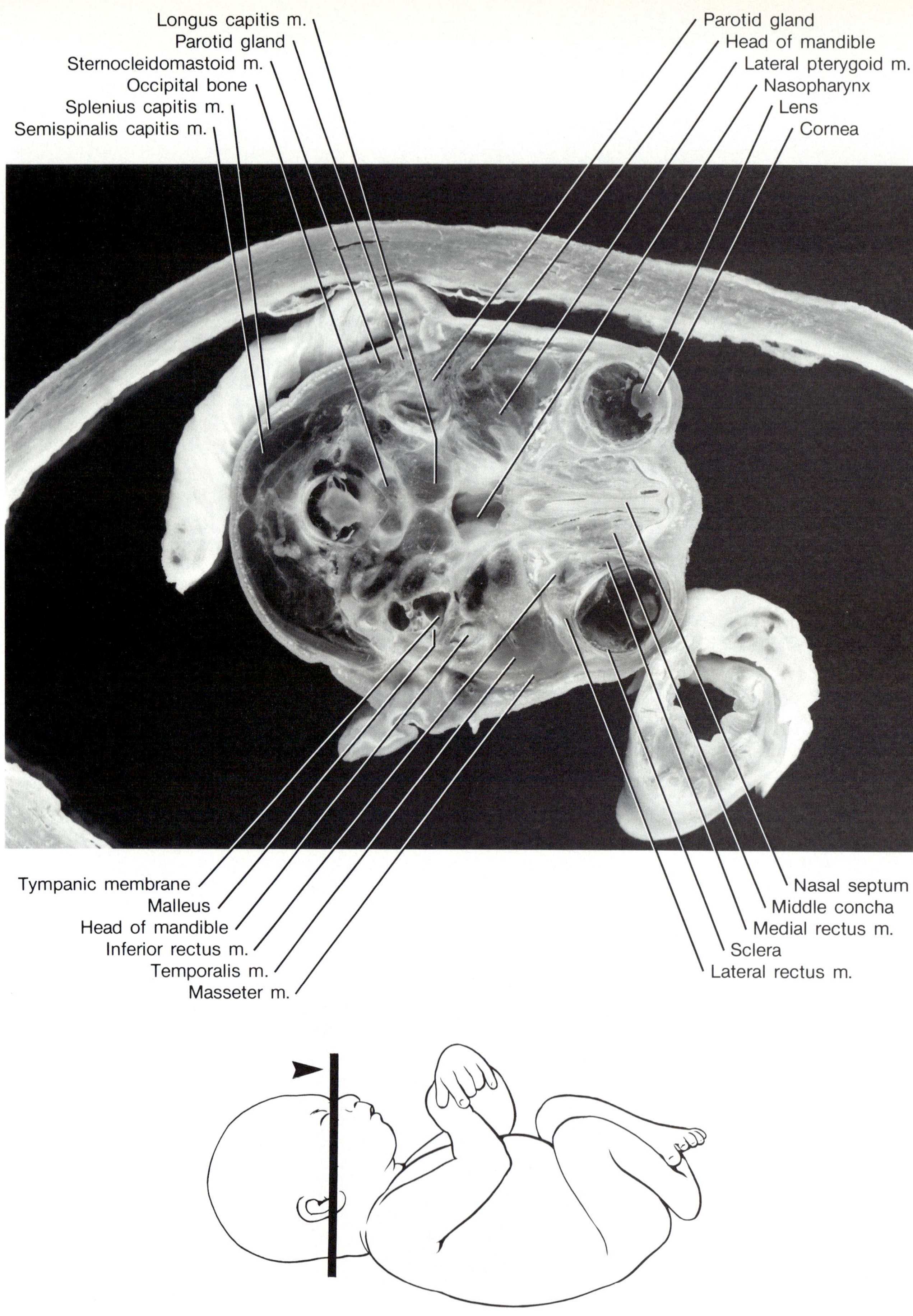

Figure 1.18

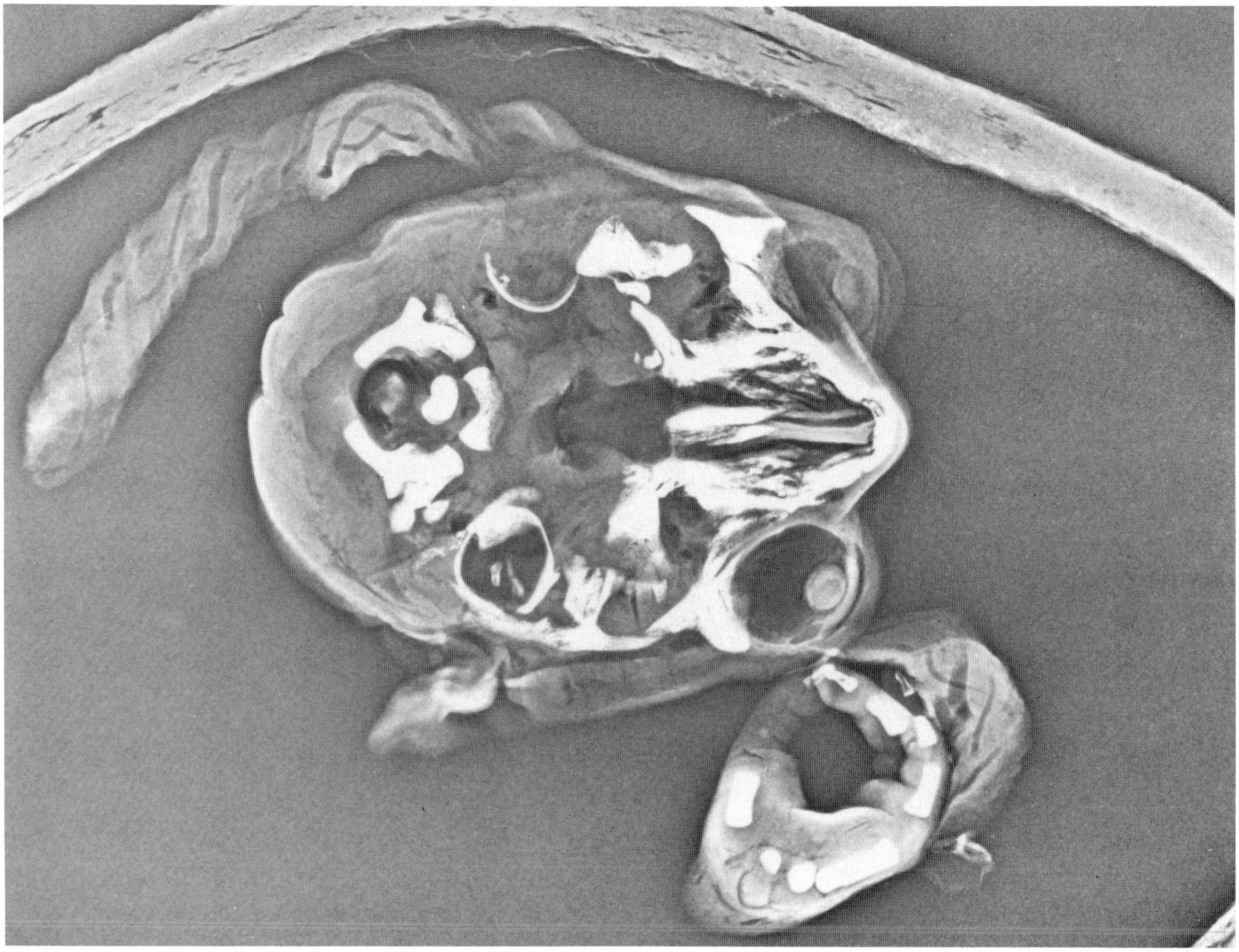

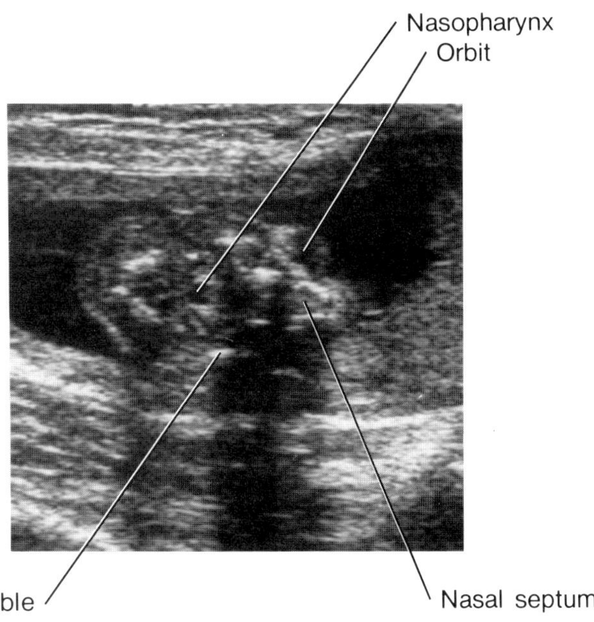

Nasopharynx
Orbit
Mandible
Nasal septum

Retromandibular v.
Parotid gland
Medial pterygoid m.
Masseter m.
Hard palate
Tooth bud
Maxilla
Perpendicular plate of ethmoid
Stylohyoid m.
Internal carotid a.
Posterior belly of digastric m.
Sternocleidomastoid m.
Internal jugular v.
Arch of atlas
2nd cervical vertebra
Trapezius m.
Pisiform
Triangular
Lunate
Scaphoid
Inferior concha
Nasolacrimal duct
Sclera
Vertebral a.
Longus capitis m.
Pharynx
Uvula

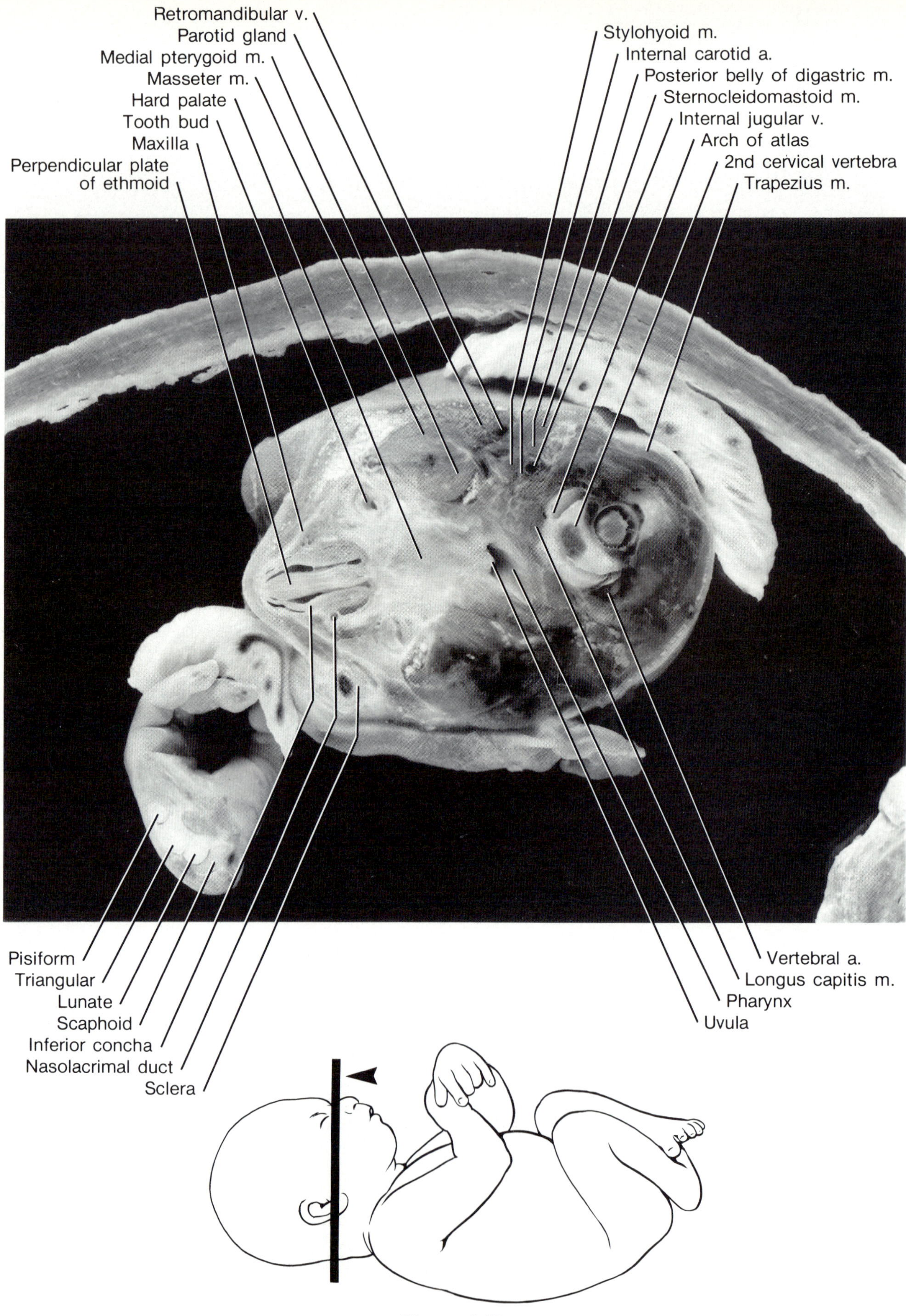

Figure 1.19

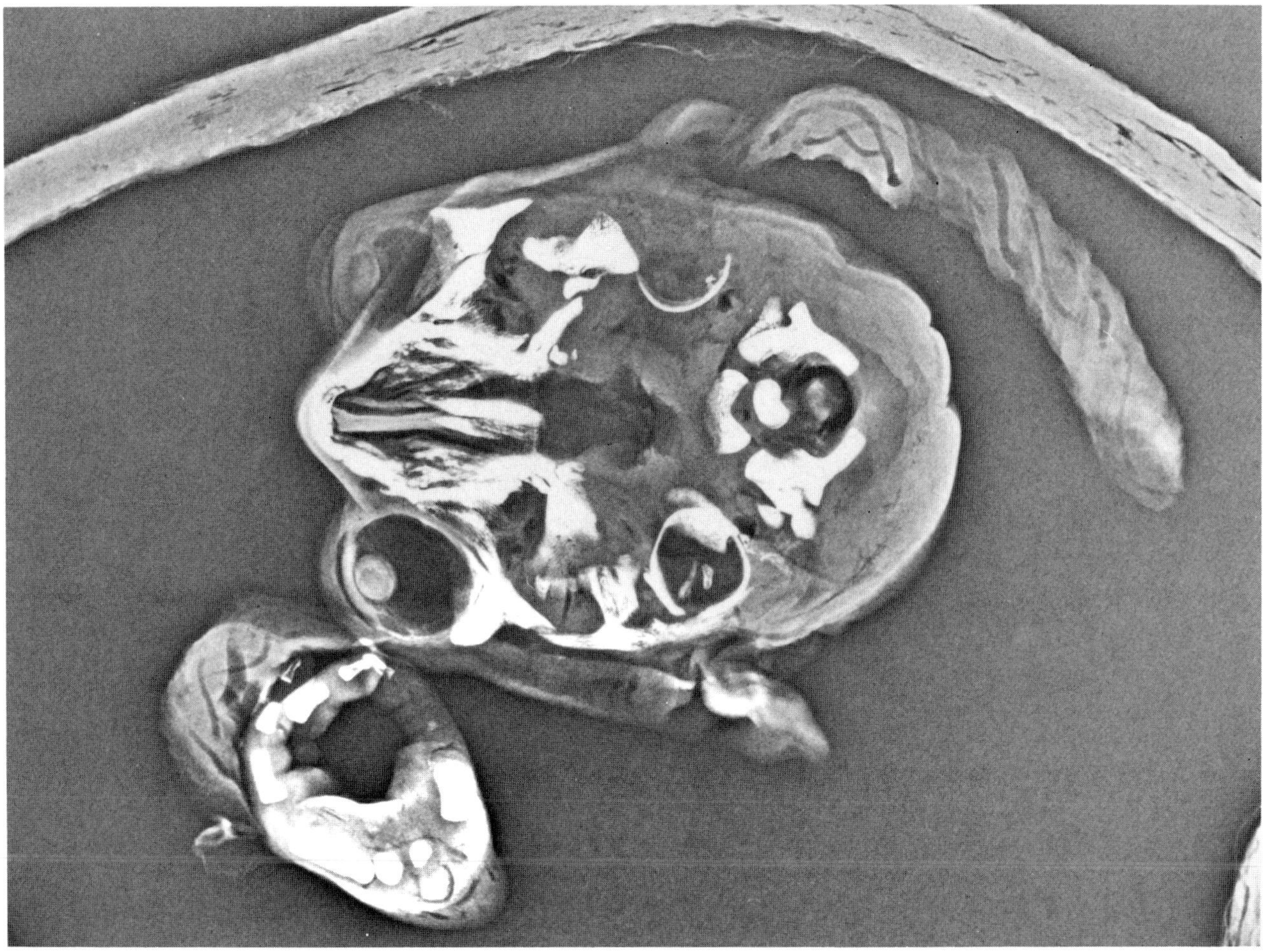

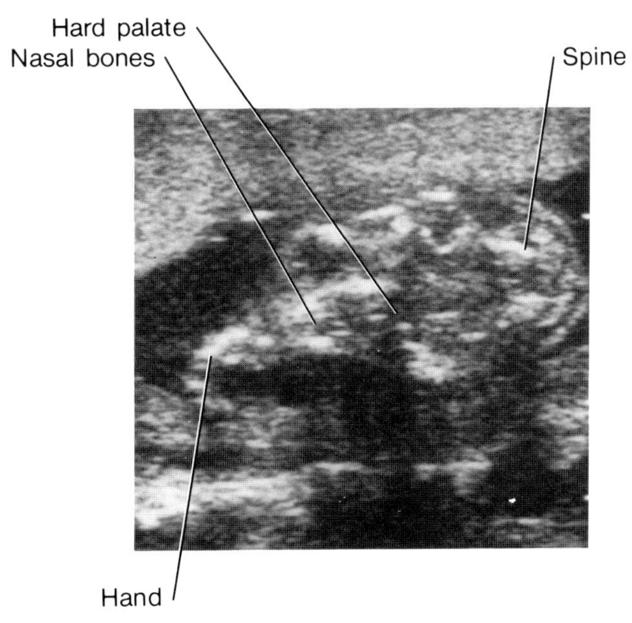

Hard palate
Nasal bones
Spine
Hand

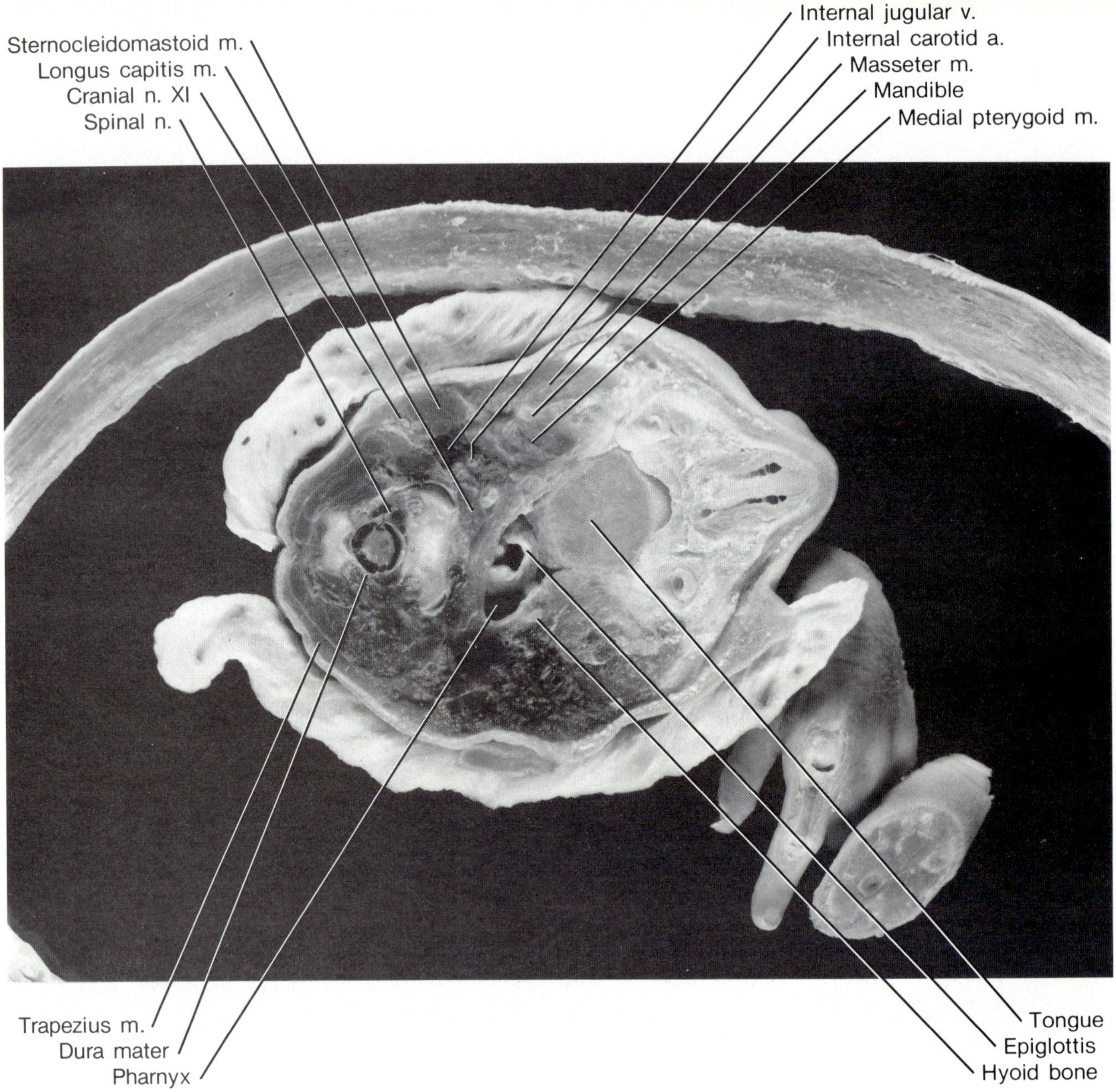

Sternocleidomastoid m.
Longus capitis m.
Cranial n. XI
Spinal n.
Internal jugular v.
Internal carotid a.
Masseter m.
Mandible
Medial pterygoid m.
Trapezius m.
Dura mater
Pharnyx
Tongue
Epiglottis
Hyoid bone

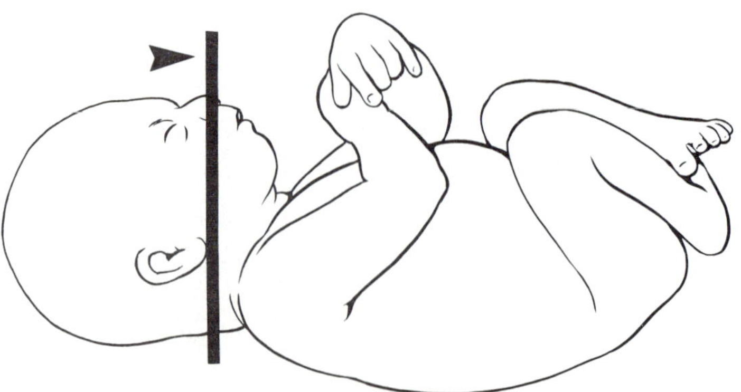

Figure 1.20

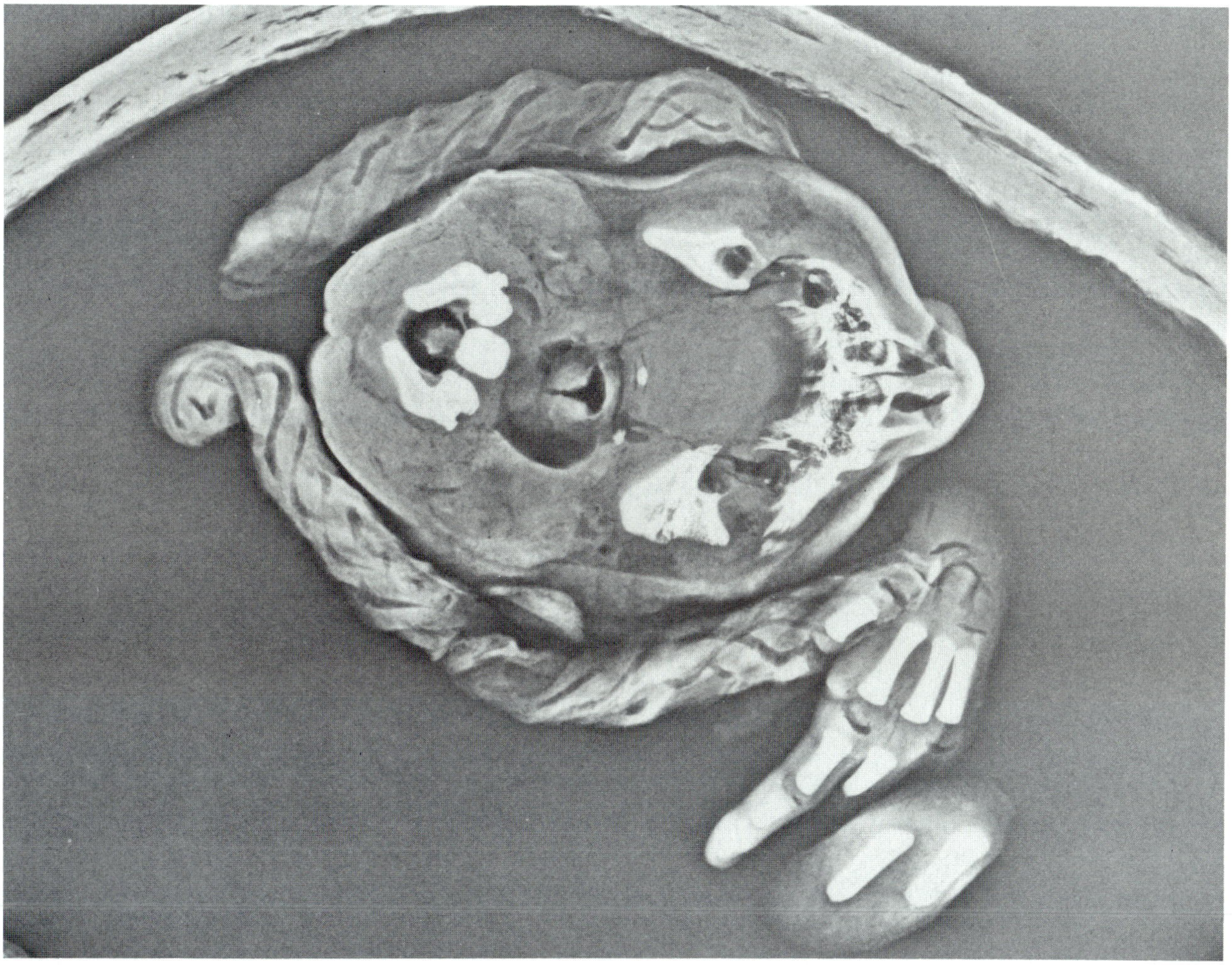

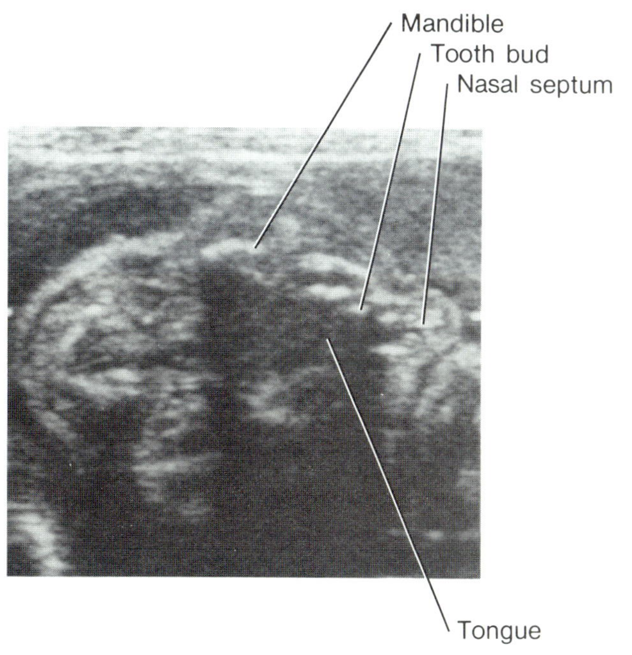

Mandible
Tooth bud
Nasal septum
Tongue

Genioglossus m.
Tongue
Tooth buds
Maxilla
Trapezium
Radius
Scaphoid
Capitate
Hamate
Sublingual gland
Transverse m.
Hyoid cartilage
Submandibular gland
Thyroid cartilage
Cricoid cartilage
Sternocleidomastoid m.
Body of vertebra
Adductor pollicis m.
Mandible
Masseter m.
Pharynx
Thyroarytenoid m.
Styloglossus m.

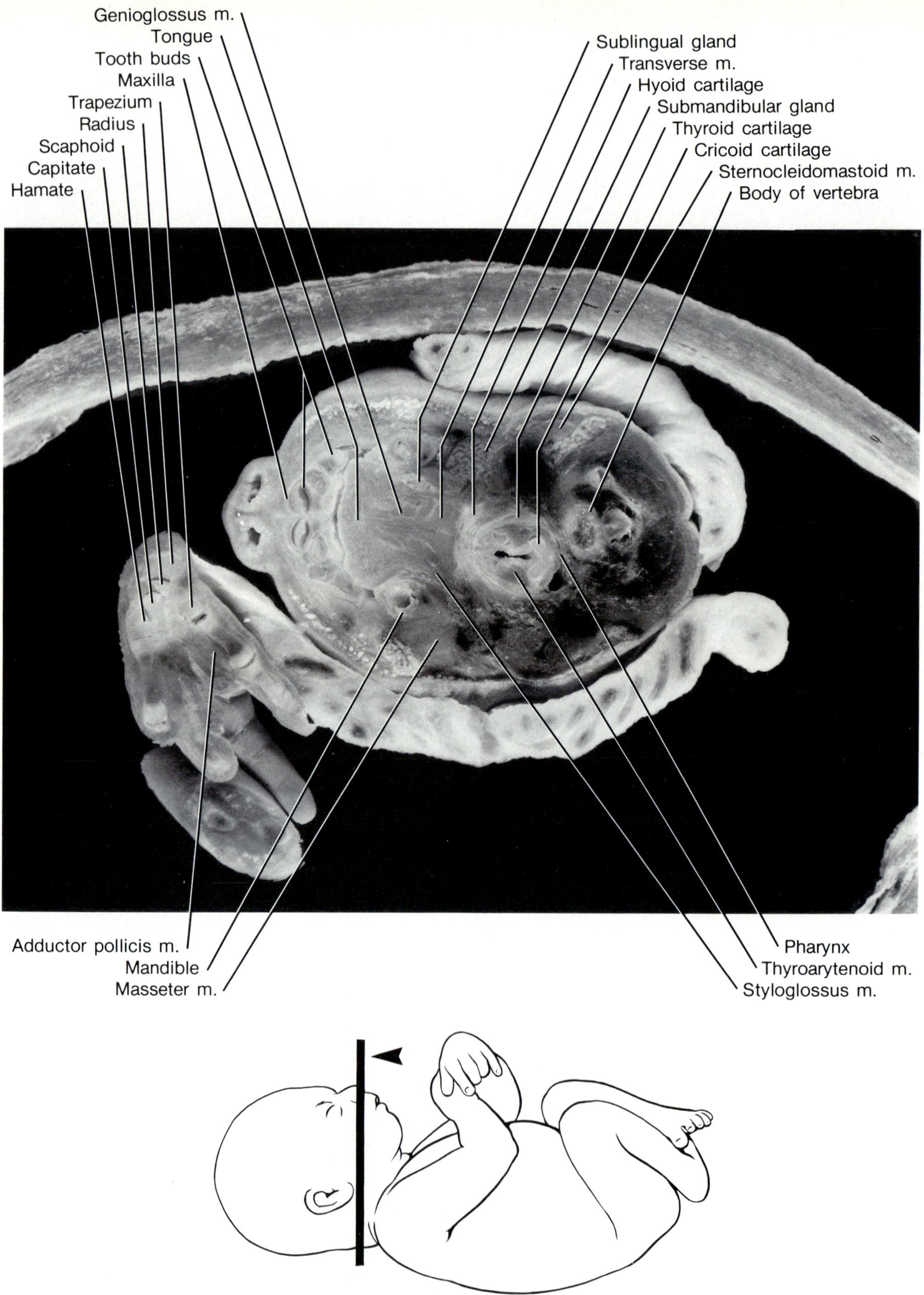

Figure 1.21

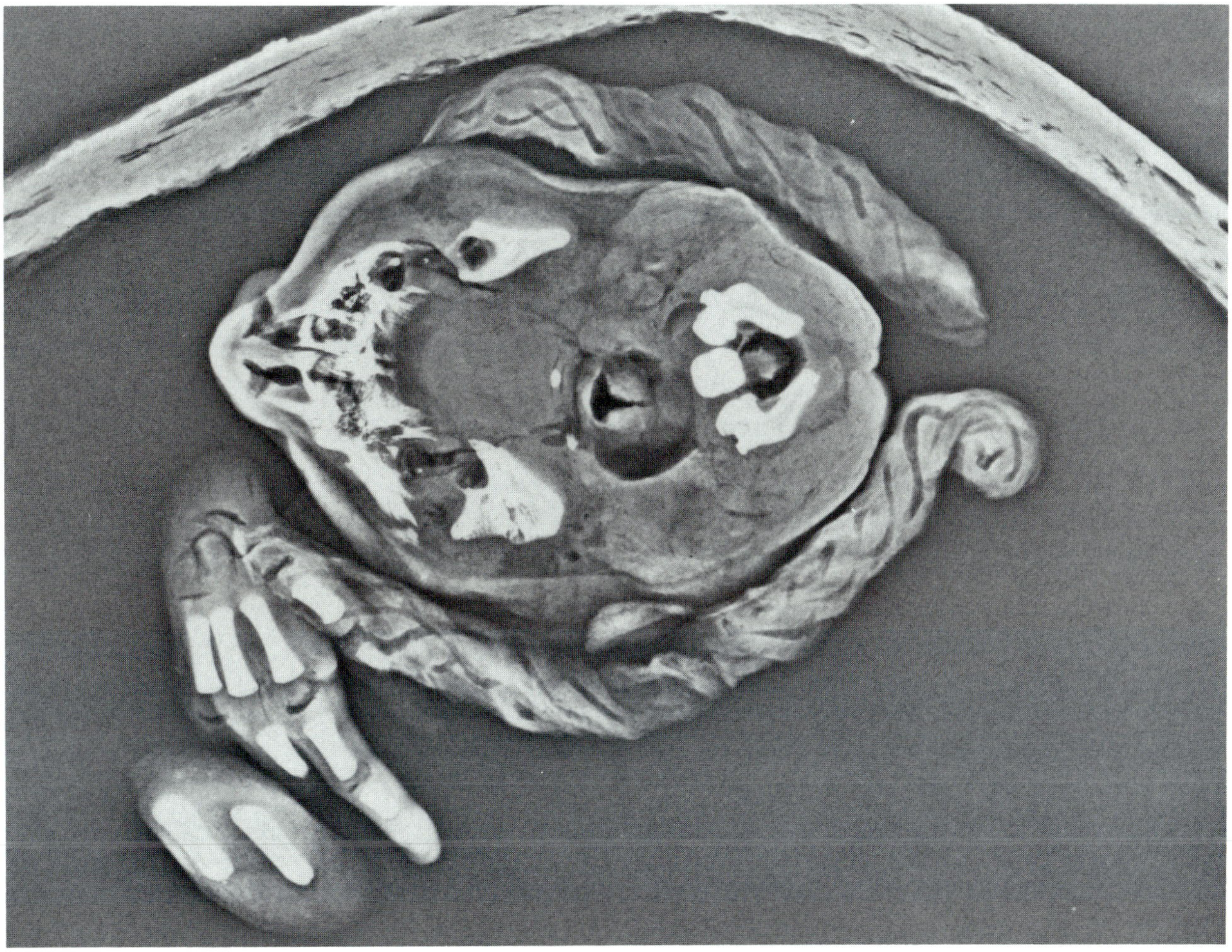

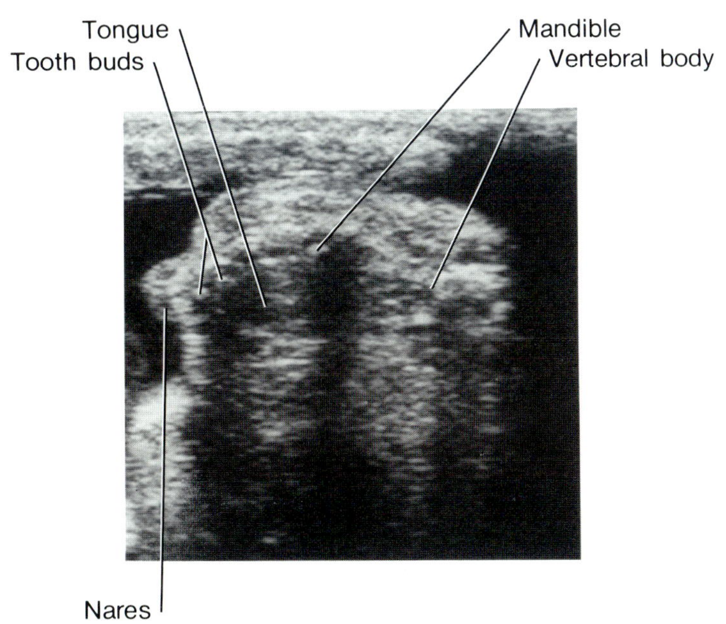
Tongue
Tooth buds
Mandible
Vertebral body
Nares

Carotid a.
Internal jugular v.
Sternocleidomastoid m.
Spinal cord
Parotid gland
Mandible
Geniohyoid m.
Tongue
Maxilla
Trapezius m.
Dura mater
Vertebral a.
Pharynx
Cricoid cartilage
Submandibular gland
Hyoid cartilage
Thyroid cartilage
Vocal cord

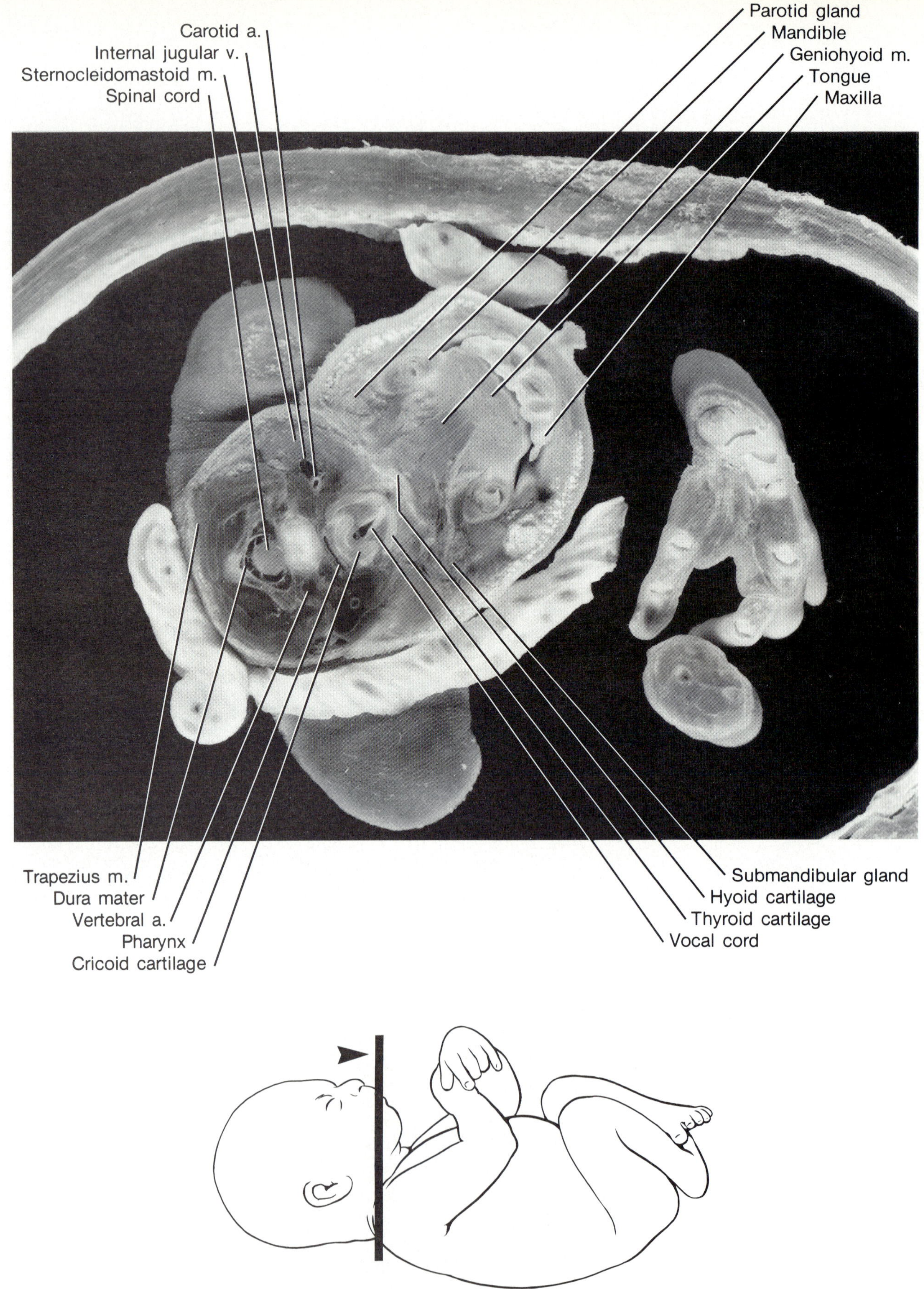

Figure 1.22

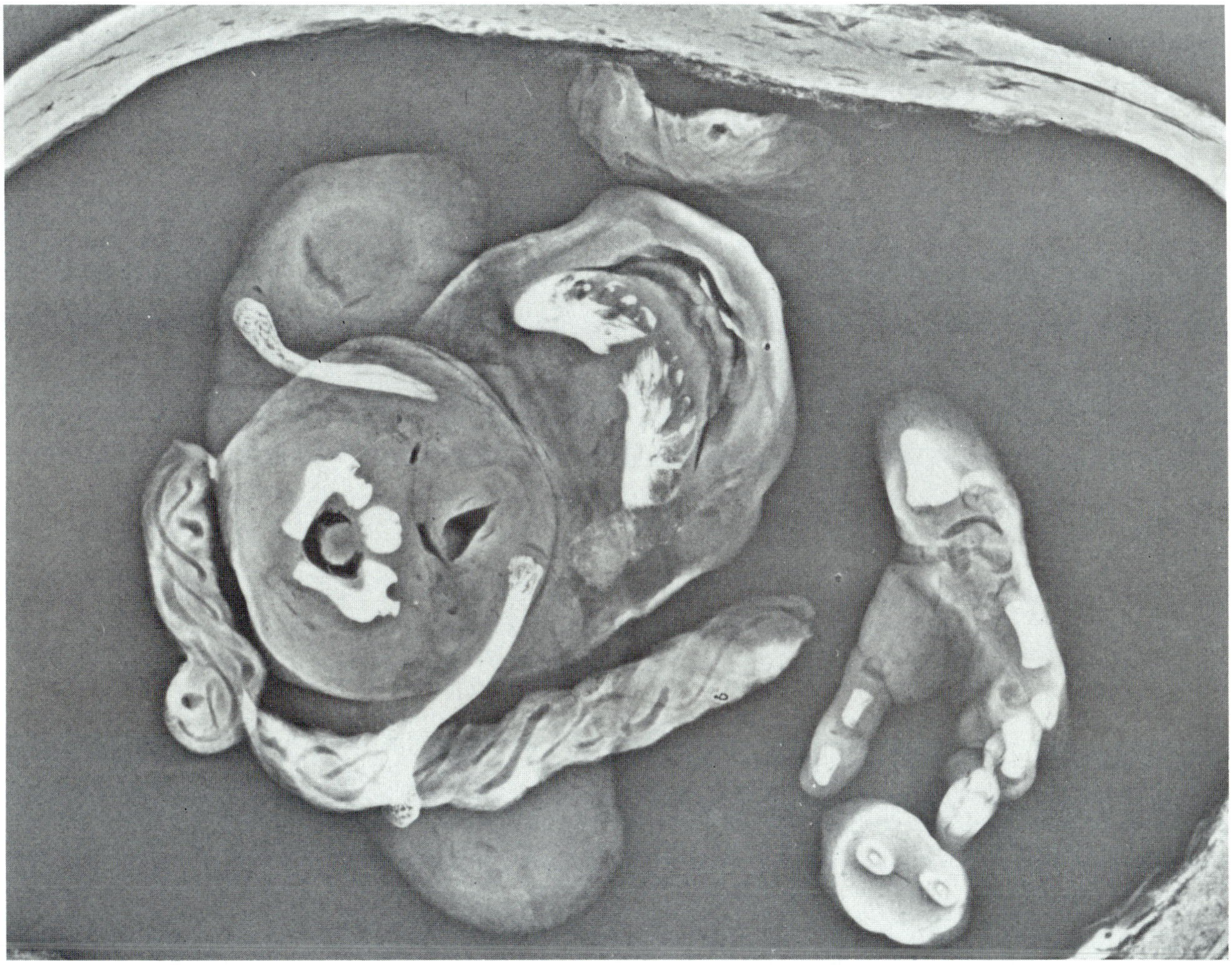

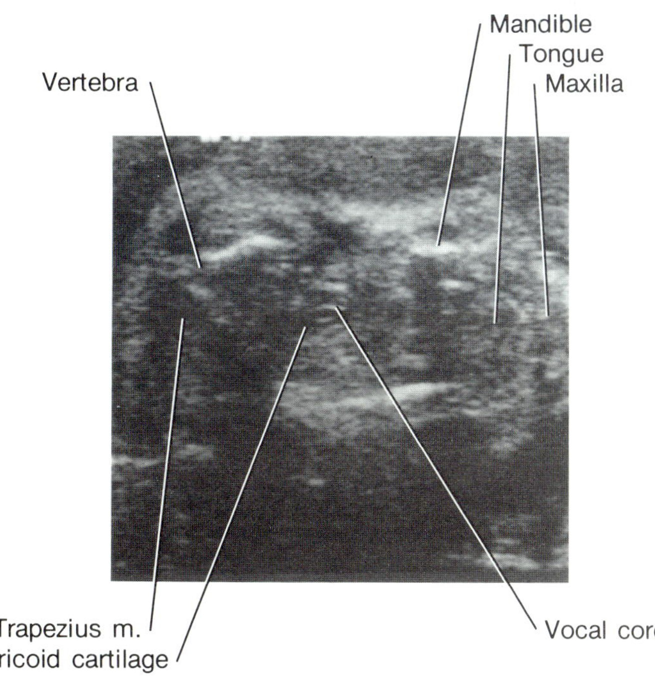

Mandible
Tongue
Maxilla
Vertebra
Trapezius m.
Cricoid cartilage
Vocal cord

Sternocleidomastoid m.
Geniohyoid m.
Tooth buds
Mandible
Tongue
Deltoid m.
Thyroid gland
Clavicle
Articulating facets
Spinous process
Trapezius m.
Buccinator m.
Anterior belly of digastric m.
Mylohyoid m.
Sternoclavicular joint
Trachea
Dura mater
Spinal cord
Acromioclavicular joint
Esophagus
Internal jugular v.

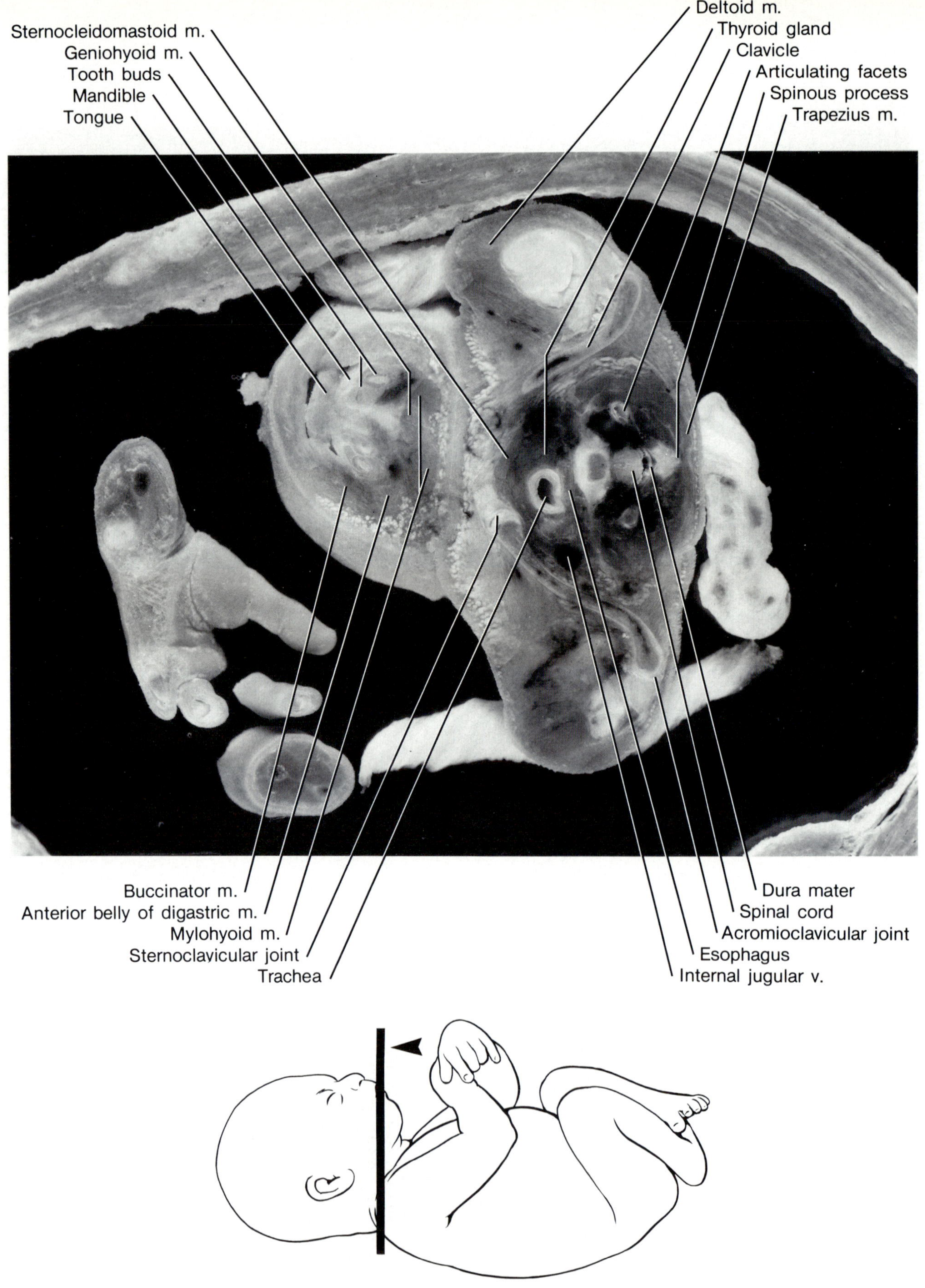

Figure 1.23

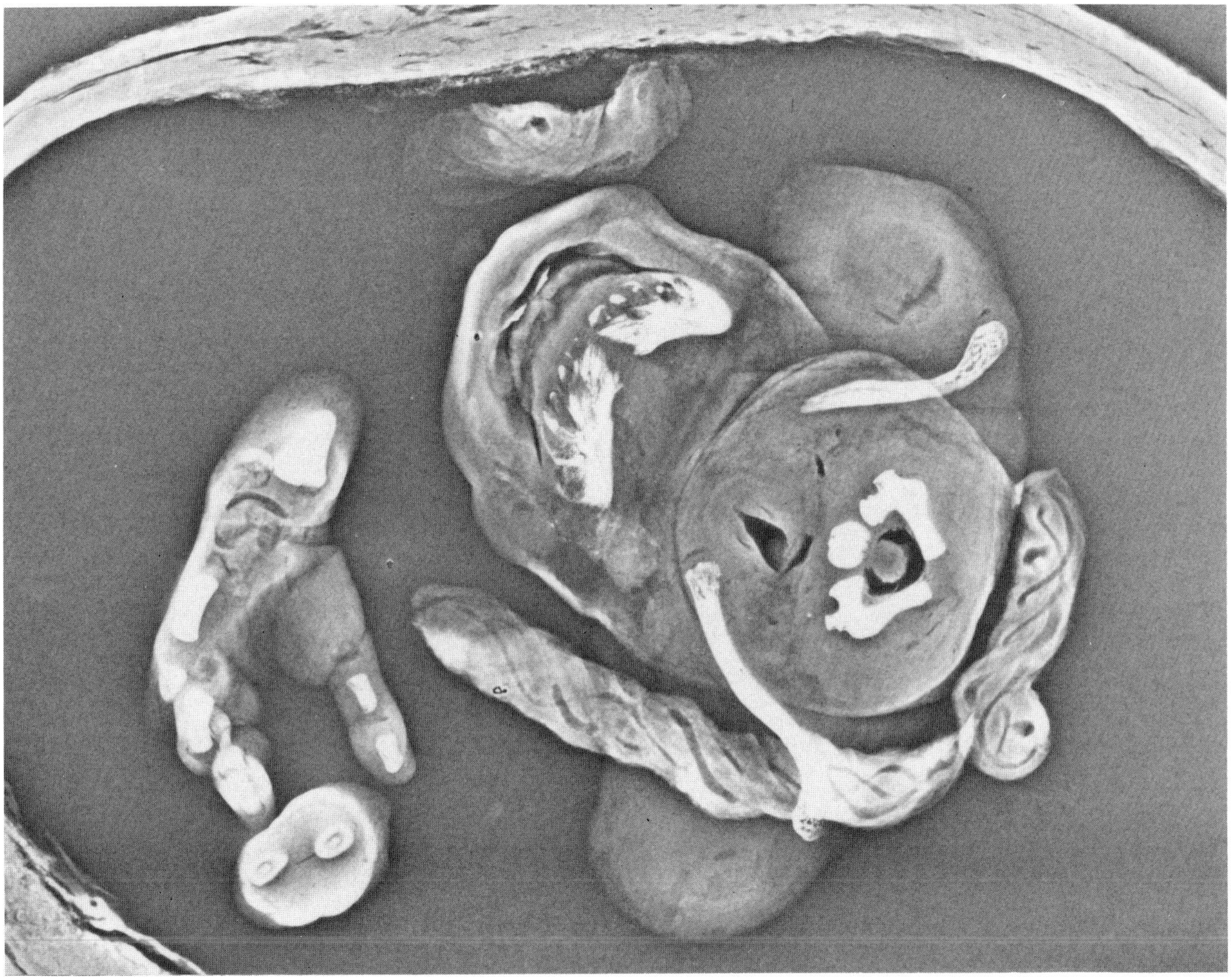

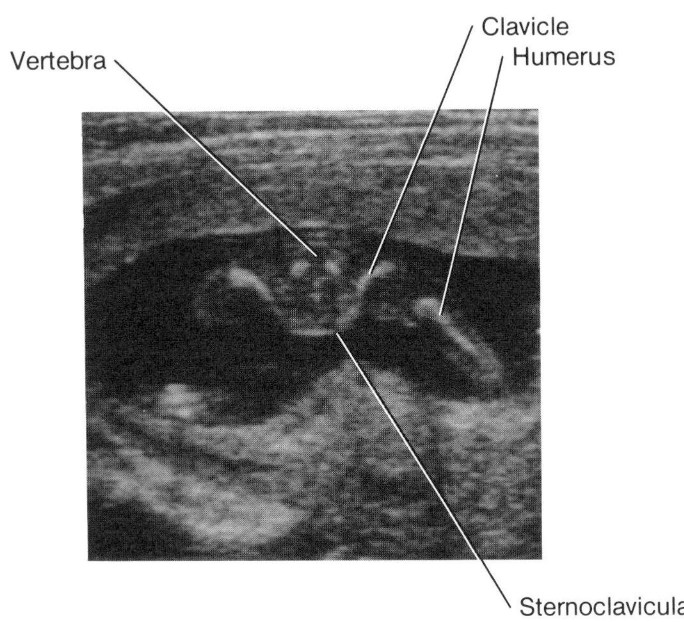

Vertebra
Clavicle
Humerus
Sternoclavicular joint

Esophagus
Vertebral body
Lamina
Spinous process
Head of humerus
Clavicle
Thyroid gland
Manubrium
Trapezius m.
Internal vertebral plexus of veins
Spinal nerves
Sternoclavicular joint
Pectoralis major m.
"Strap" muscles
Trachea

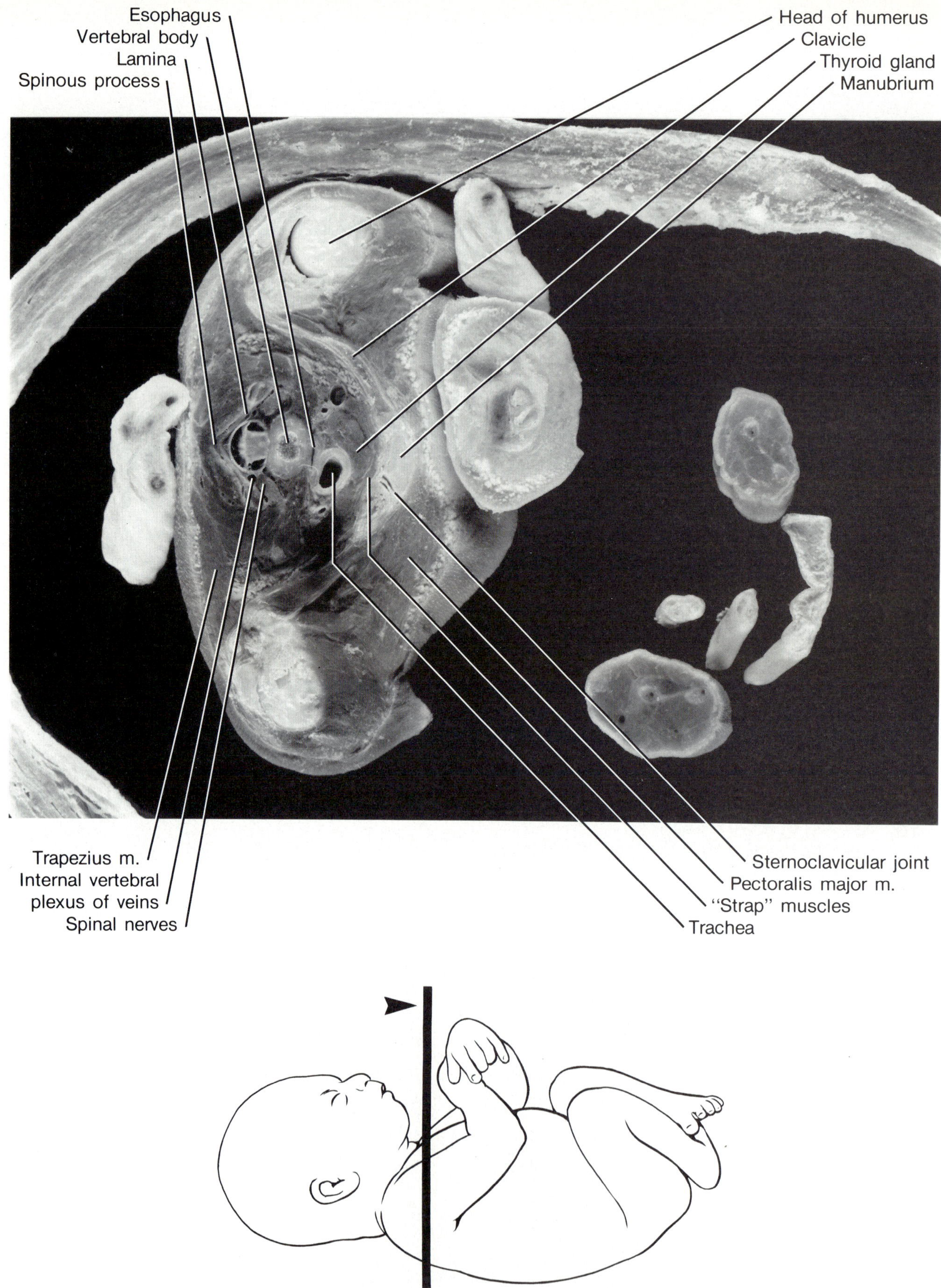

Figure 1.24

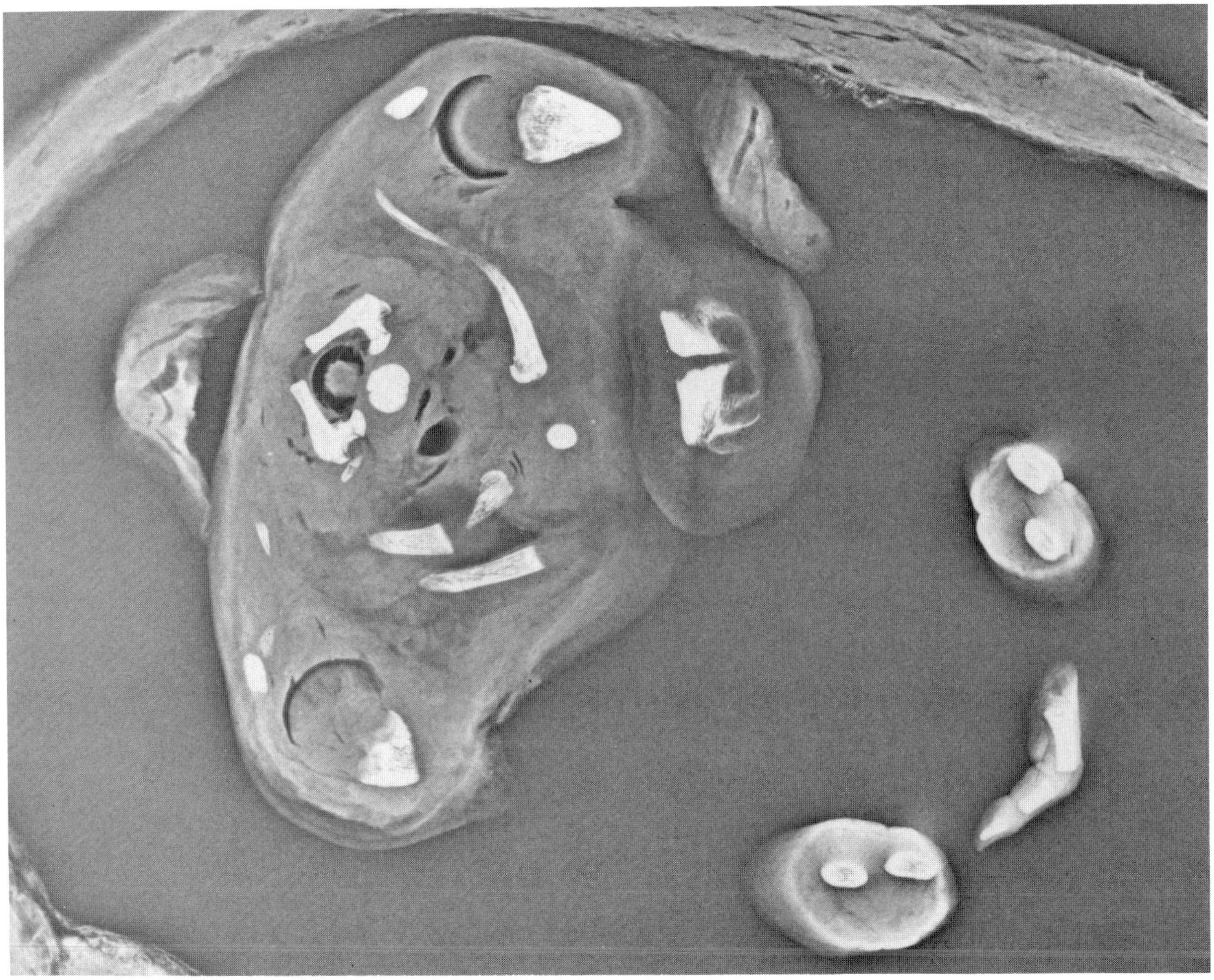

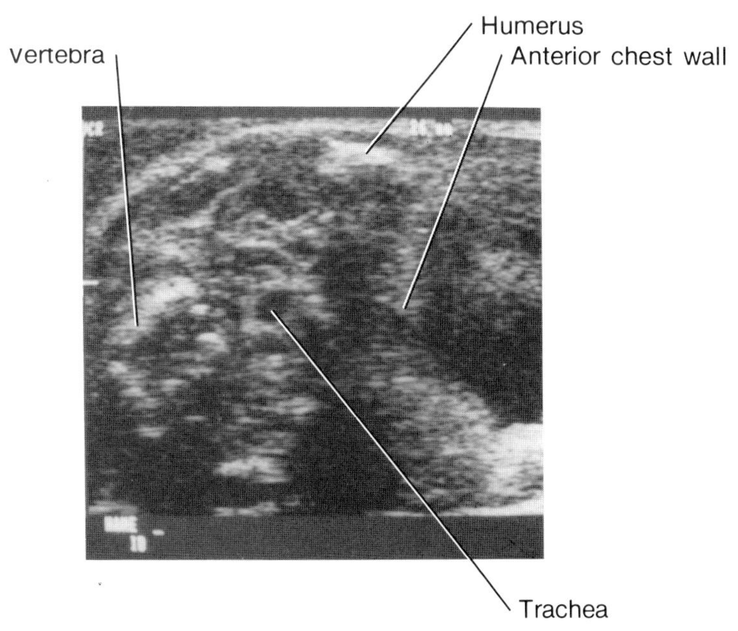

vertebra
Humerus
Anterior chest wall
Trachea

Axillary a.
Subclavian v.
Thymus
Radius
Ulna
Head of humerus
Brachial plexus
Carotid a.
Esophagus
Dura mater
Pectoralis major m.
Common carotid a.
Internal thoracic a.
Pectoralis minor m.
Axillary v.
Trachea
Left subclavian a.
First rib
Axillary a.
Deltoid m.

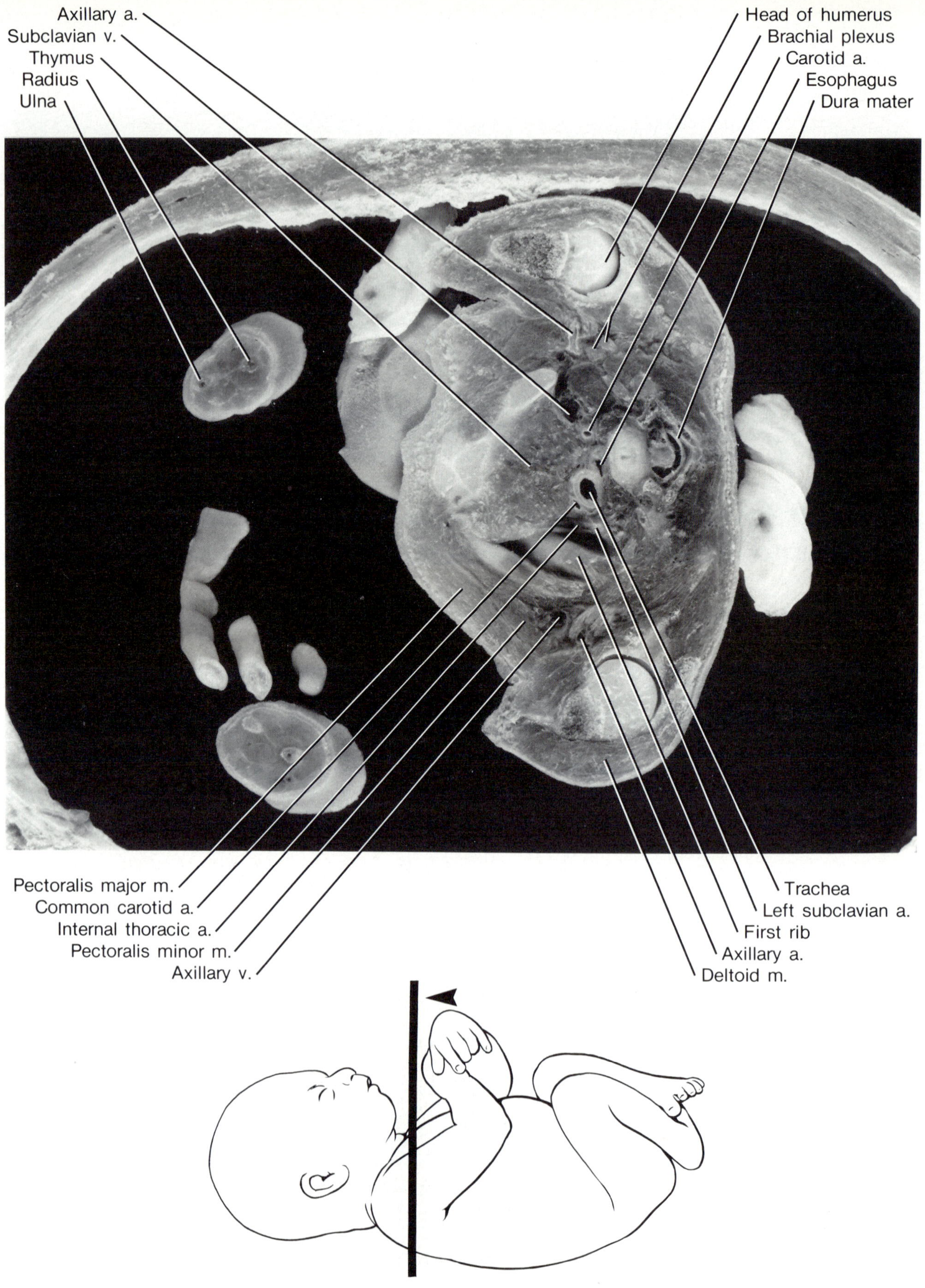

Figure 1.25

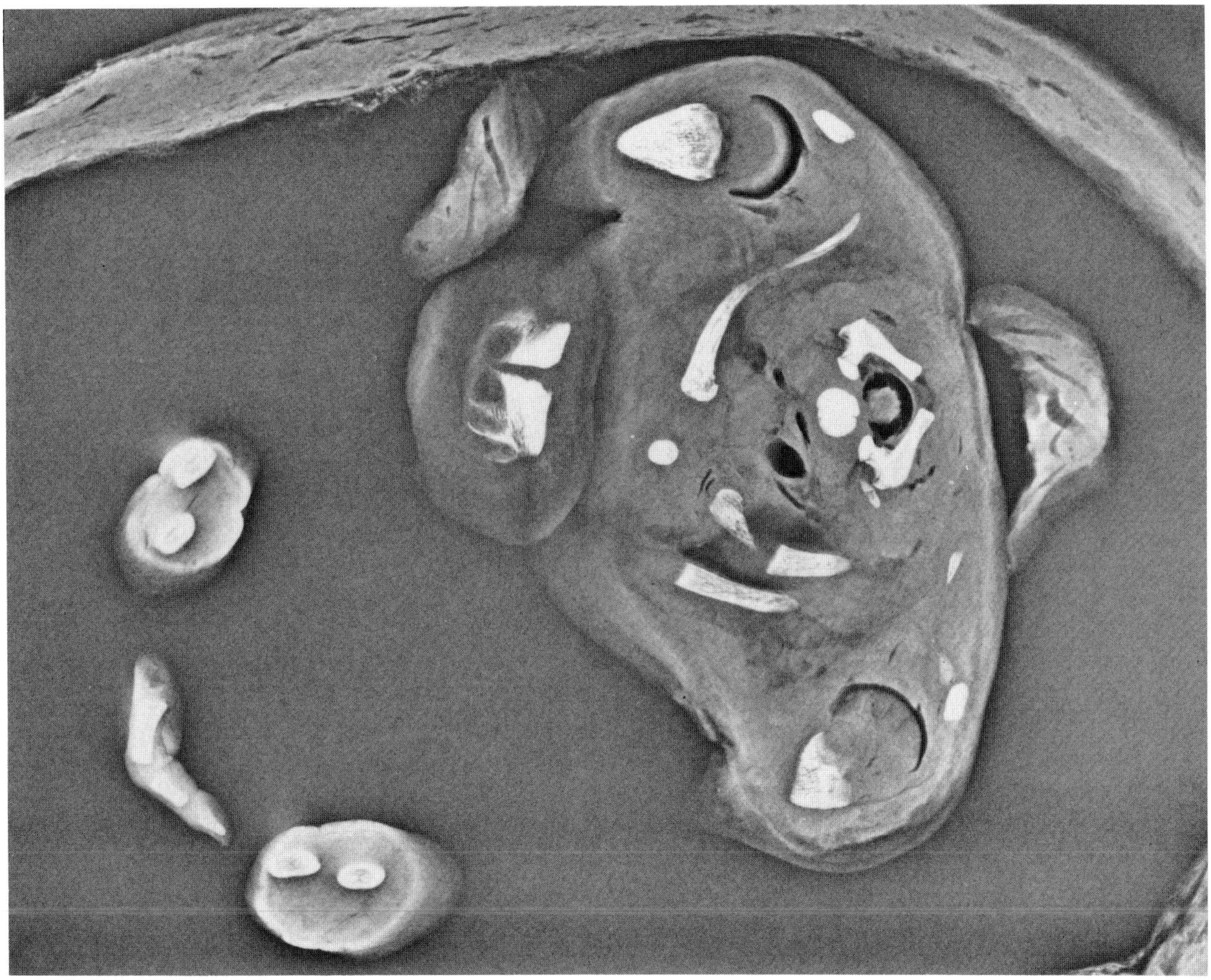

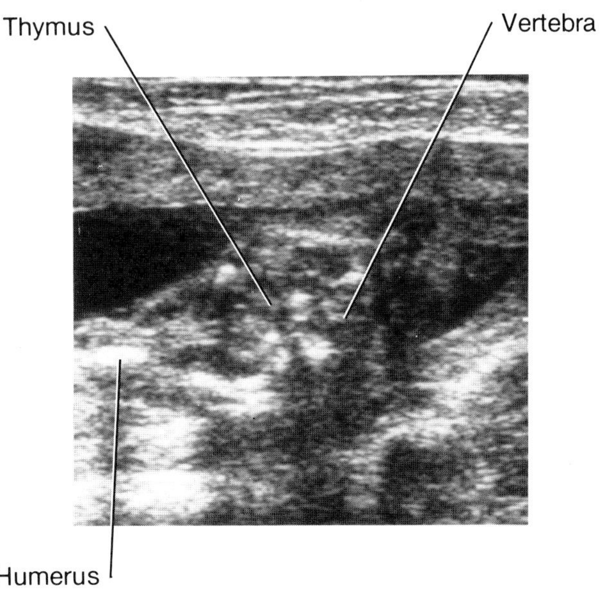

Thymus
Vertebra
Humerus

Esophagus
Vertebral body
Lamina
Brachial plexus
Left common carotid a.
Left brachiocephalic v.
Supraspinatus m.
Longus colli m.
Trachea
Head of humerus
Axillary vessels
Pectoralis major m.
Thymus
Right common carotid a.
Right subclavian a.

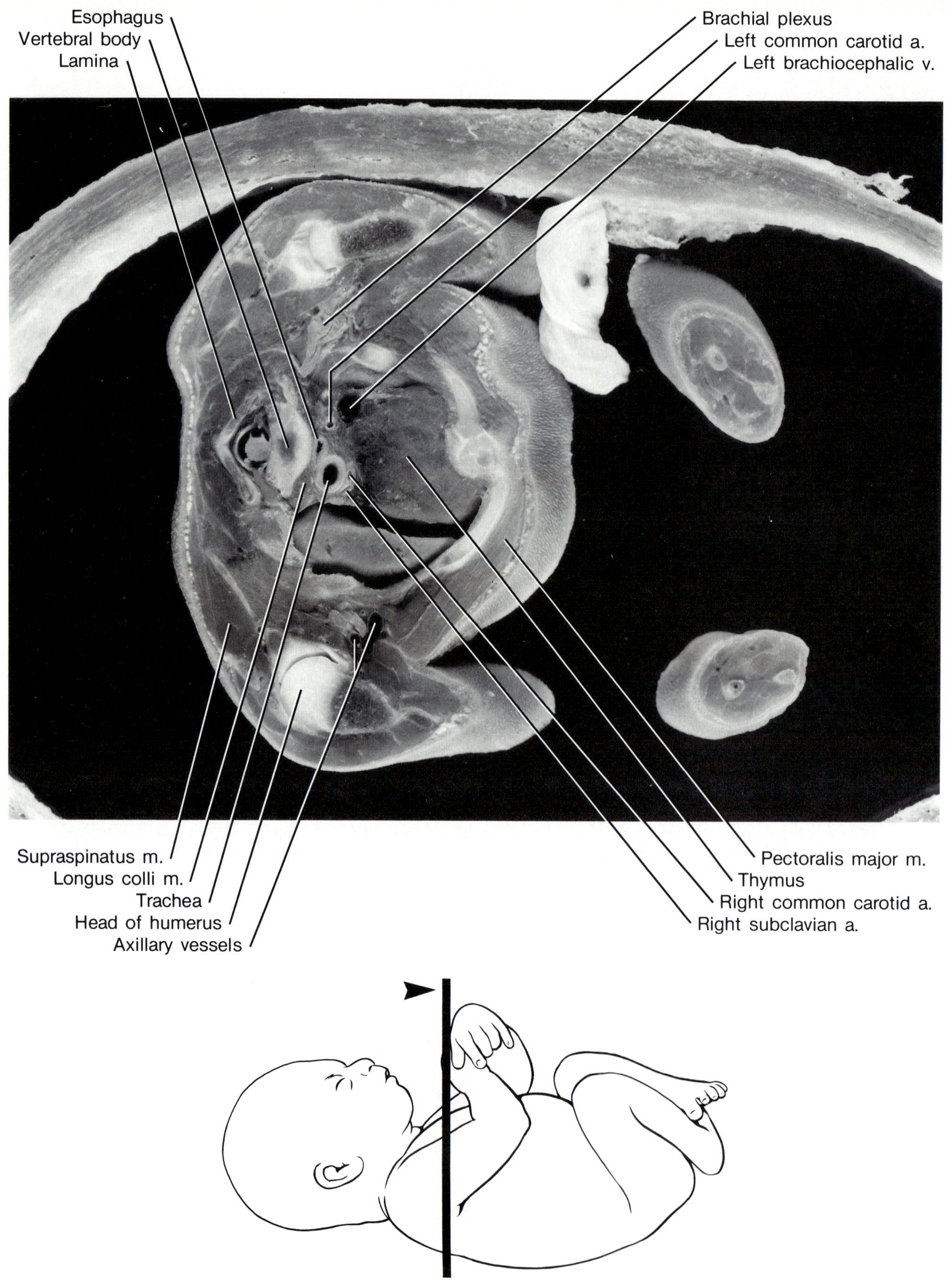

Figure 1.26

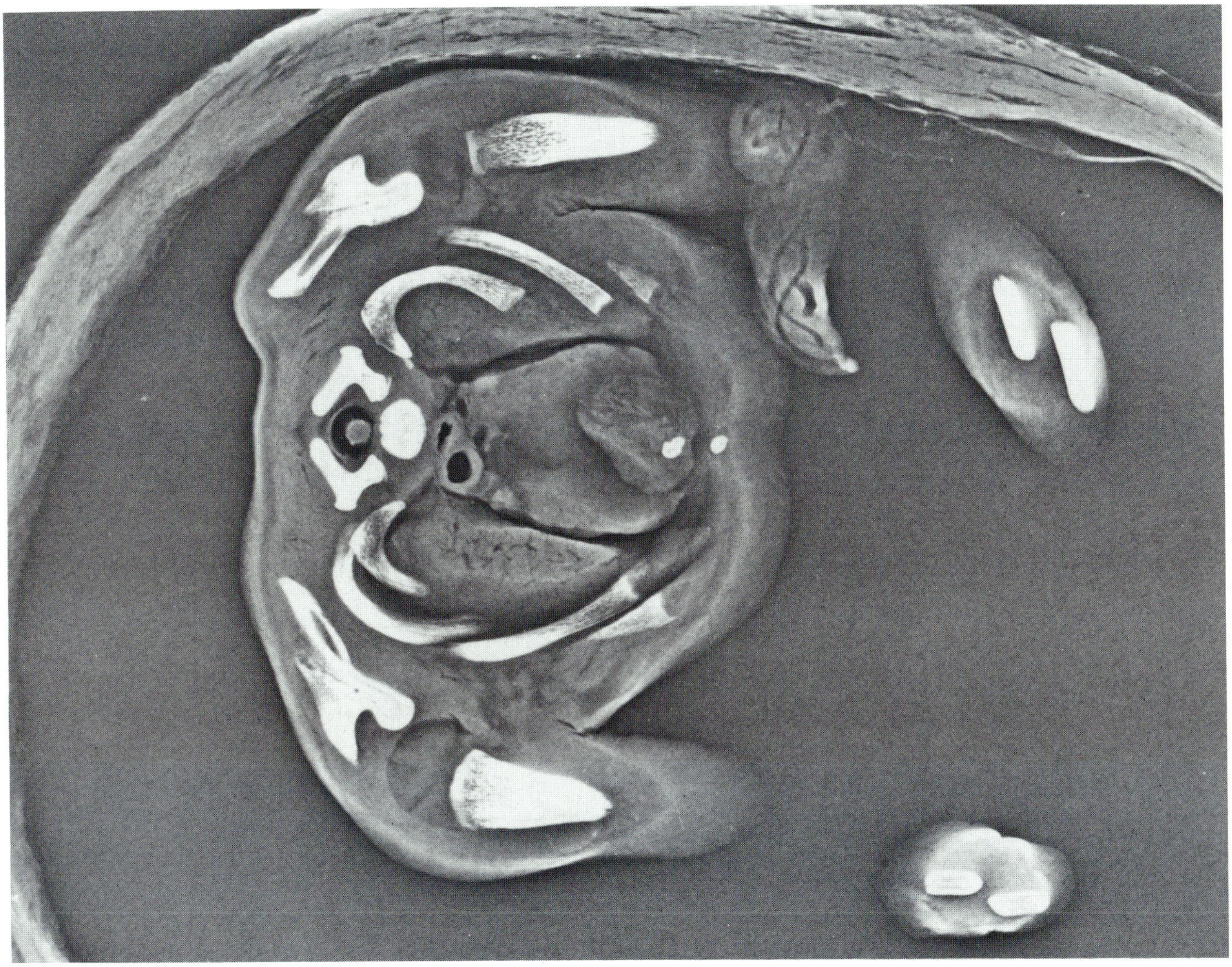

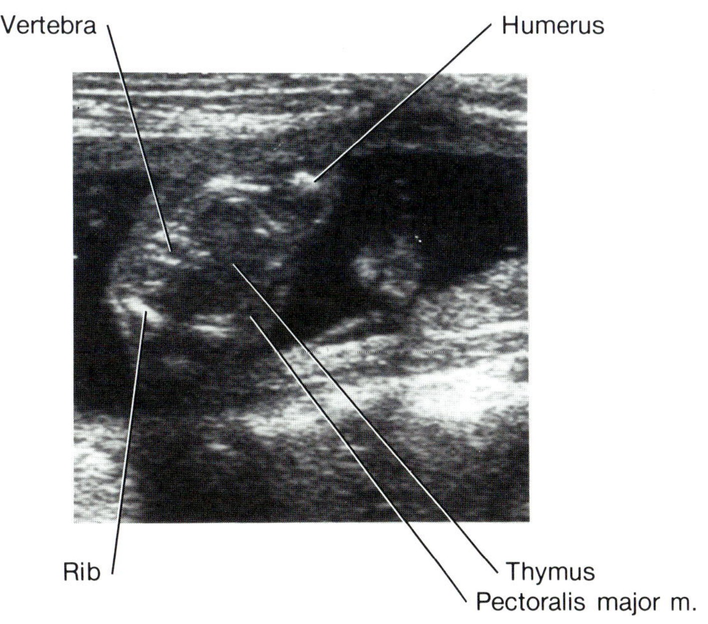

Vertebra
Humerus
Rib
Thymus
Pectoralis major m.

Humerus
Pericardium
Remnant of
right ventricle
Radius
Ulna
Brachiocephalic a.
Left common carotid a.
Thymic a.
Left subclavian a.
Lung
Intervertebral canal
Manubrium
Right atrium
Thymus
Brachiocephalic v.
Superior vena cava
Dura mater
Sympathetic ganglia
Esophagus
Trachea
Pleural cavity

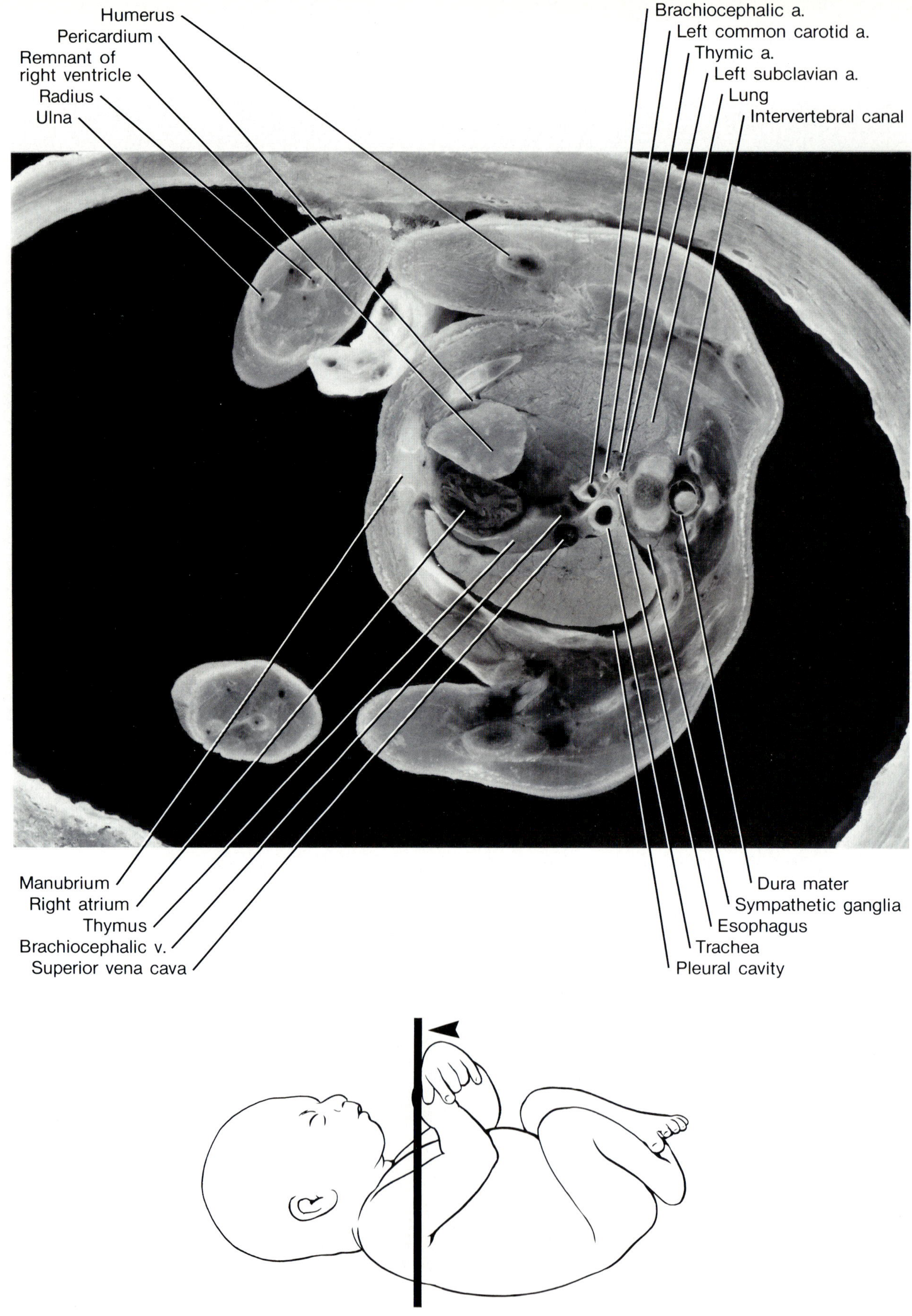

Figure 1.27

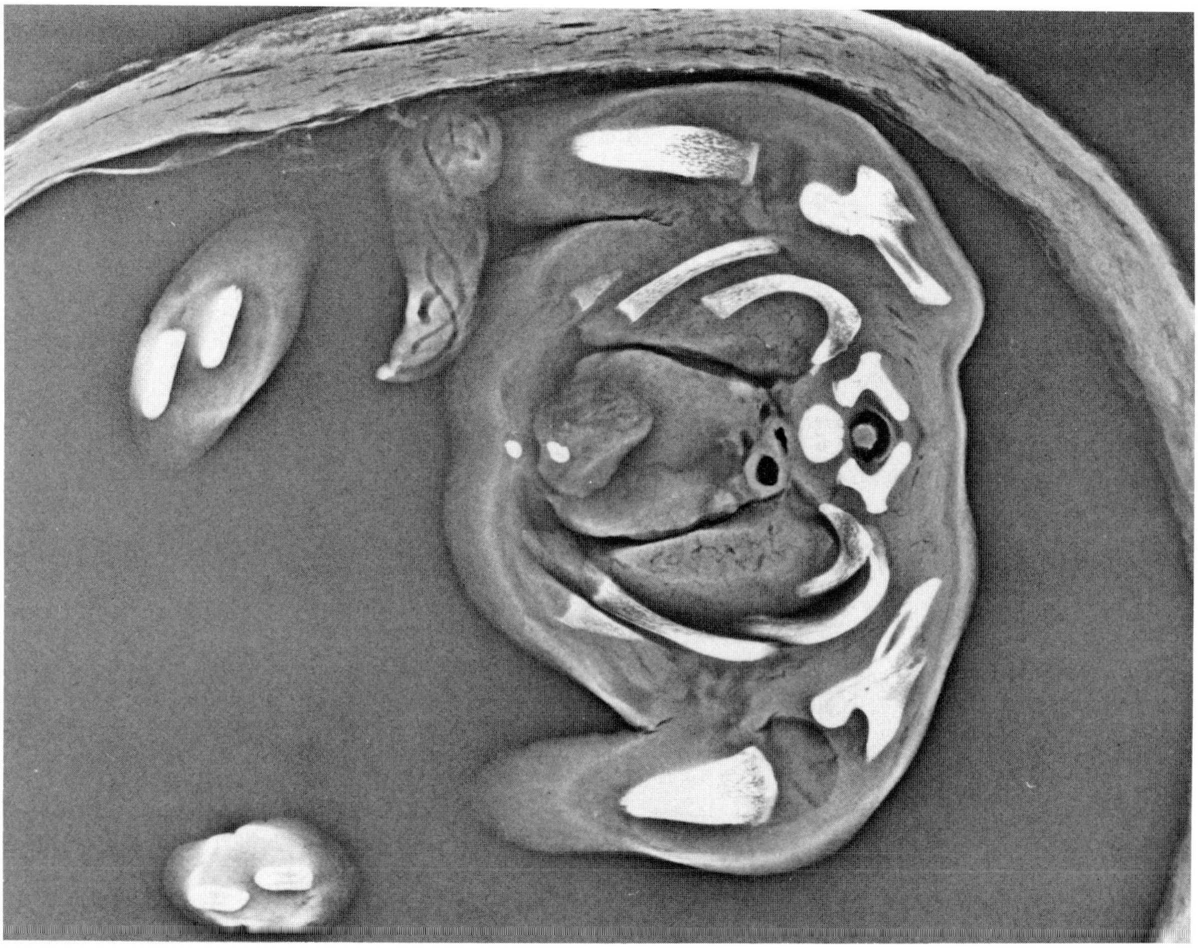

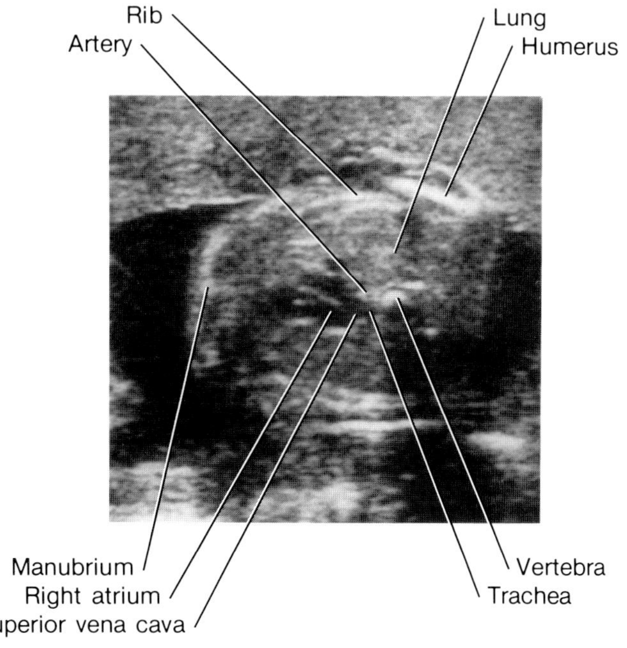

Rib
Artery
Lung
Humerus
Manubrium
Right atrium
Superior vena cava
Vertebra
Trachea

Pulmonary trunk
Thymus
Brachiocephalic a.
Pericardium
Right ventricle
Esophagus
Lung
Arch of aorta
Right atrium
Wall of right atrium
(pectinate muscle)
Superior vena cava

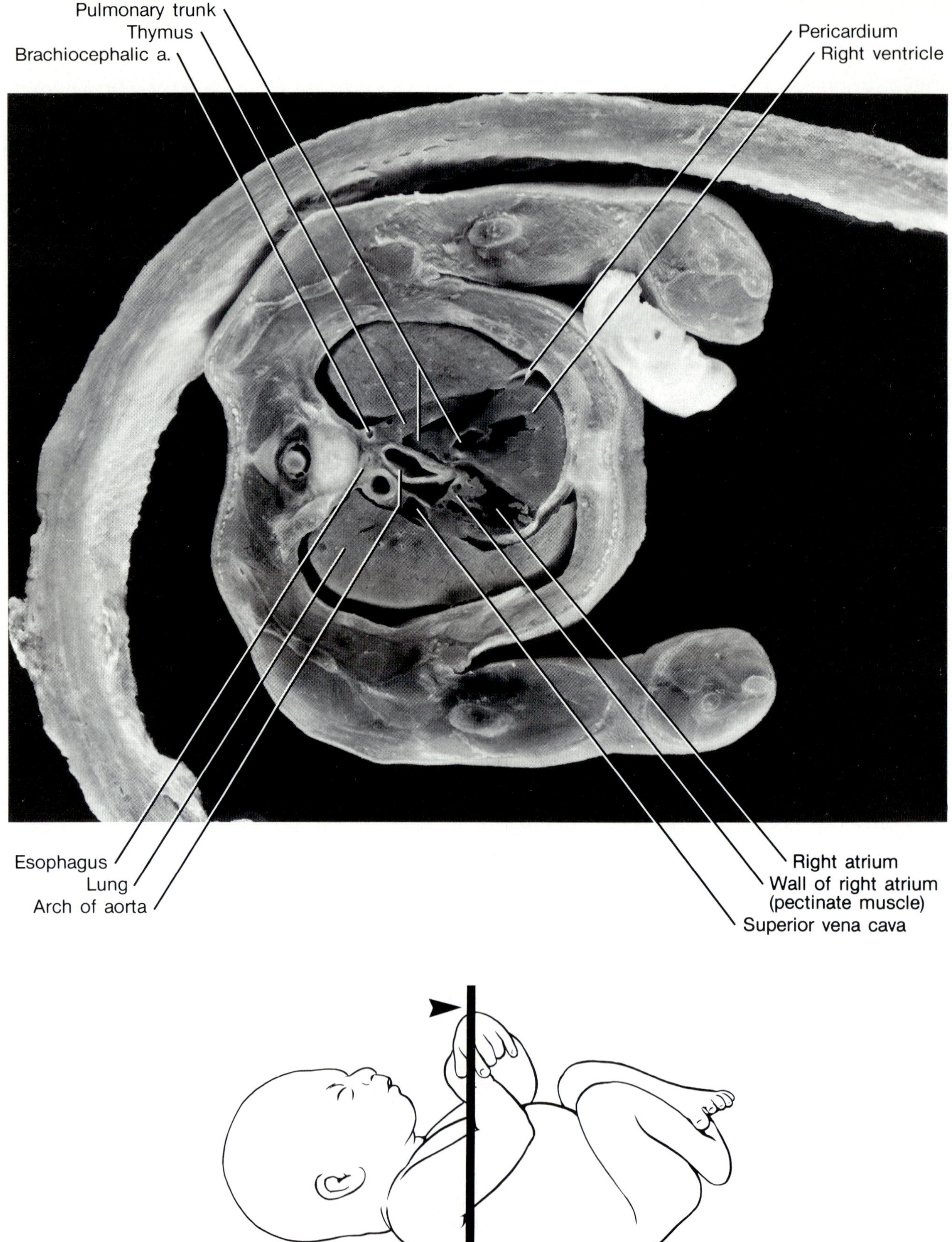

Figure 1.28

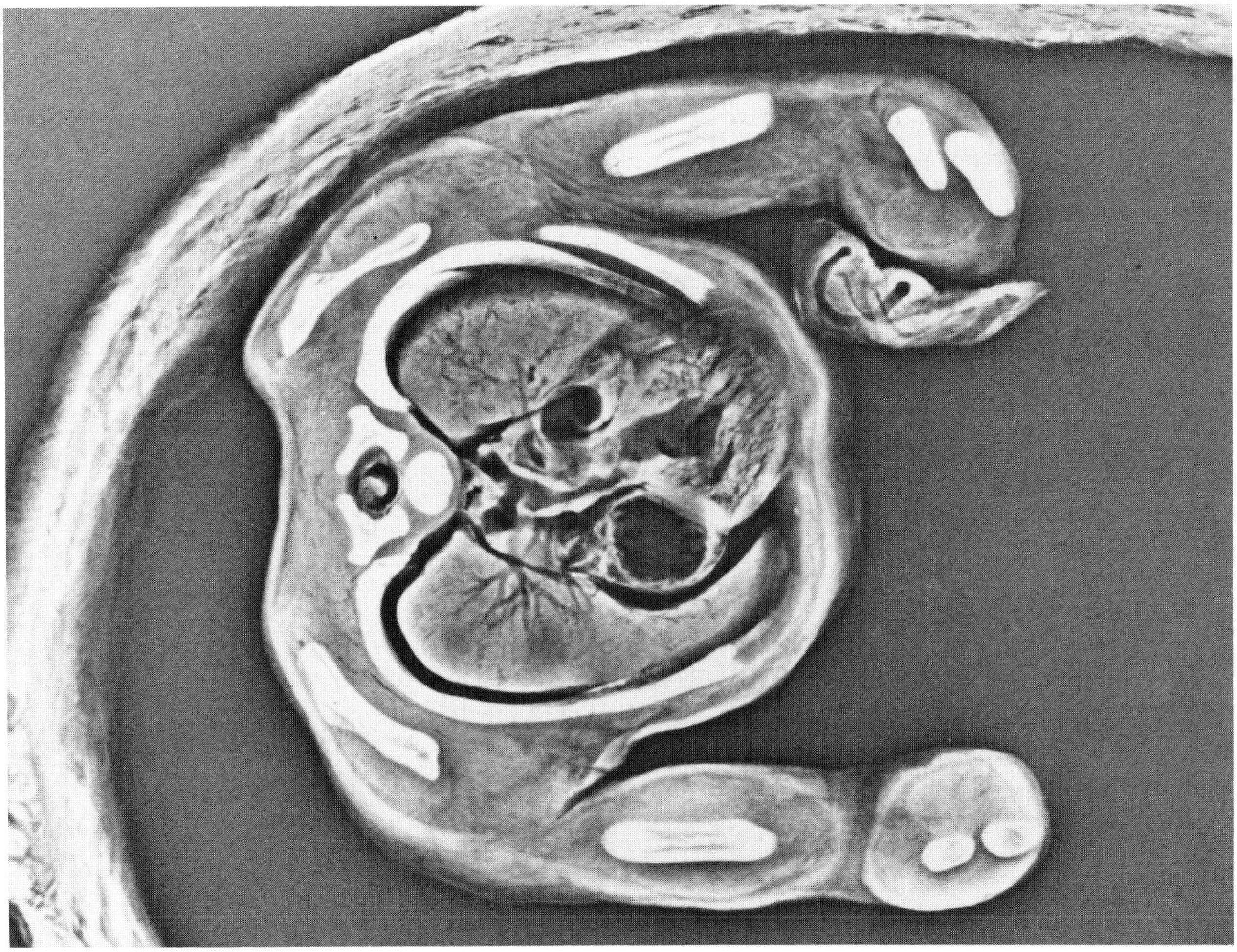

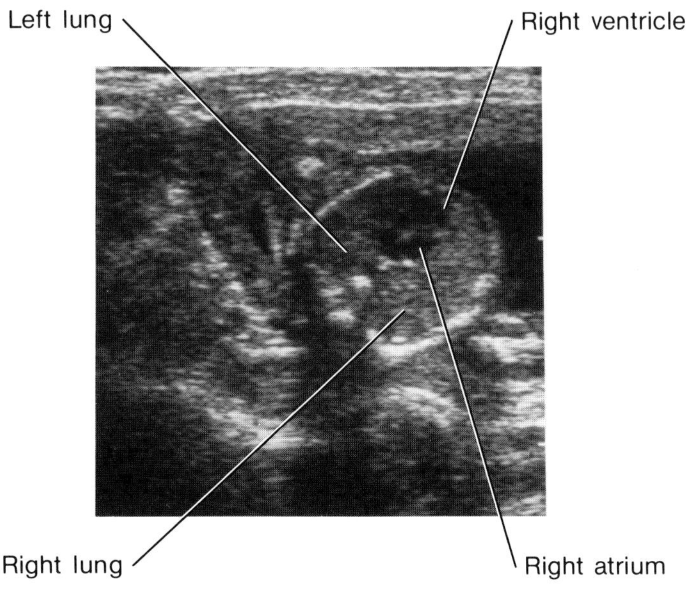
Left lung
Right ventricle
Right lung
Right atrium

Left atrium
Aortic valves
Left ventricle
Chordae tendineae
Humerus
Radius
Ulna
Wall of left atrium
Left pulmonary a.
Lung
Aorta
Thoracic duct
Pericardium
Anterior papillary m.
Tricuspid valve
Right atrium
Superior vena cava
Scapula
Esophagus
Azygos v.
Bifurcation of trachea
Triceps m.

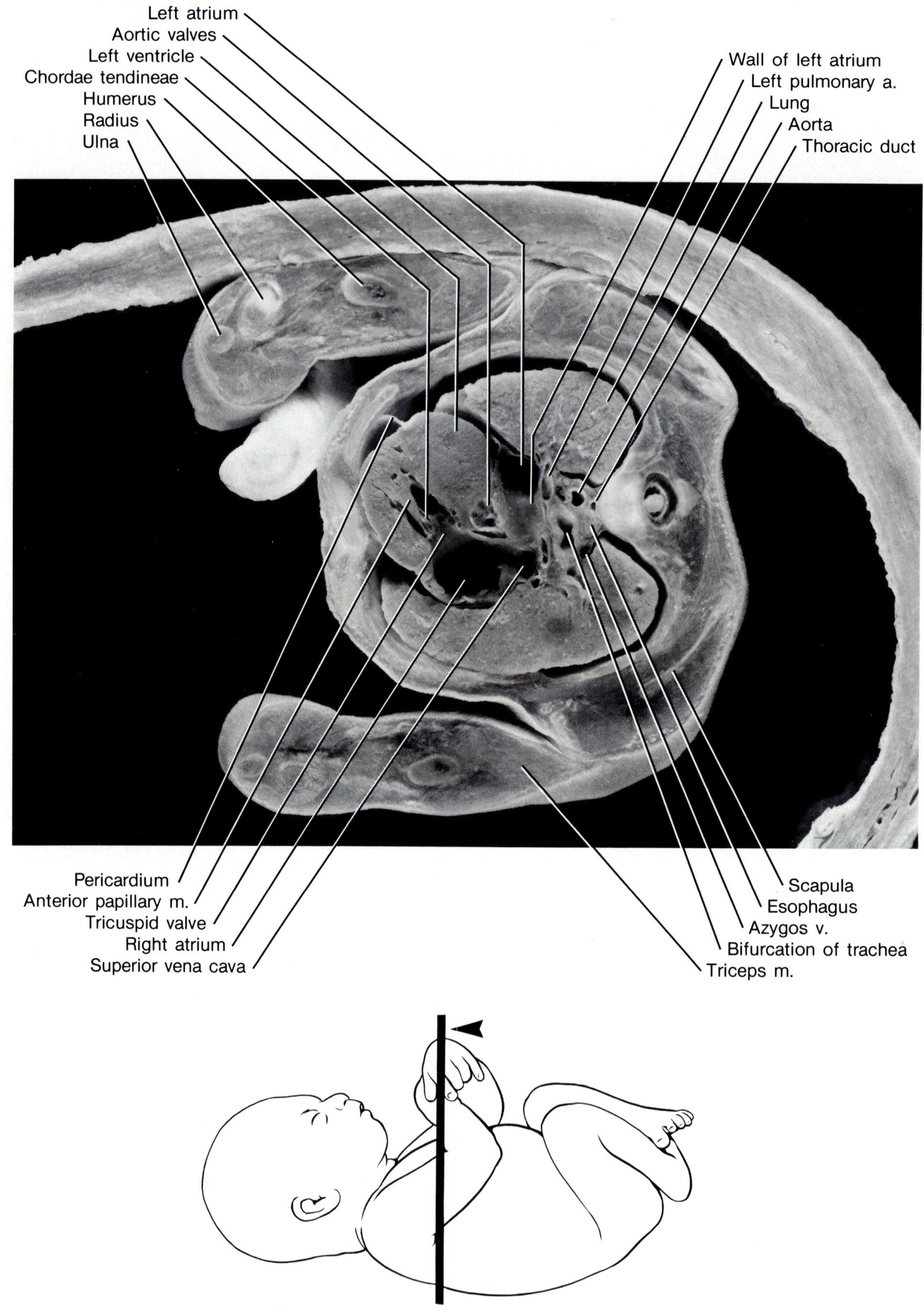

Figure 1.29

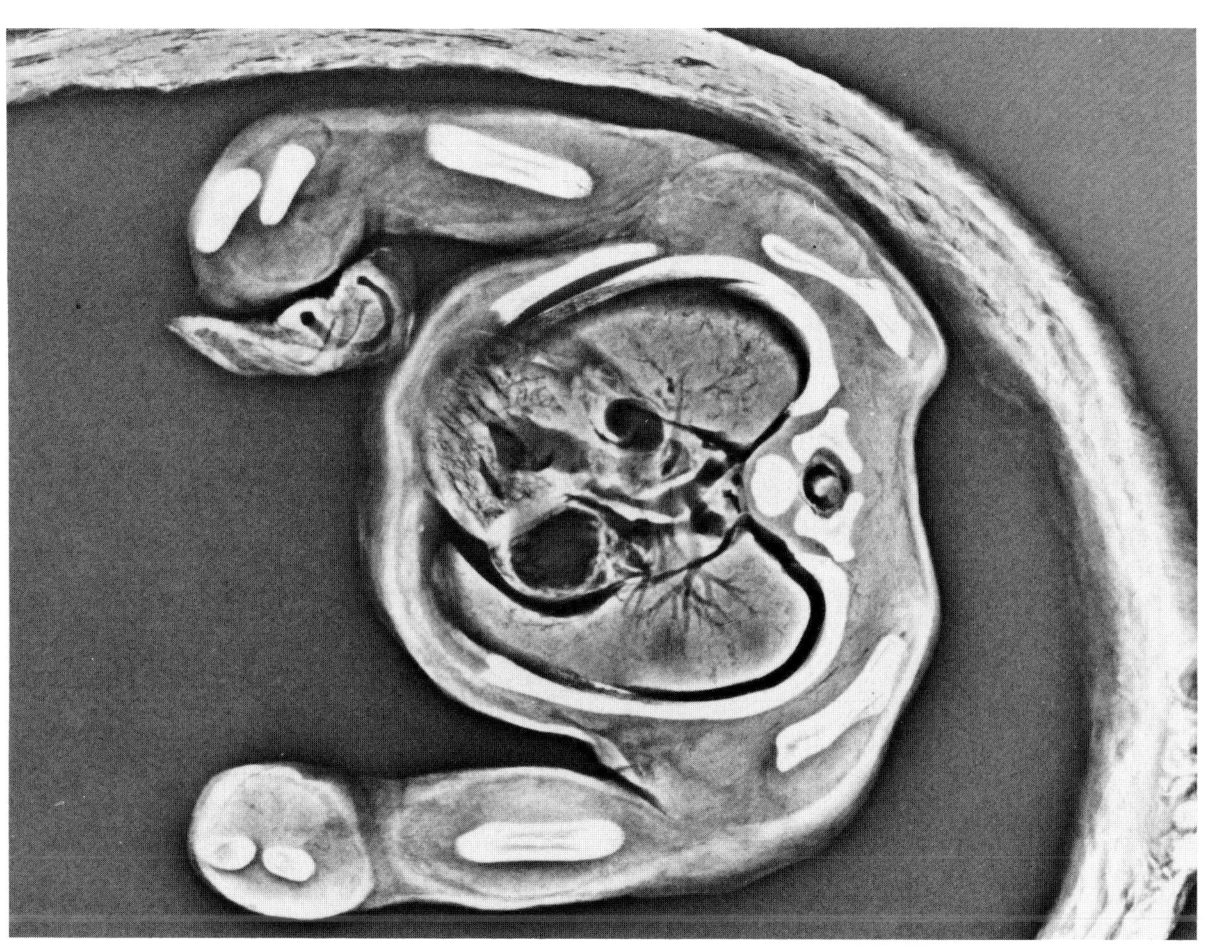

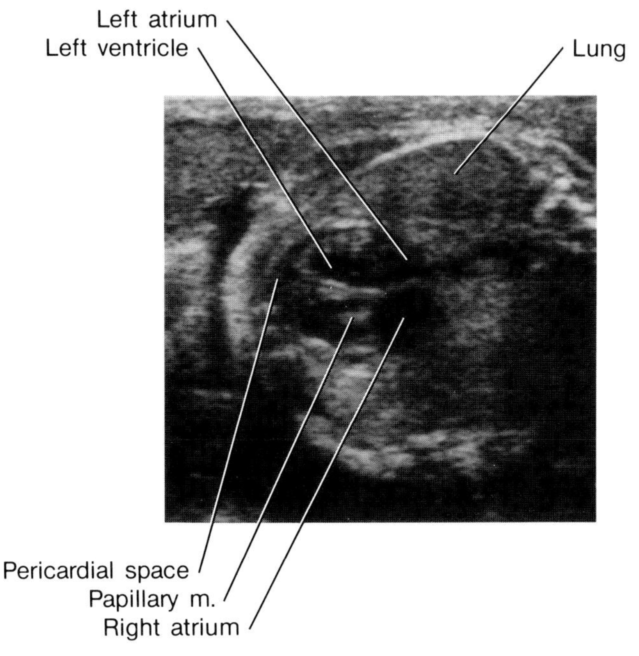

Left atrium
Left ventricle
Lung
Pericardial space
Papillary m.
Right atrium

Aortic valve
Auricle of left atrium
Left atrium
Scapula
Aorta
Esophagus
Left ventricle
Triceps m.
Right ventricle
Humerus
Radius
Ulna
Body of vertebra
Upper lobe of lung
Azygos v.
Bifurcation of trachea
Pulmonary a.
Pulmonary v.
Diaphragm
Chordae tendineae
Tricuspid valve
Right atrium
Interatrial septum

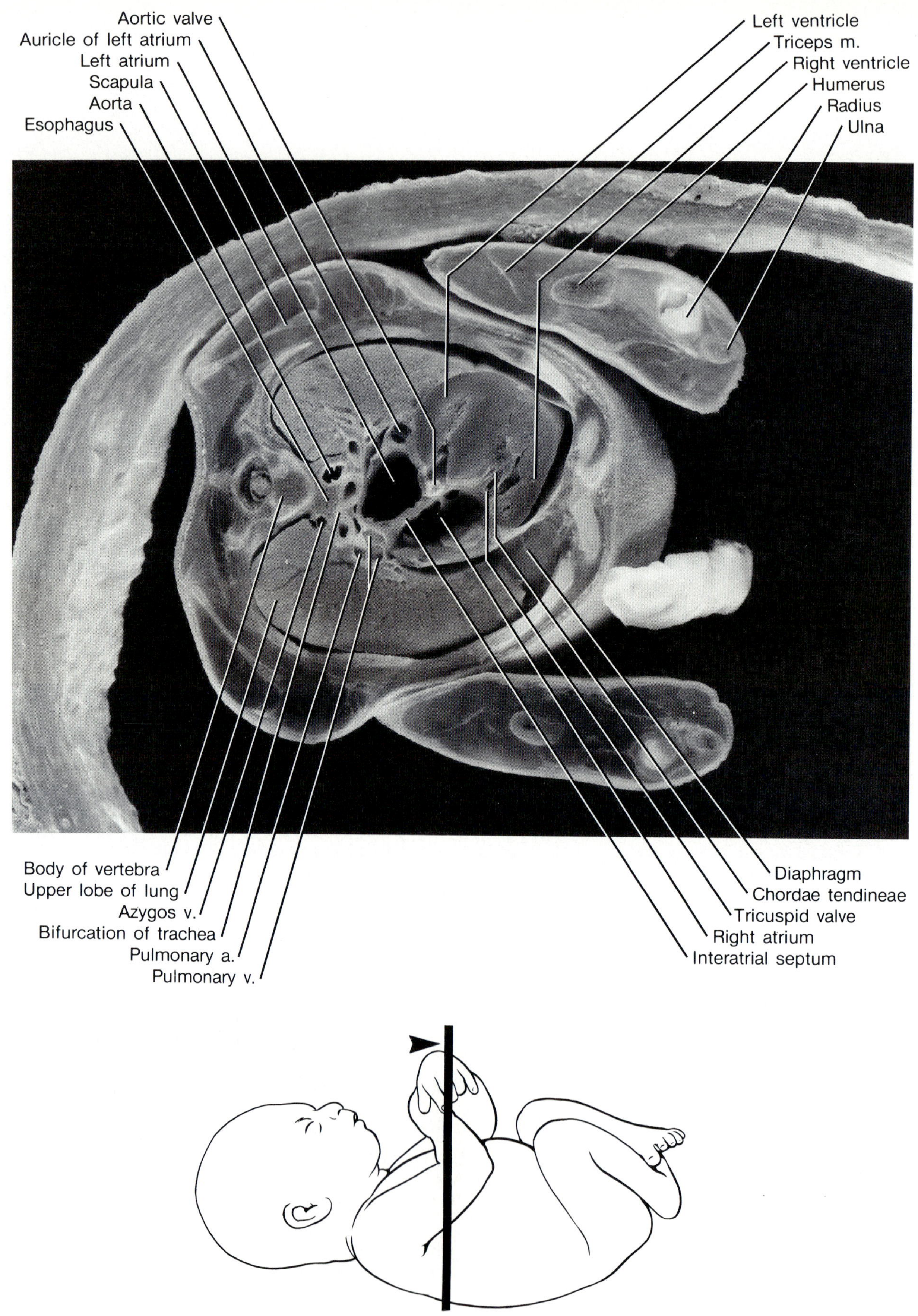

Figure 1.30

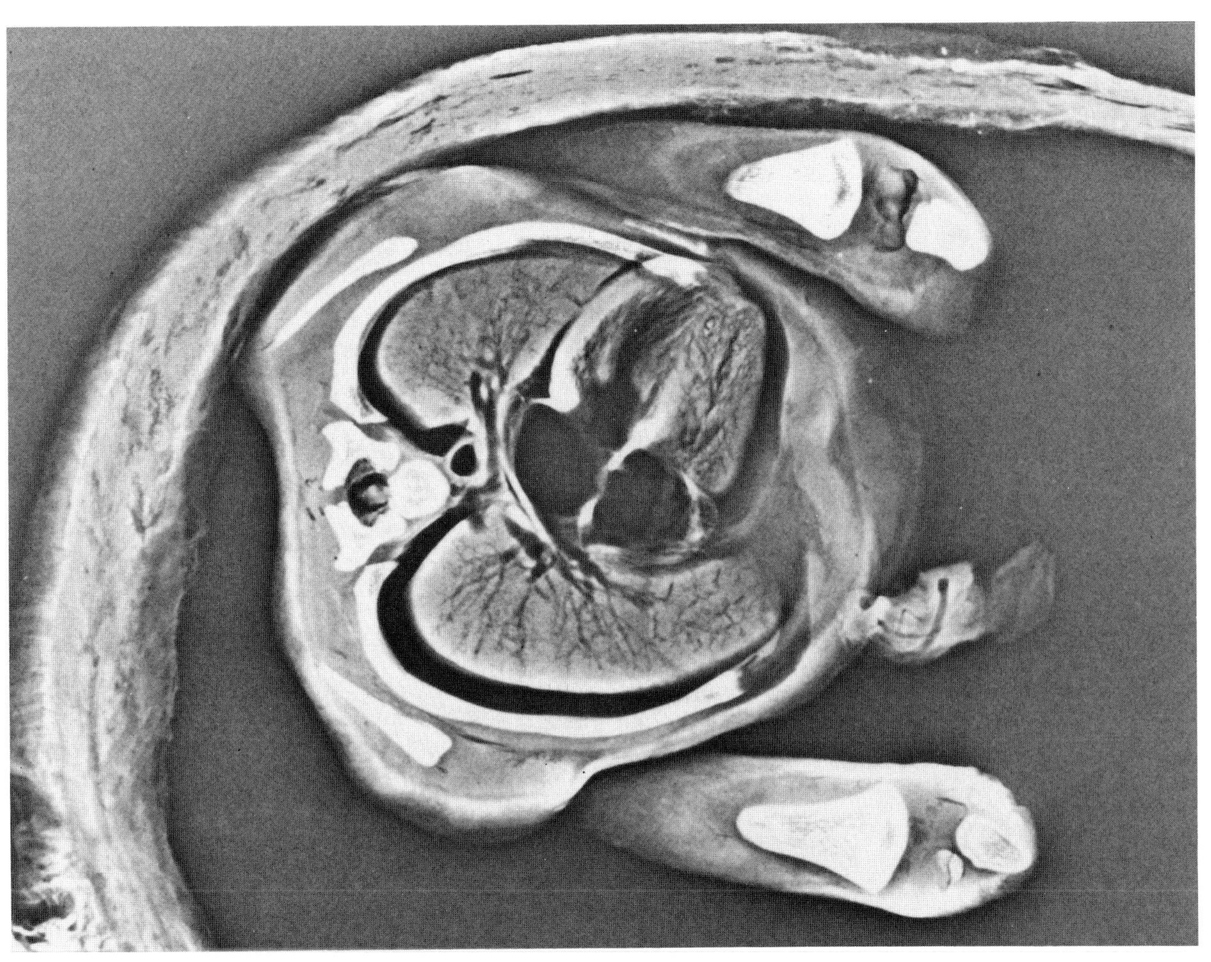

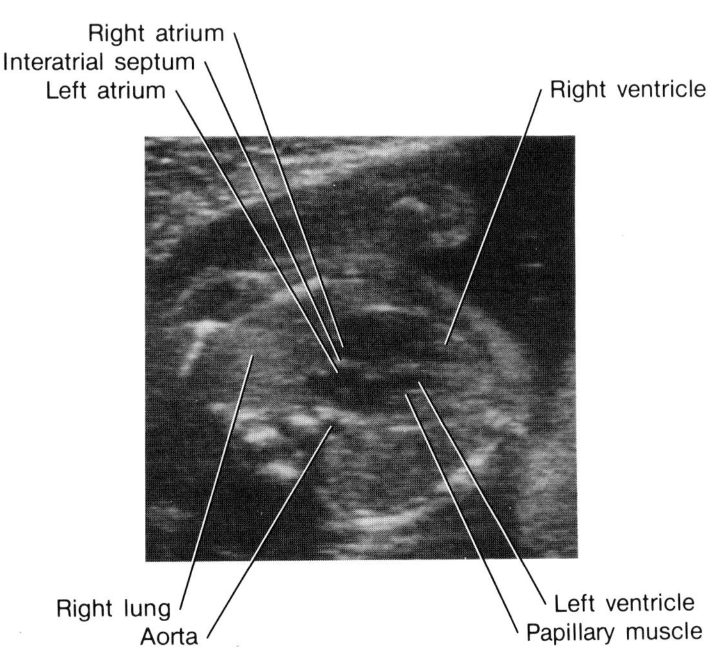

Right atrium
Interatrial septum
Left atrium
Right ventricle
Right lung
Aorta
Left ventricle
Papillary muscle

Bronchi
Mitral valve
Left ventricle
Anterior papillary m.
Pericardium
Infraspinatus m.
Aorta
Lower lobe of lung
Scapula
Thoracic duct
Liver
Opening of corononary sinus
Right atrium
Azygos v.
Esophagus
Pulmonary a.
Left atrium

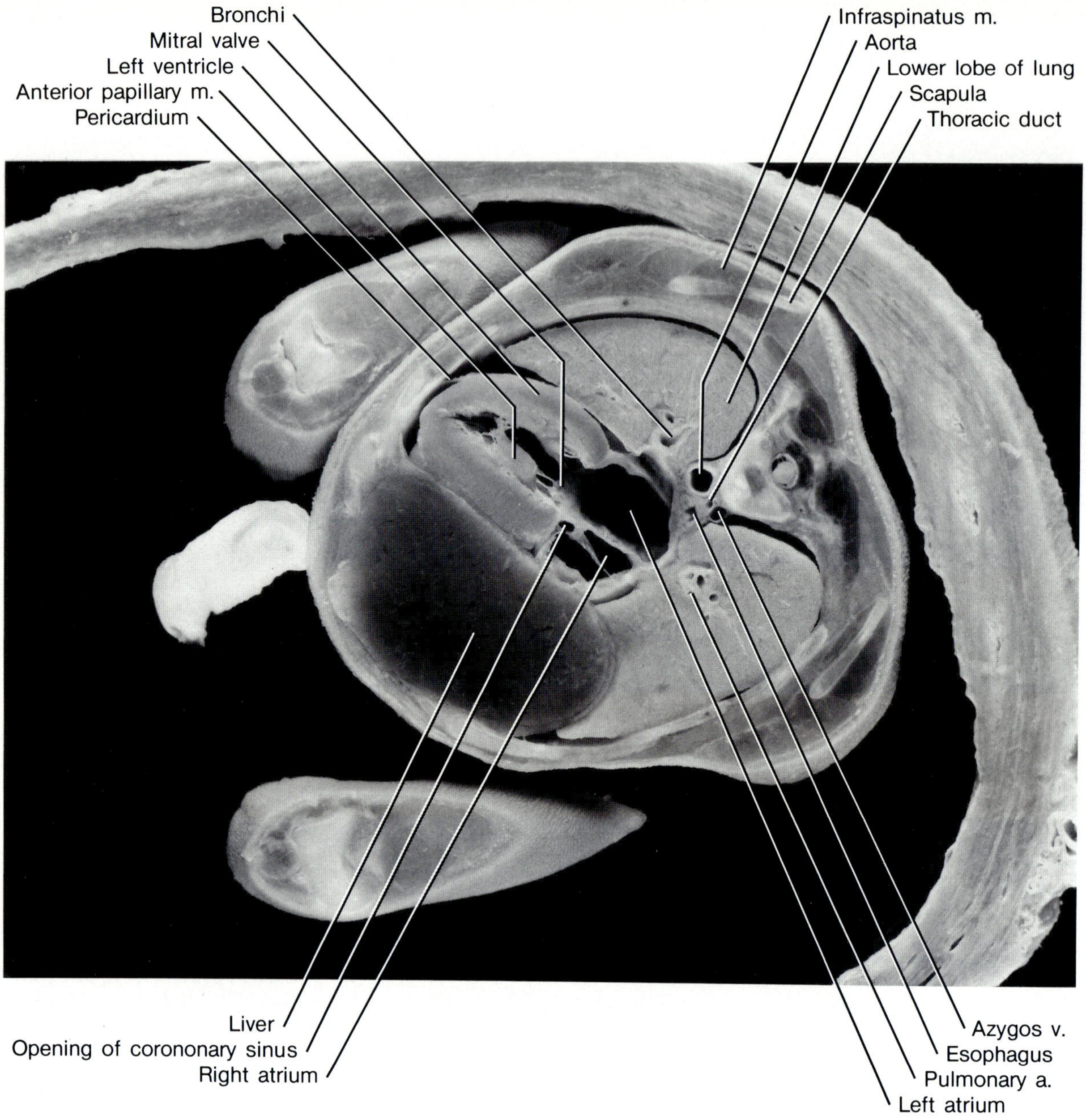

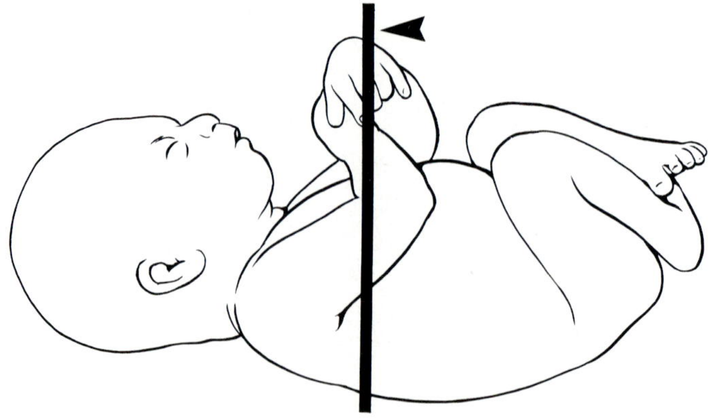

Figure 1.31

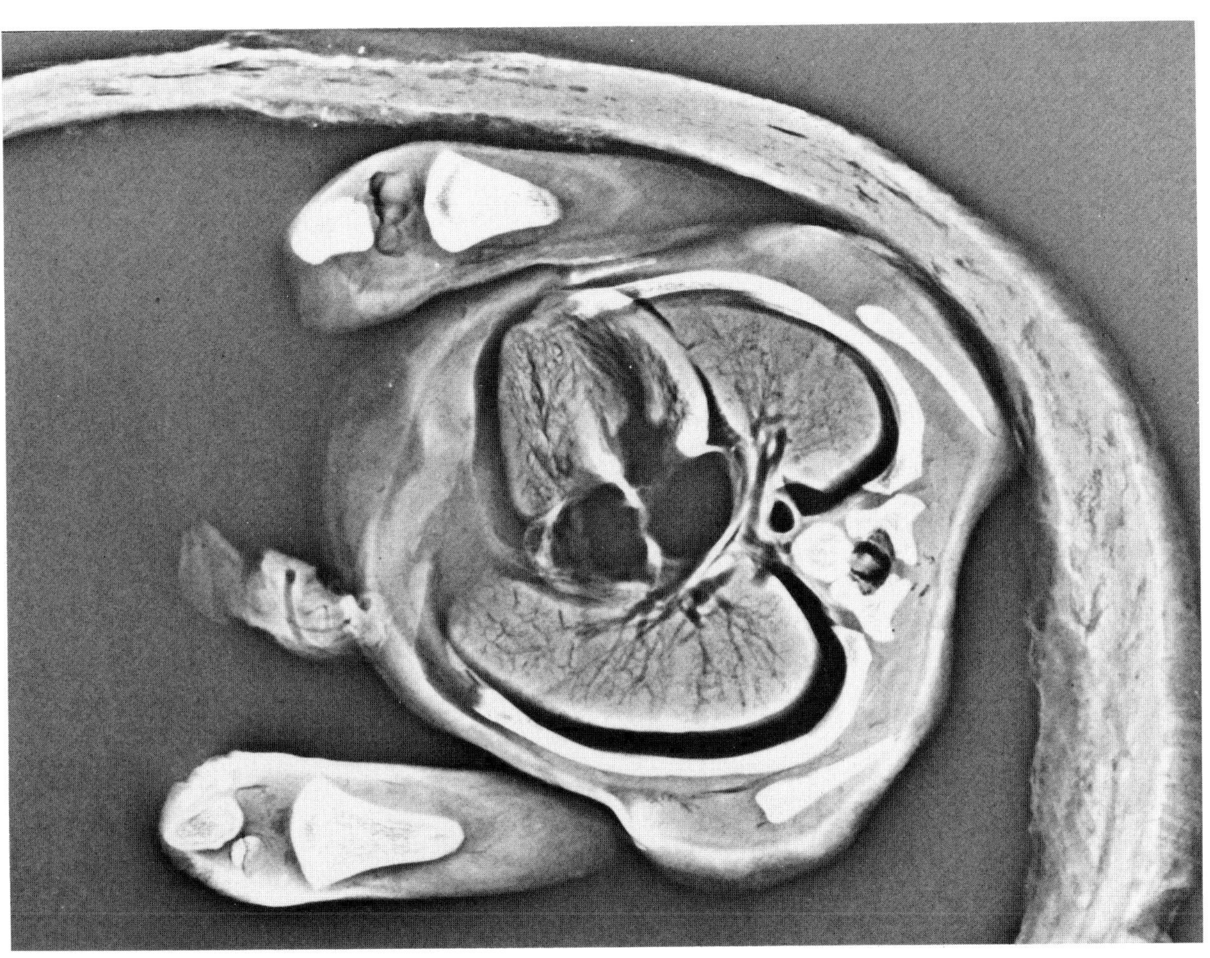

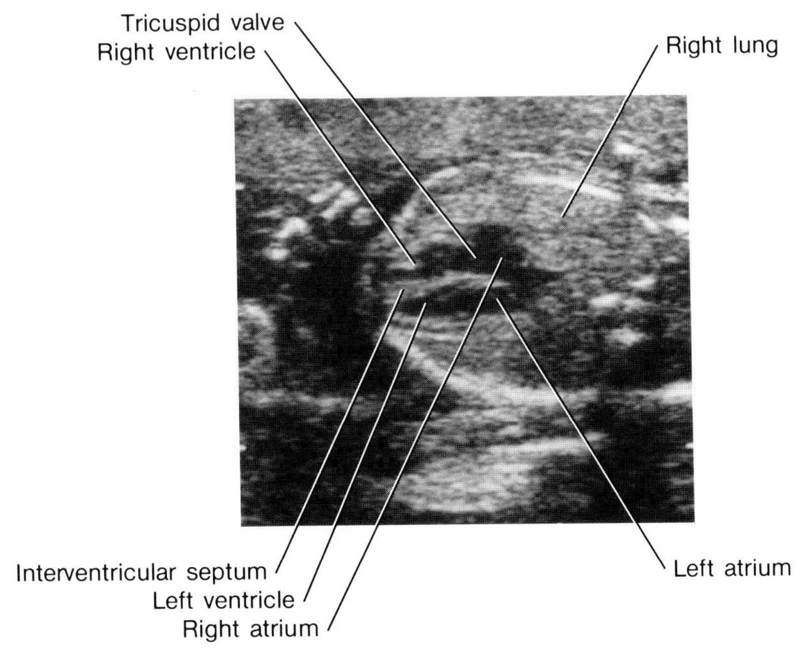

Tricuspid valve
Right ventricle
Right lung
Interventricular septum
Left ventricle
Right atrium
Left atrium

Wall of left atrium
Bronchus
Pulmonary a.
Aorta
Lower lobe, left lung
Infraspinatus m.
Trapezius m.
Upper lobe, left lung
Left ventricle
Trabeculae carneae
Coronary sinus
Liver
Rectus abdominis m.
Scapula
Intervertebral disc
Lower lobe, right lung
Azygos vein
Esophagus
Right pulmonary vein
Inferior vena cava
Valve of inferior vena cava
Olecranon process
Diaphragm
Humerus

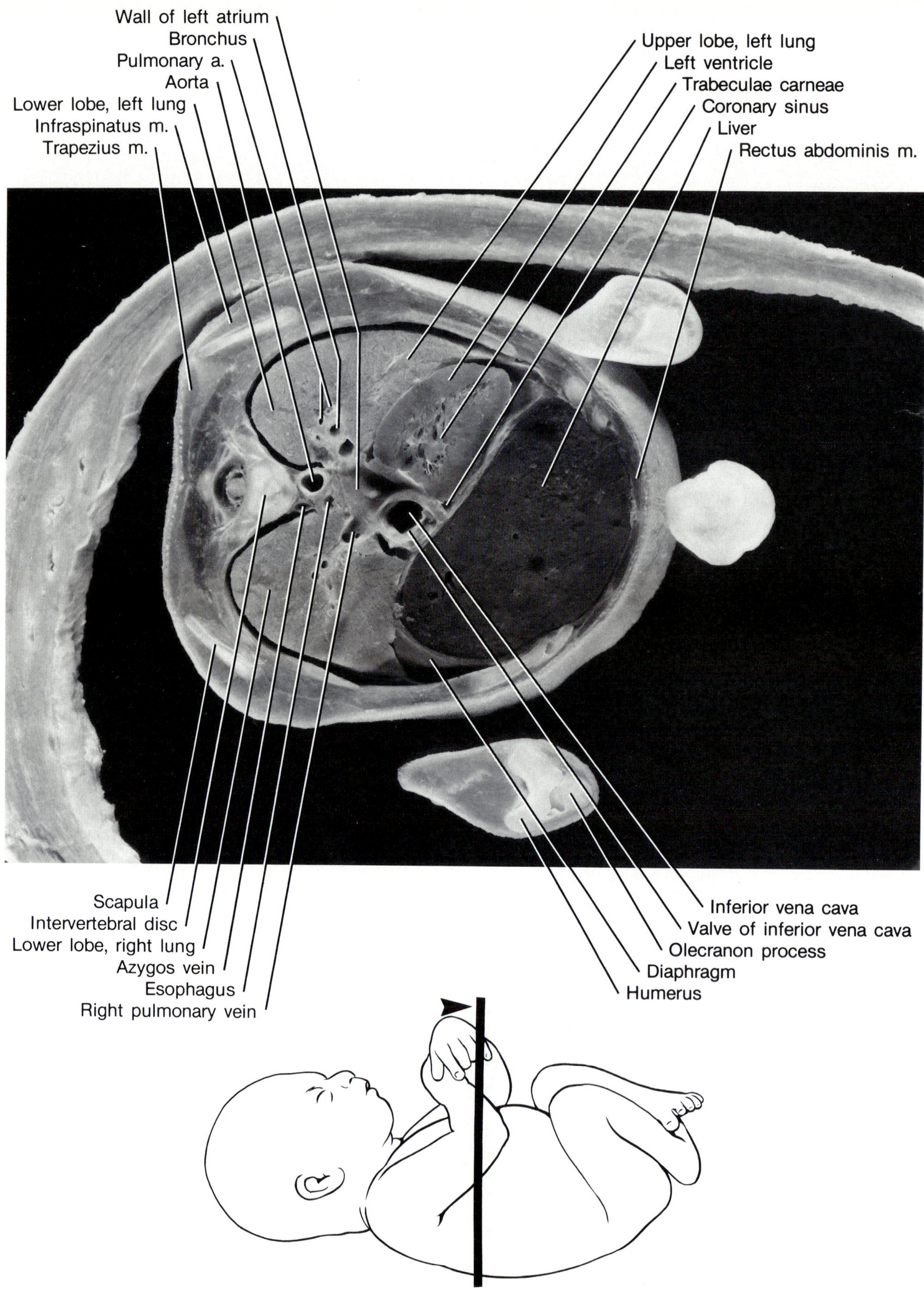

Figure 1.32

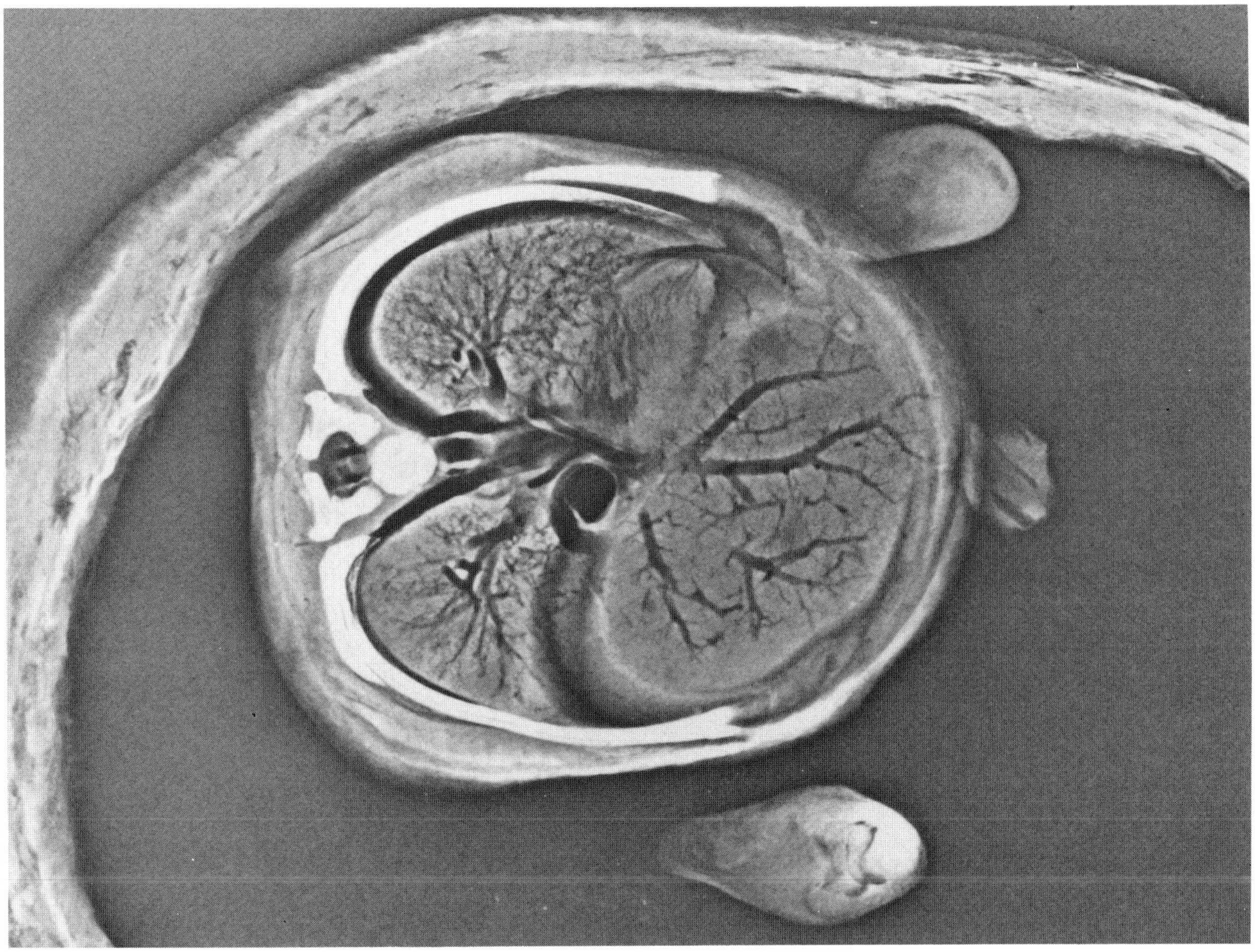

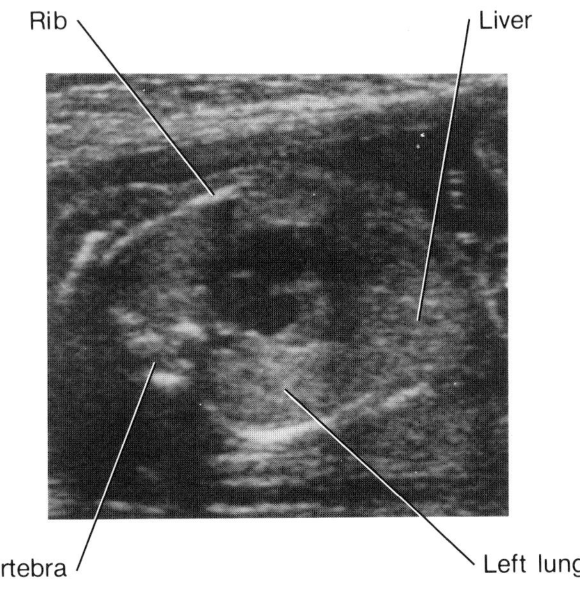

Rib
Liver
Vertebra
Left lung

Pulmonary vein
Bronchi
Pulmonary a.
Lower lobe, left lung
Esophagus
Diaphragm
Hepatic v.
Hepatic triad
Inferior vena cava
Aorta
Body of vertebra
Azygos v.

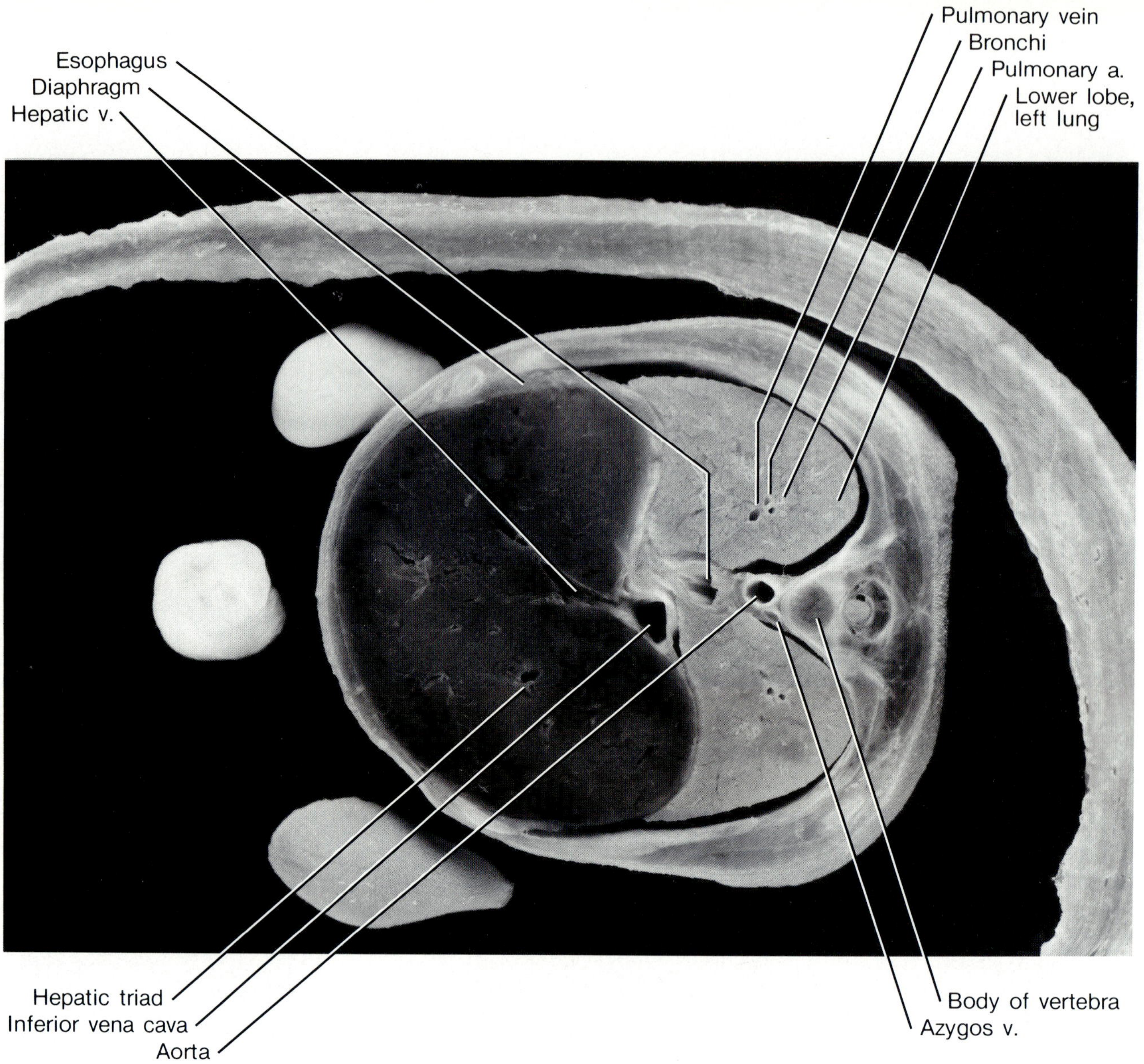

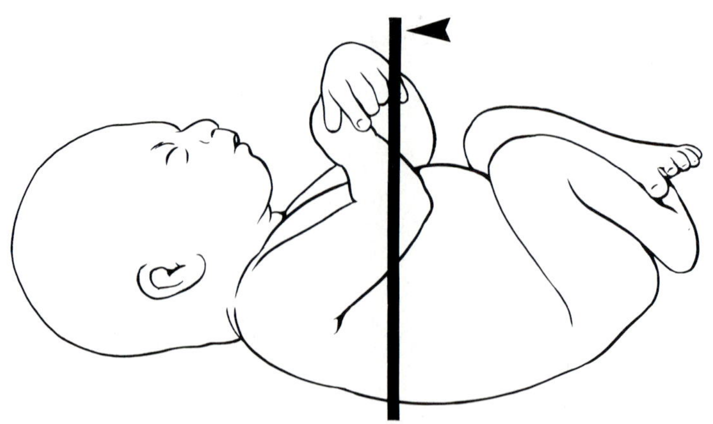

Figure 1.33

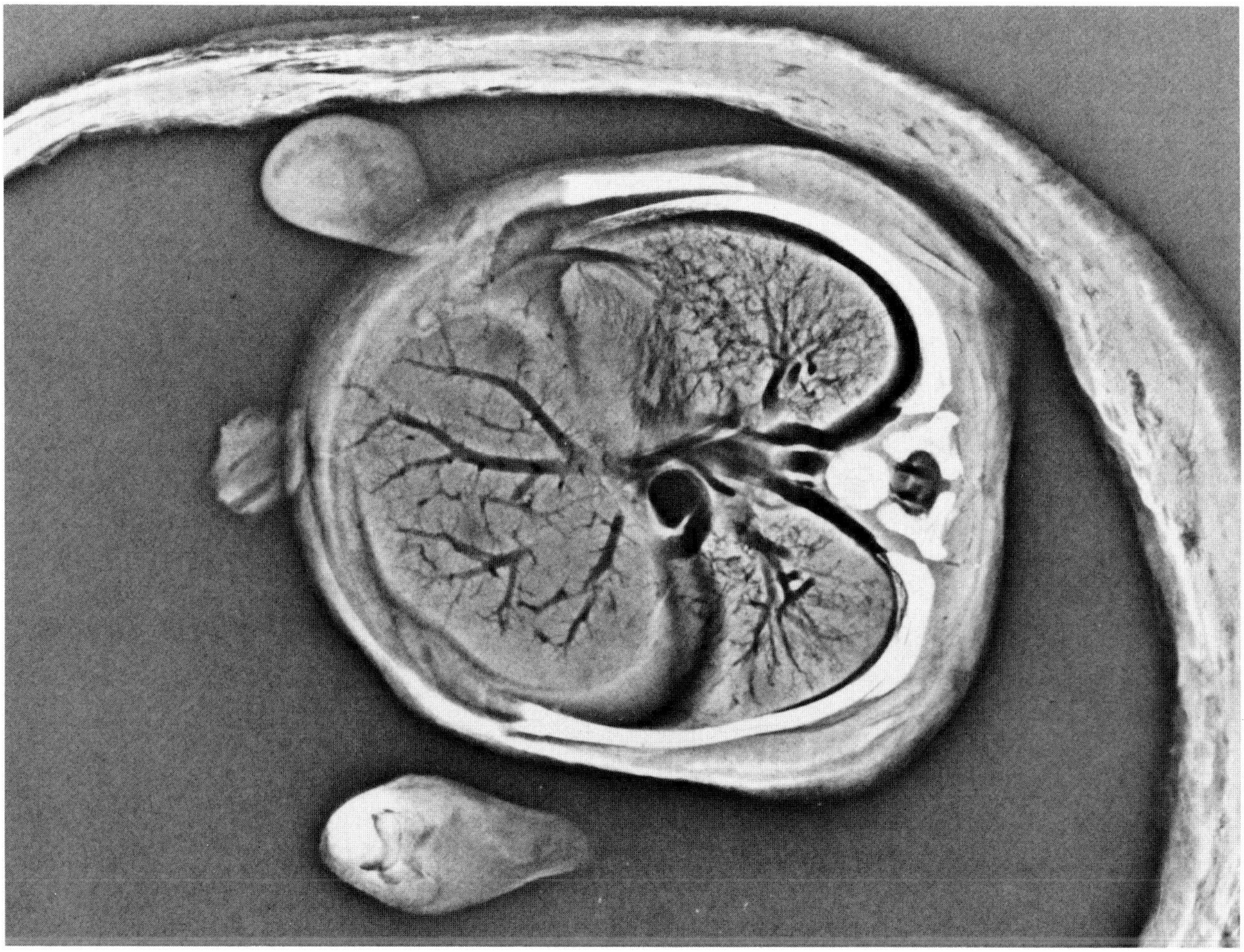

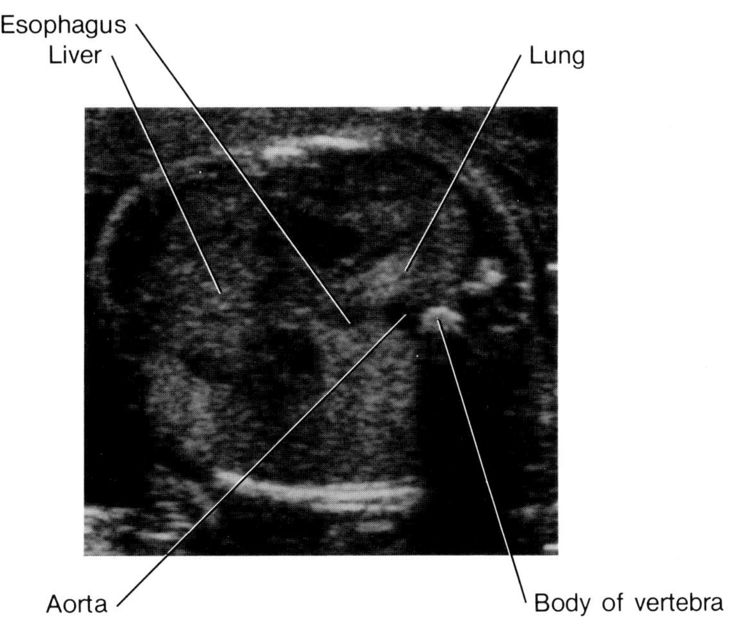

Esophagus
Liver
Lung
Aorta
Body of vertebra

Diaphragm
Lower lobe, left lung
Aorta
Sacrospinalis m.
Spleen
Stomach
Esophagus
Trapezius m.
Suprarenal gland
Inferior vena cava
Umbilical v.
Ductus venosus
Right lobe, liver

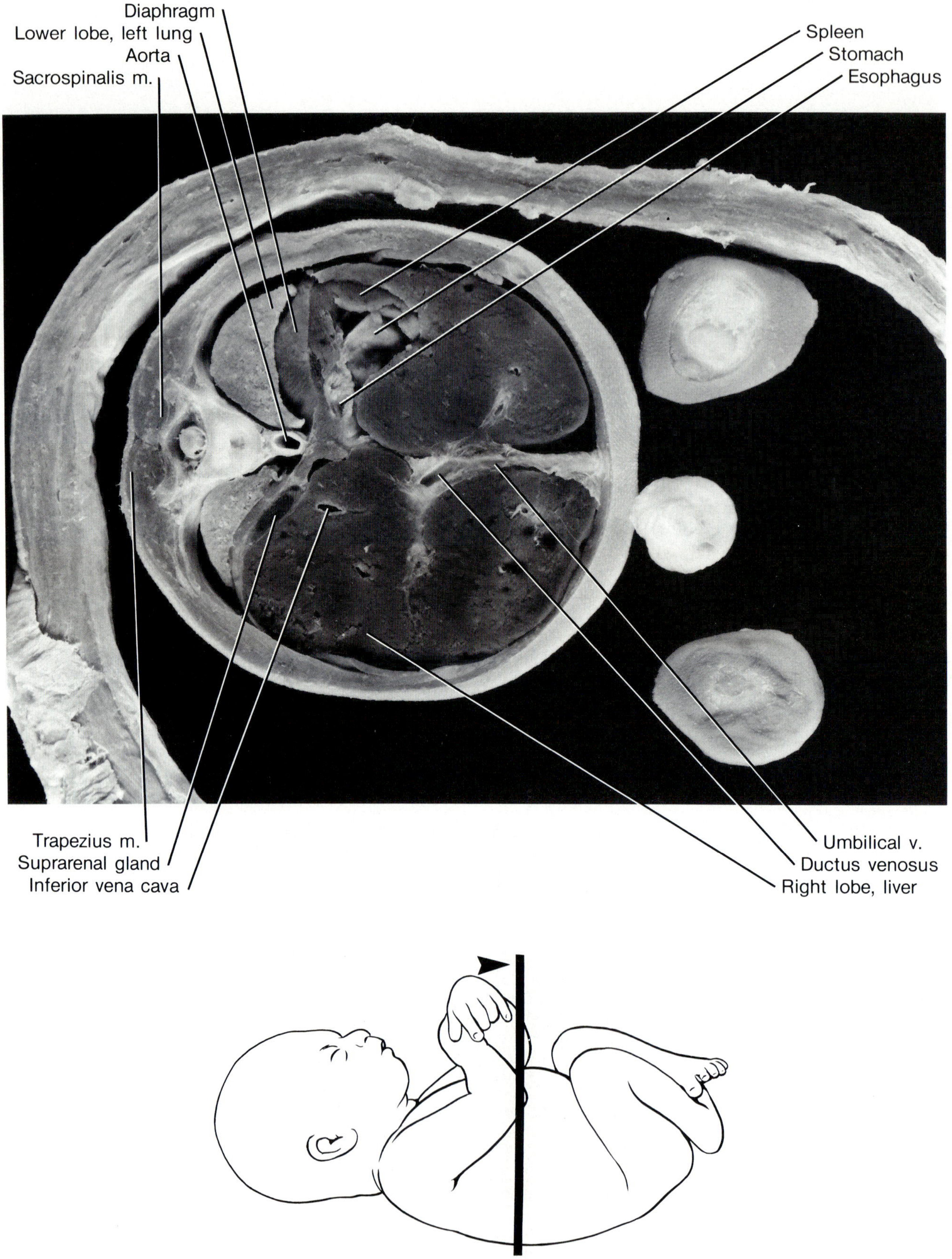

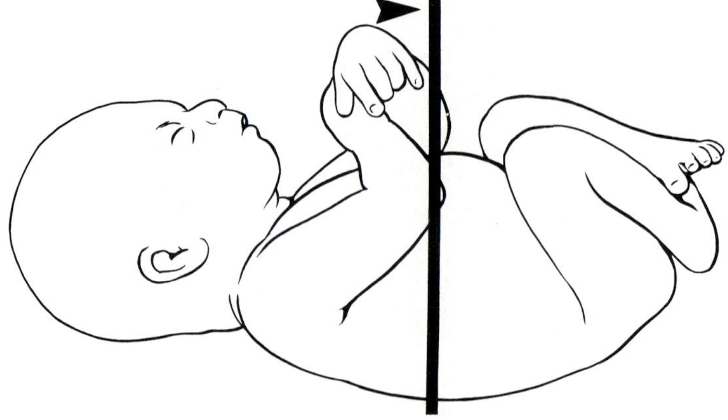

Figure 1.34

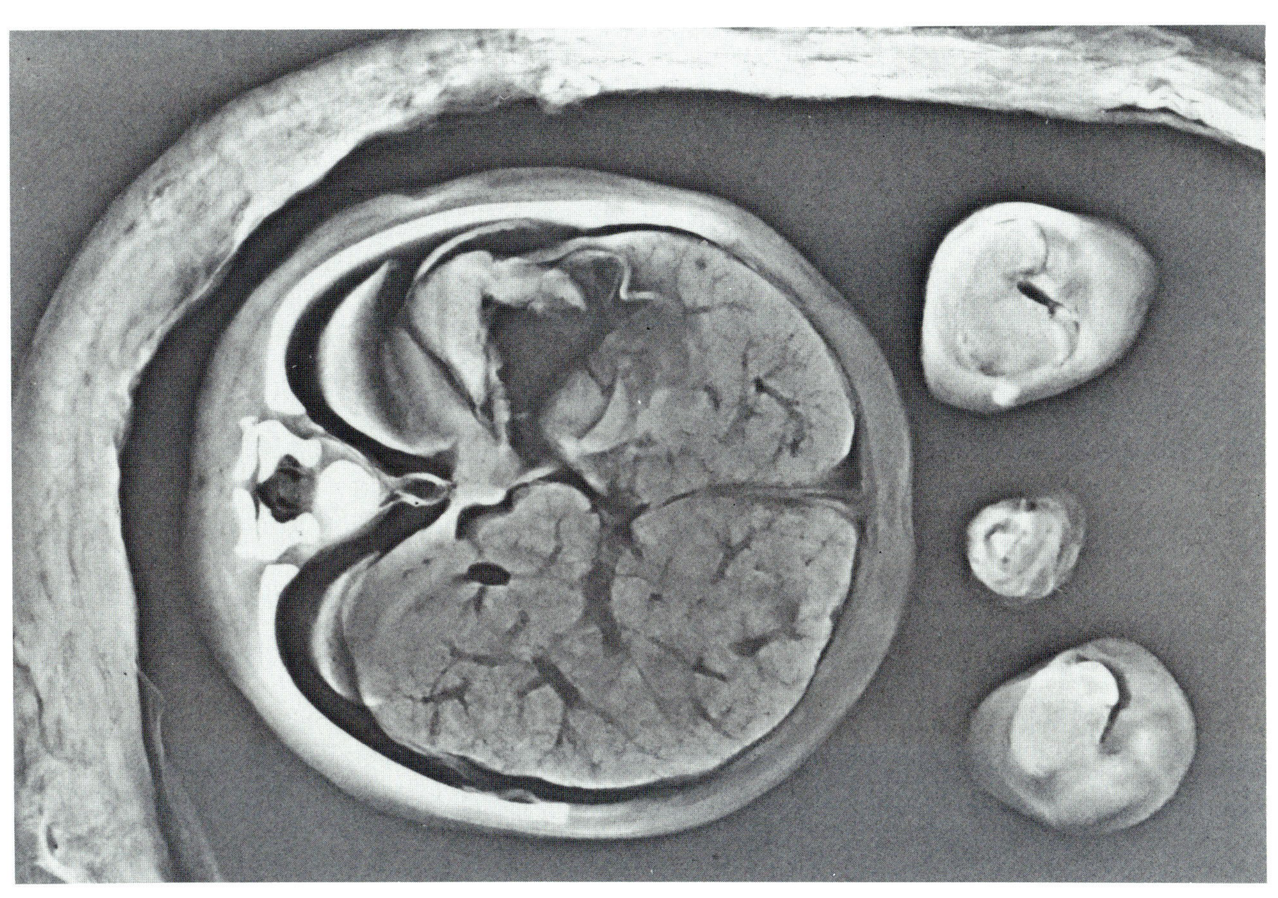

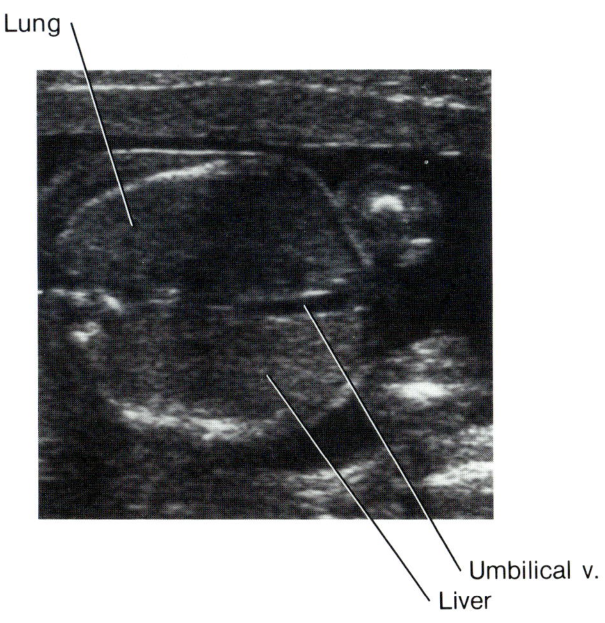
Lung
Umbilical v.
Liver

Stomach
Liver, left lobe
Knee joint
Lateral condyle
Spleen
Crura of diaphragm
Aorta
Lung
Gall bladder fossa
Liver, right lobe
Portal v.
Suprarenal gland
Inferior vena cava
Caudate lobe

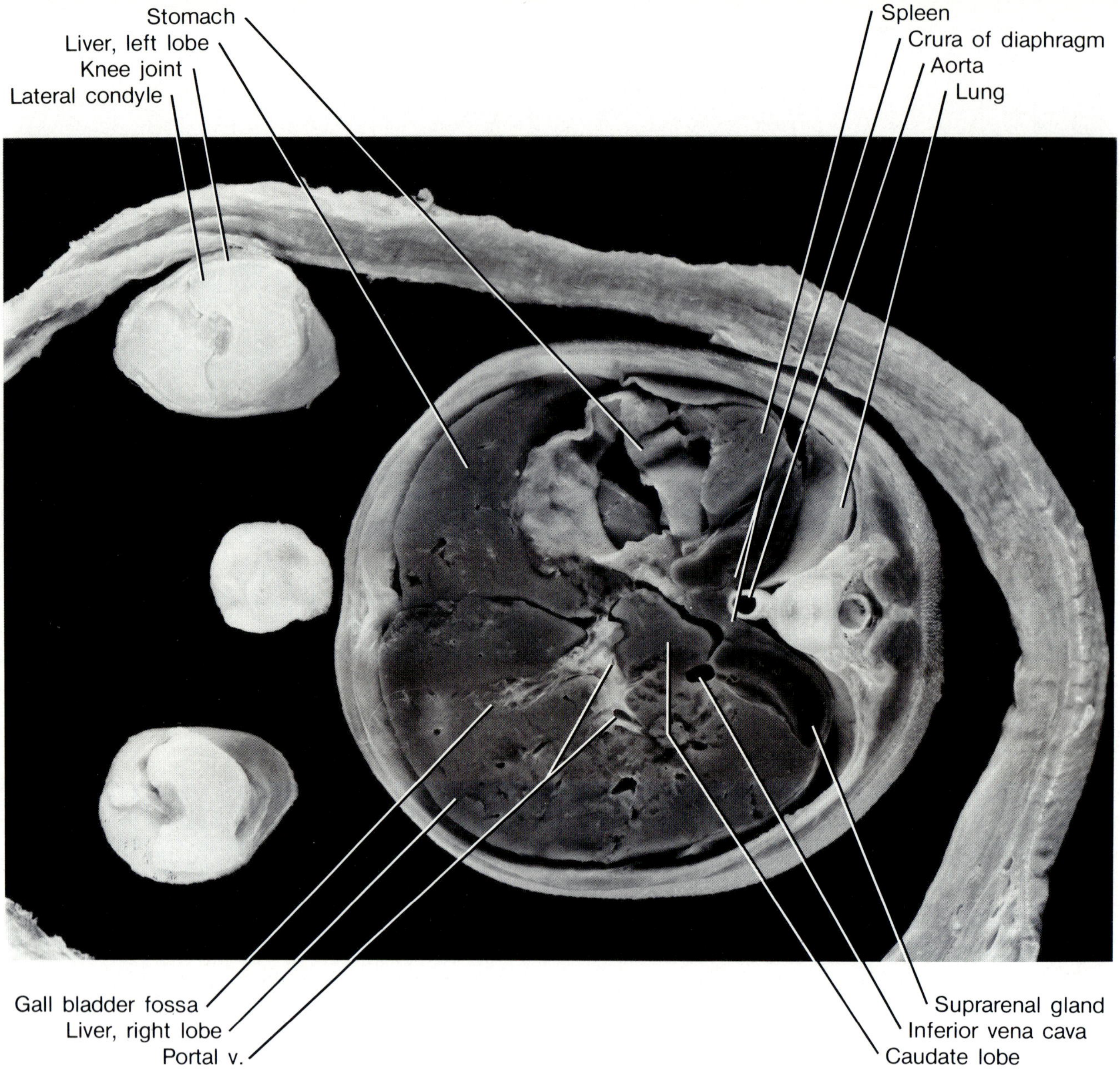

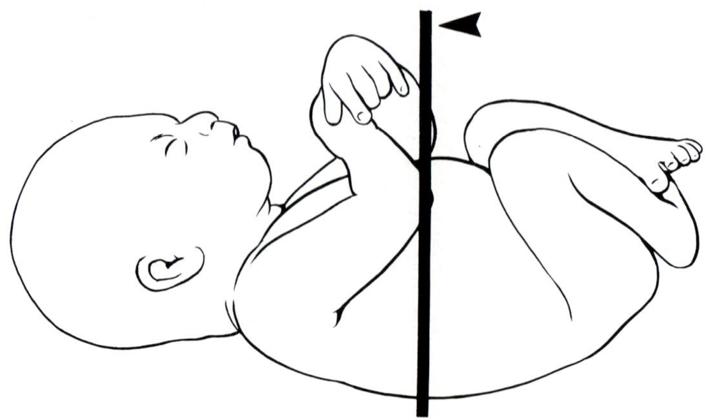

Figure 1.35

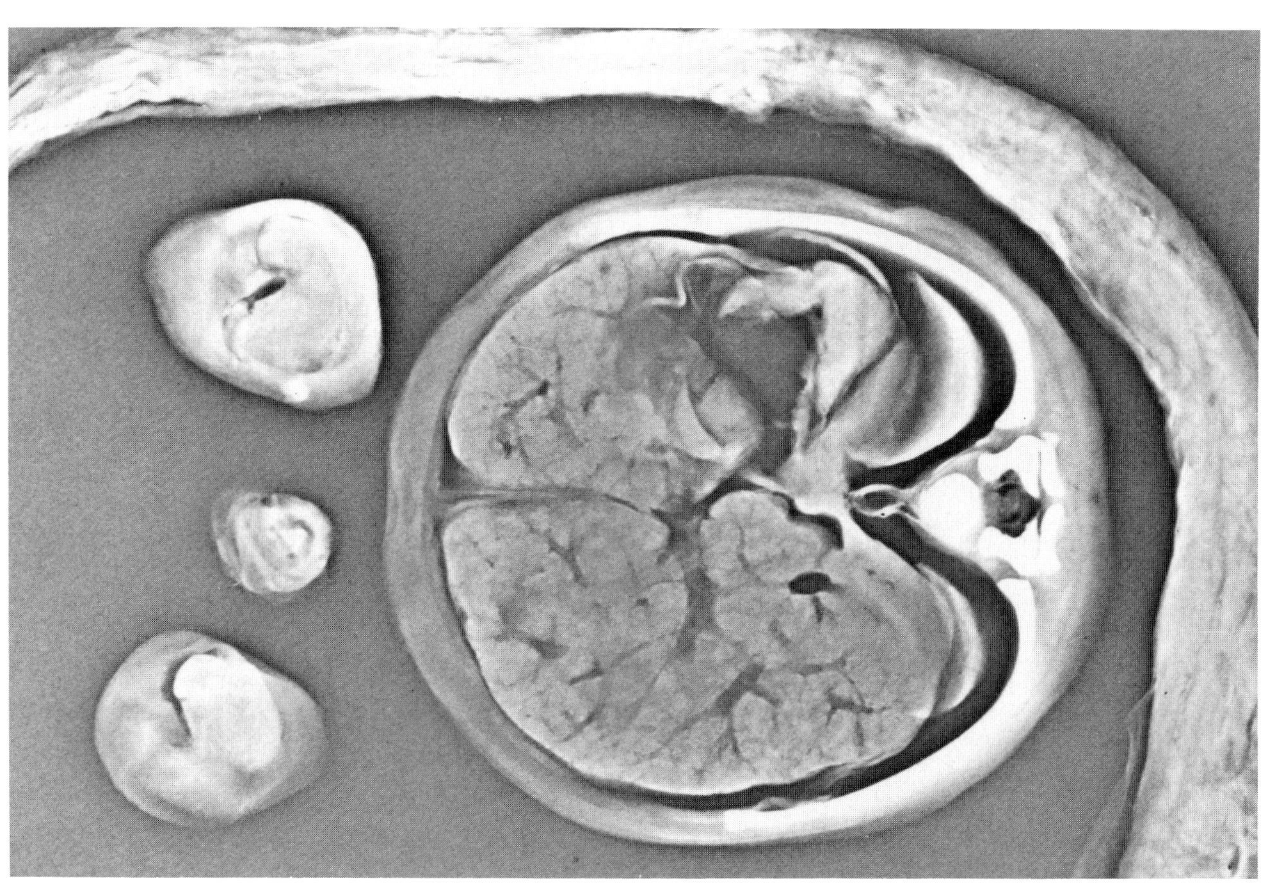

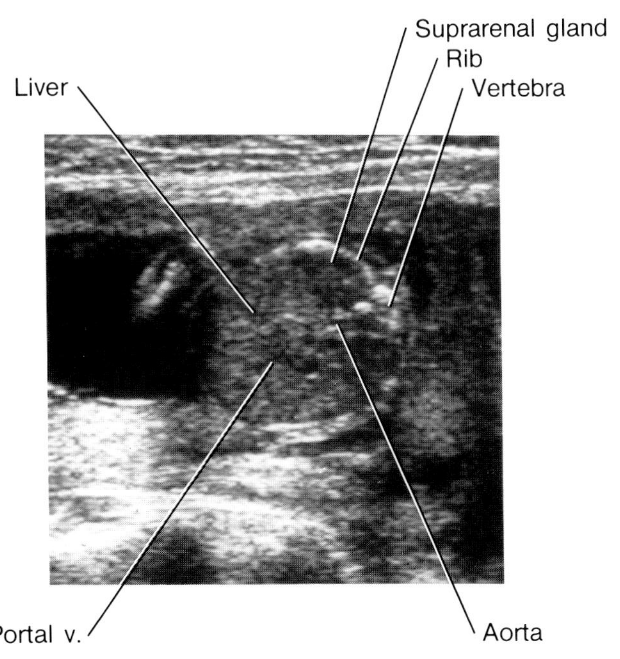
Suprarenal gland
Rib
Vertebra
Liver
Portal v.
Aorta

Lesser omentum
Body of pancreas
Spleen
Left kidney
Suprarenal gland
Stomach
Tranverse colon
Duodenum
Liver
Jejunum
Aorta
Right crus
of diaphragm
Inferior vena cava
Caudate lobe
Liver
Quadriceps m.
Quadrate lobe
Gall bladder
Cystic a.
Hepatic a.

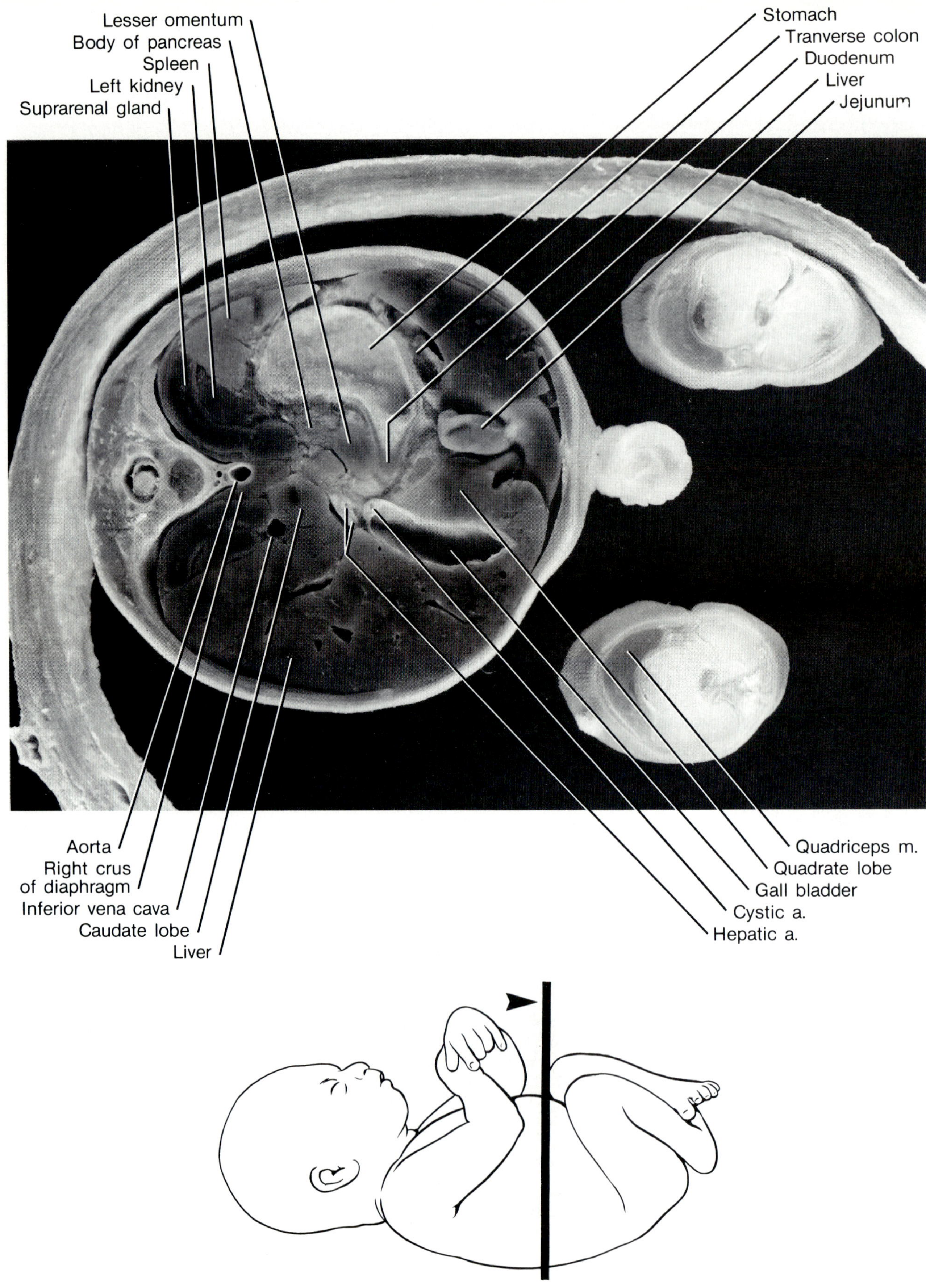

Figure 1.36

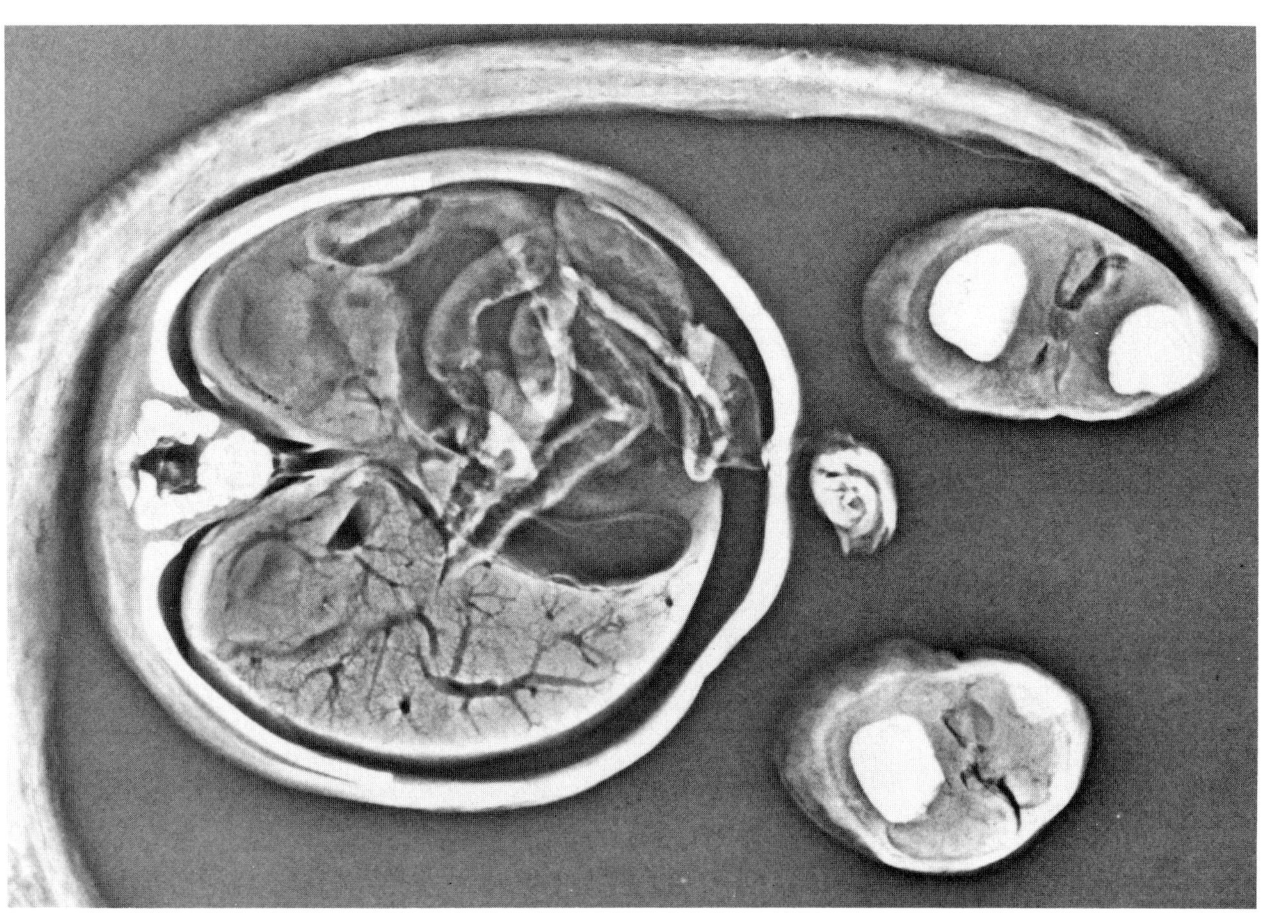

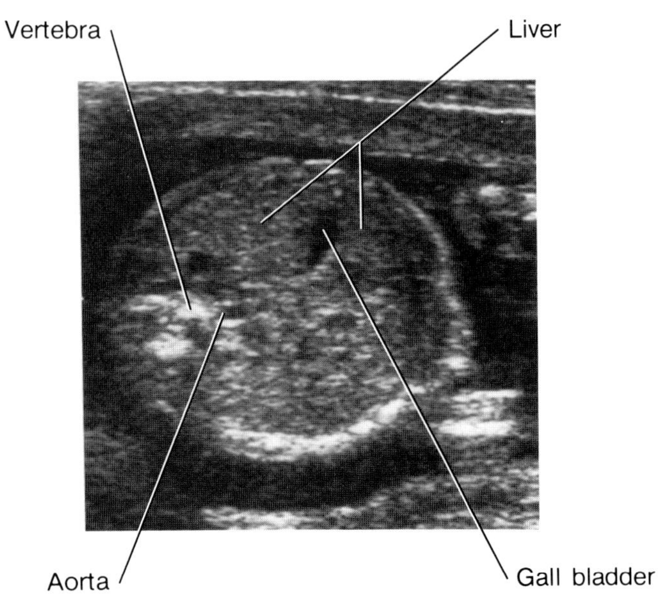

Vertebra
Liver
Aorta
Gall bladder

Jejunum
Liver
Quadriceps femoris m.
Femur
Tibia
Suprarenal gland
Celiac a.
Aorta
Kidney
Left crus
Umbilical vessels
Ileum
Transverse colon
Head of pancreas
Descending duodenum
Dura mater
Liver
Suprarenal gland
Inferior vena cava
Caudate lobe

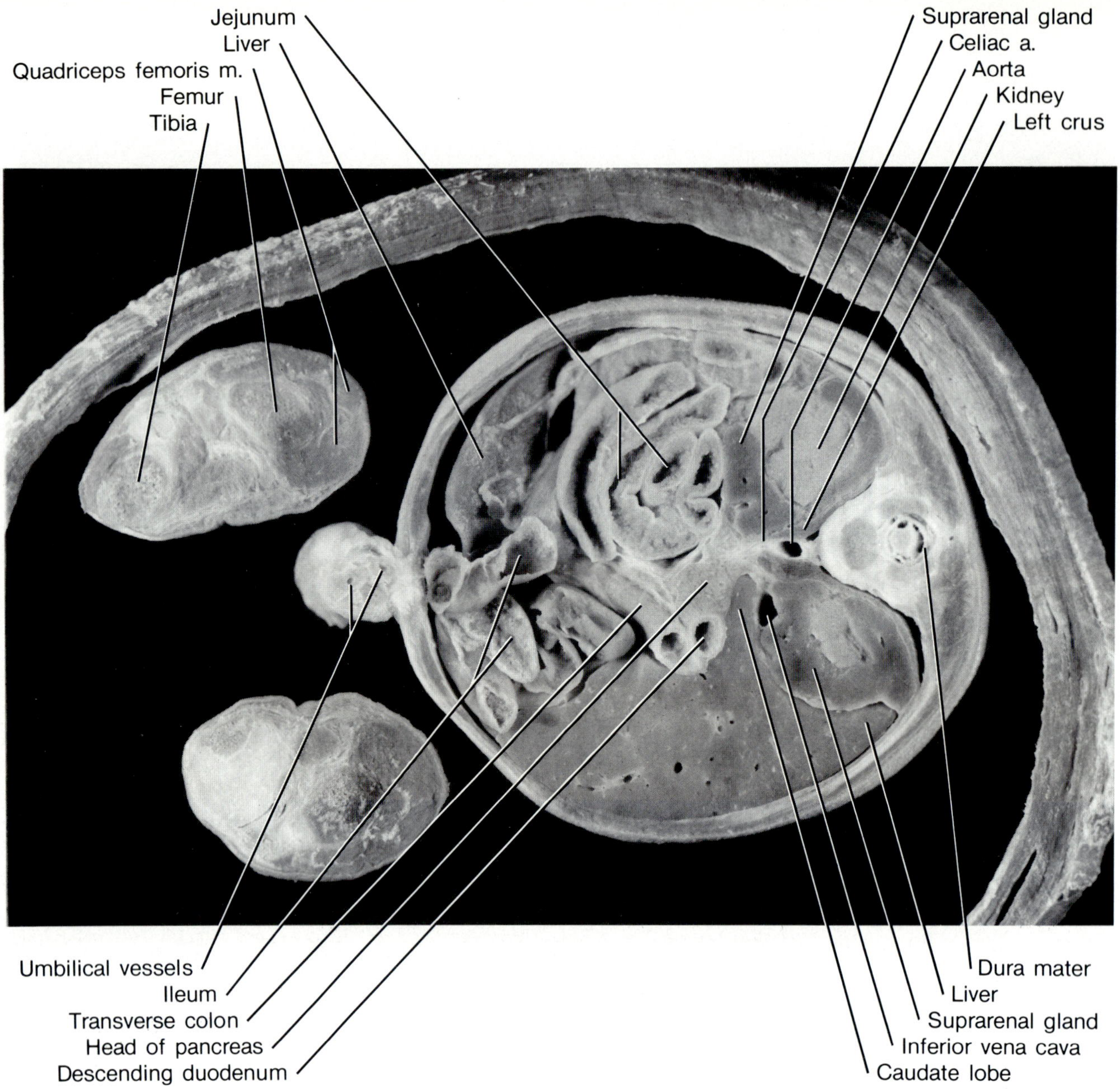

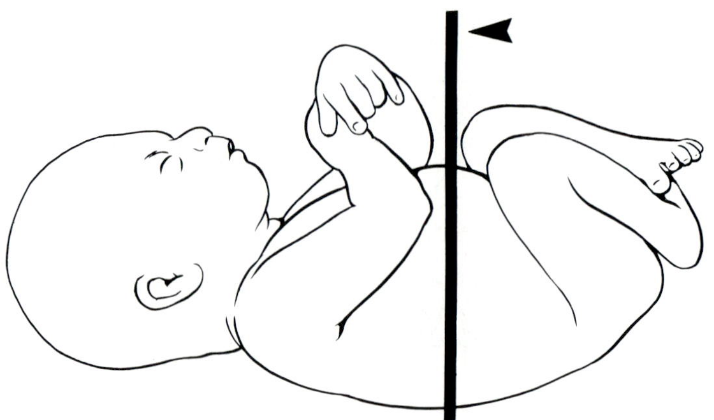

Figure 1.37

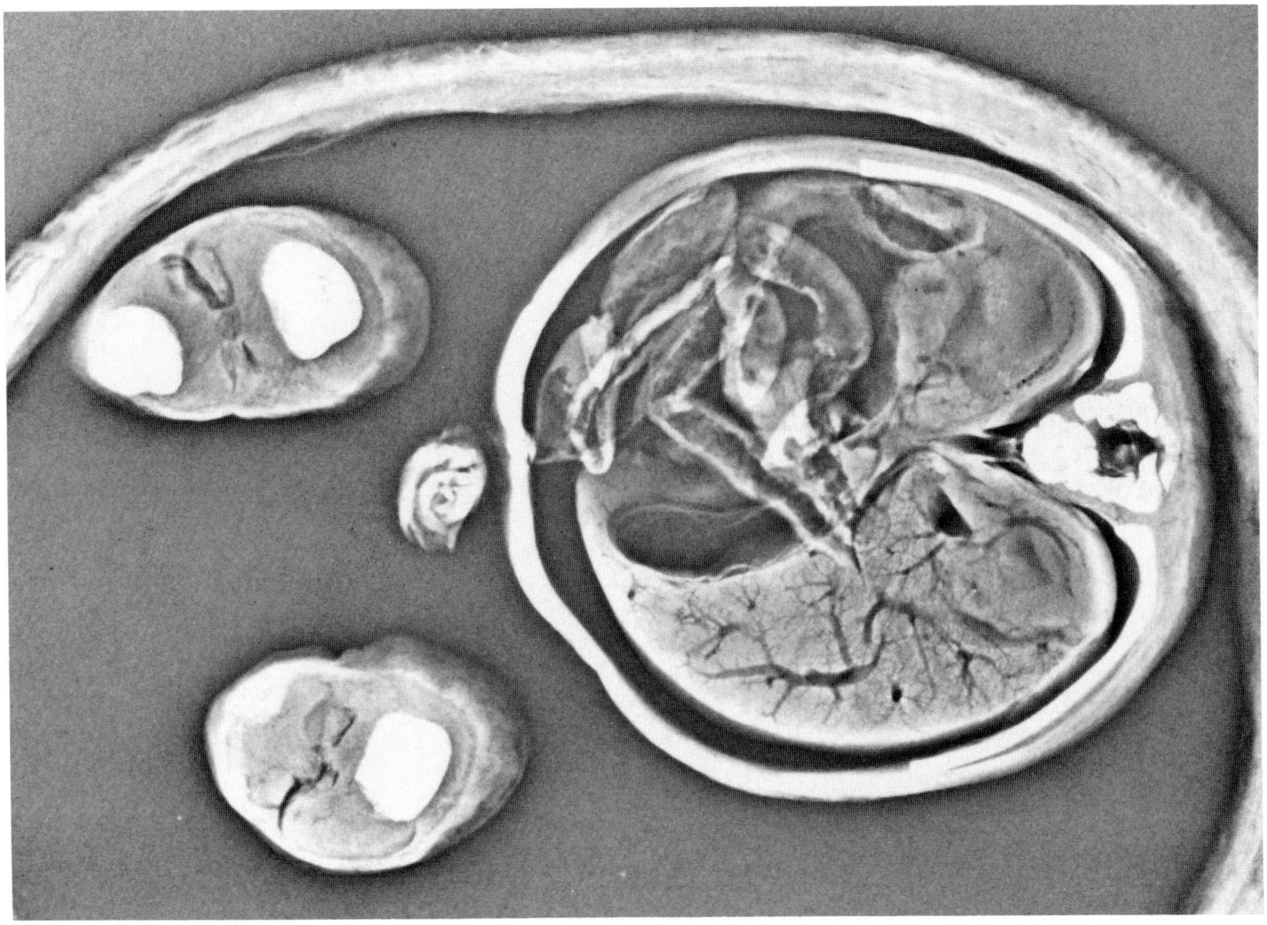

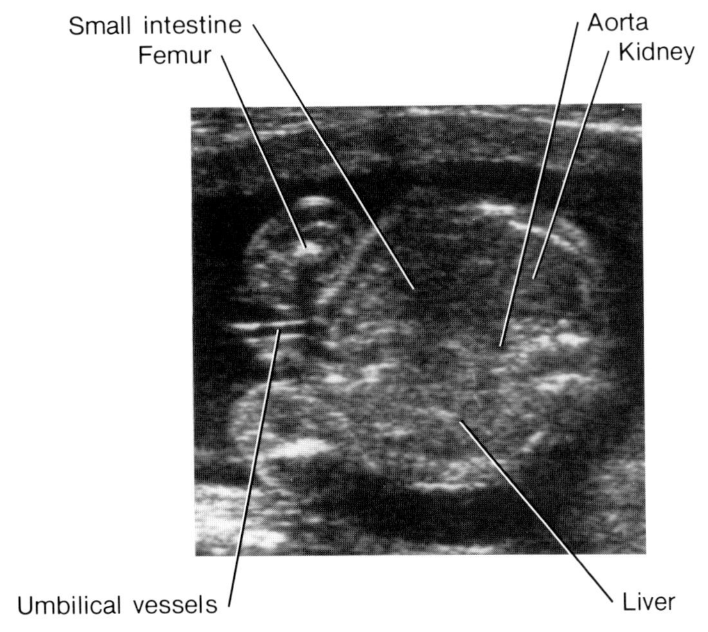

Small intestine
Femur
Aorta
Kidney
Umbilical vessels
Liver

Aorta
Right crus
Costovertebral
articulation
Dura mater
Spinal cord
Splenic flexure
Duodenum
Jejunum
Umbilical a.
Fibula
Suprarenal gland
Kidney
Inferior vena cava
Descending duodenum
Ascending colon
Liver
Tibia
Femur
Quadriceps m.
Superior mesenteric a.
Pancreas

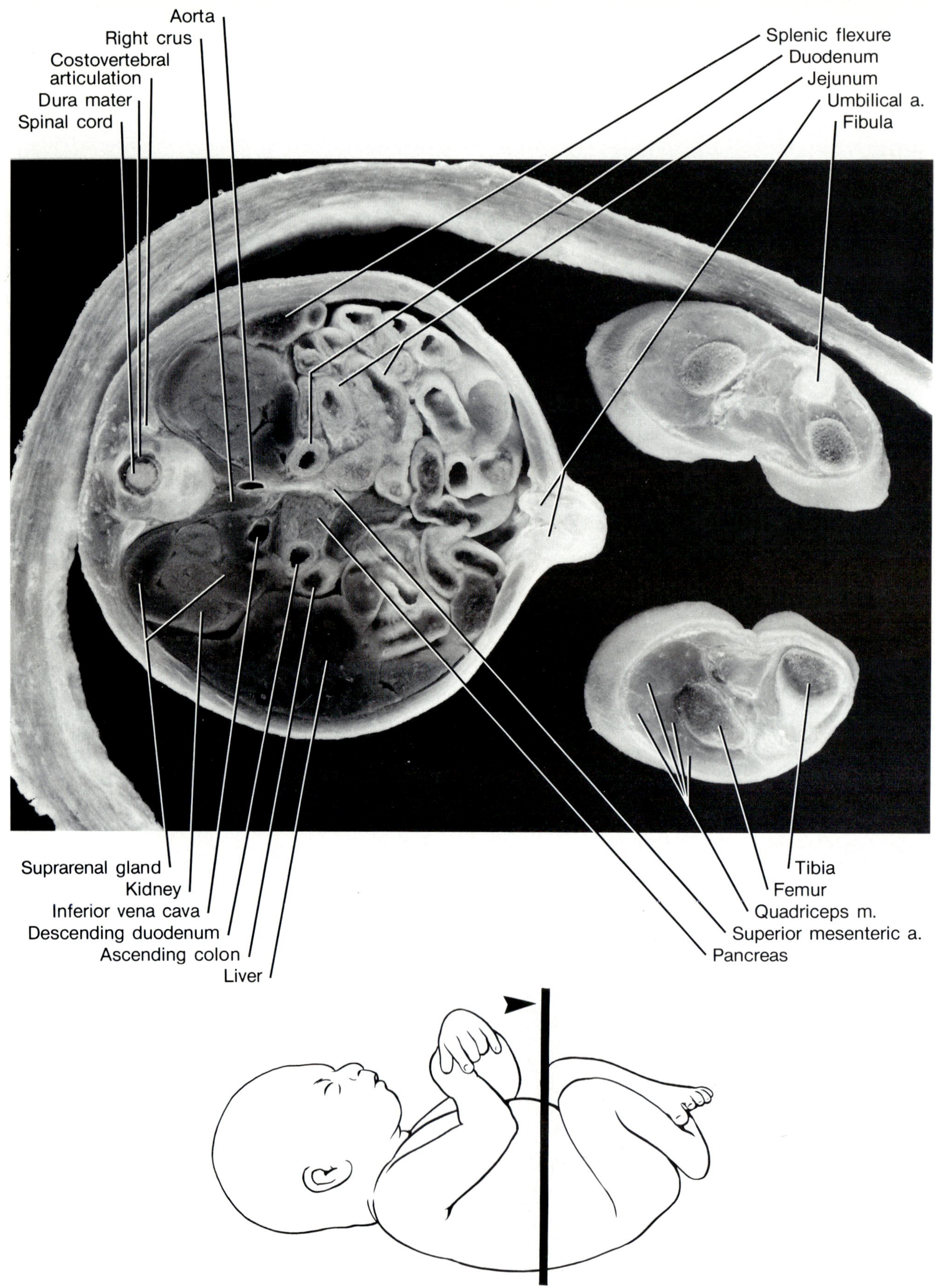

Figure 1.38

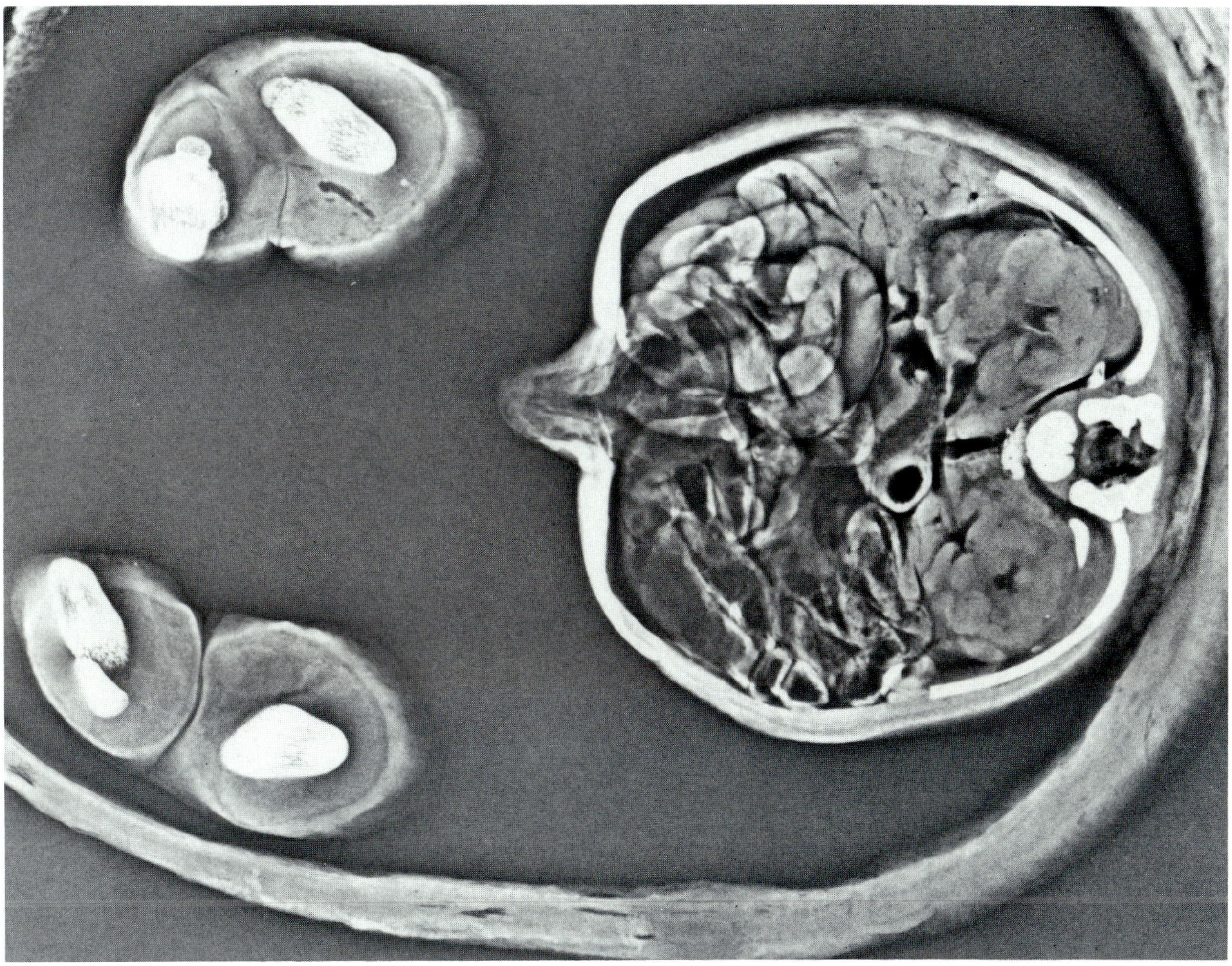

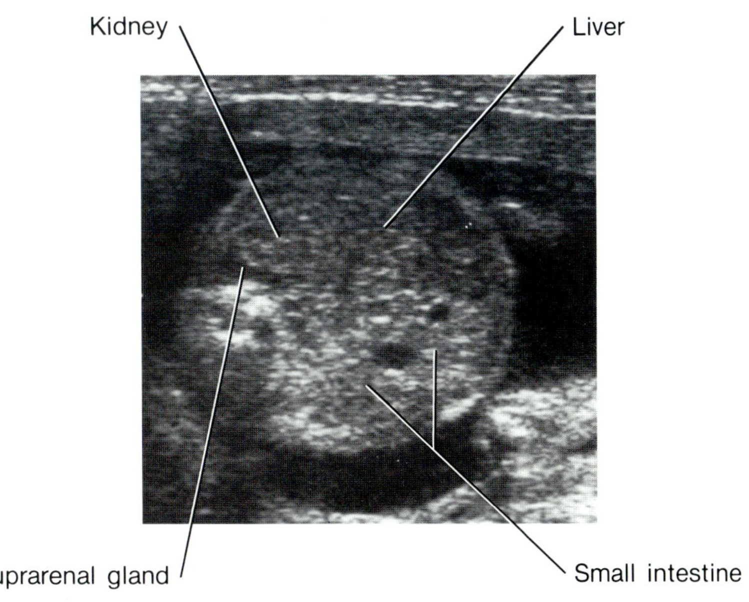

Kidney
Liver
Suprarenal gland
Small intestine

Urinary bladder
Rectus abdominis m.
Rectus femoris m.
Femur
Gastrocnemius m.
Fibula
Tibia
Mesentery of
small intestine
Suprarenal gland
Descending colon
Left renal v.
Aorta
Kidney
Body of vertebra
Umbilical a.
Transverse duodenum
Inferior vena cava
Right renal v.
Liver
Ascending colon
Internal vertebral
plexus of veins
Dura mater
Pyramid
Minor calyx
Right crus of diaphragm

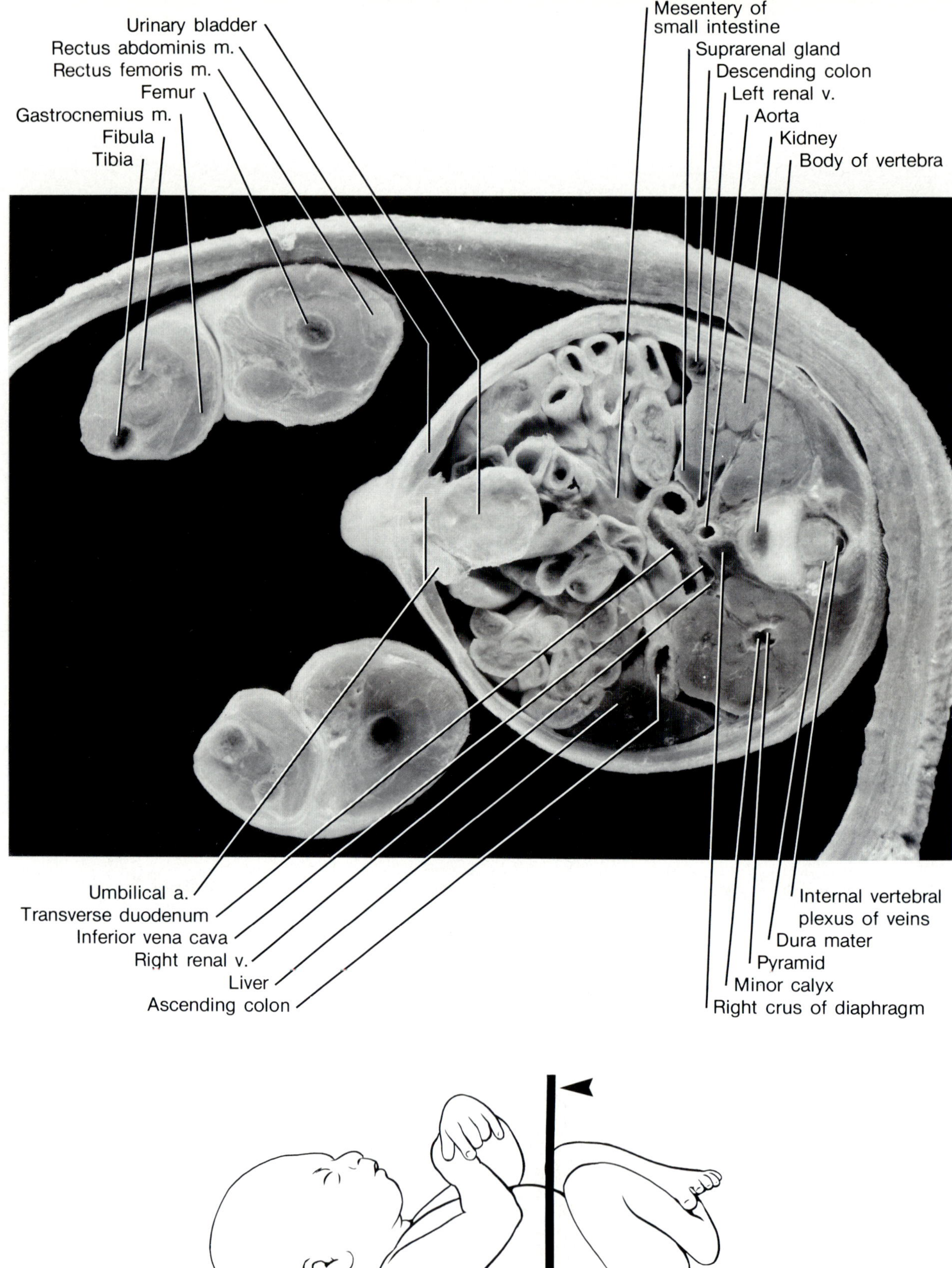

Figure 1.39

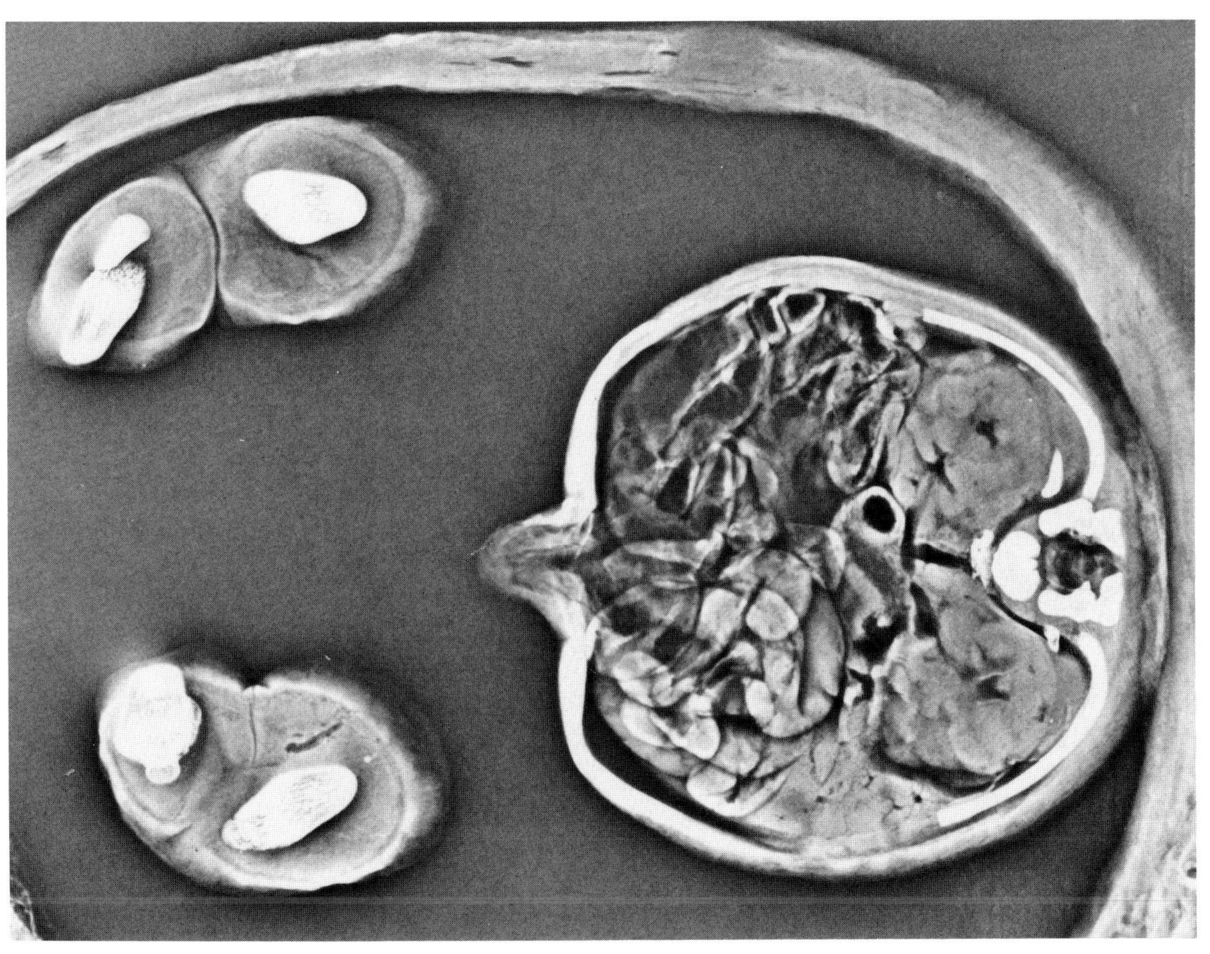

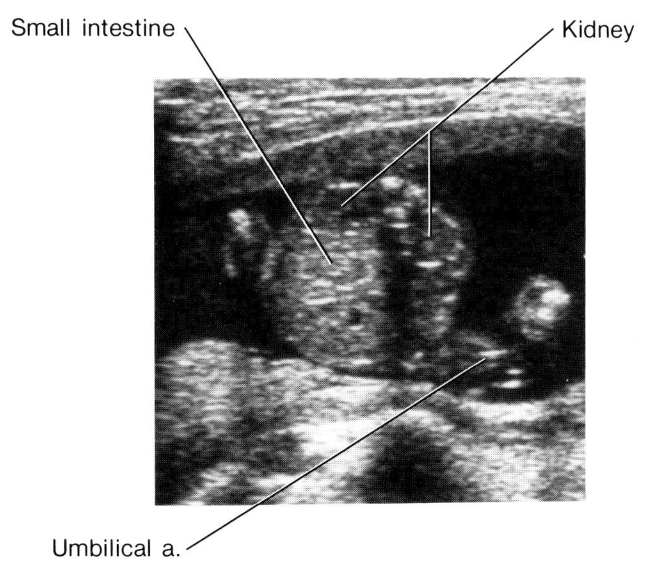
Small intestine
Kidney
Umbilical a.

Psoas m.
Right crus
Body of vertebra
Right renal a.
Descending colon
Thoracic duct
Aorta
Duodeno-jejunal junction
Kidney
Liver
Inferior vena cava
Large intestine, sigmoid colon
Tibia
Extensor m.
Fibula
Flexor m.
Sciatic nerve
Femur
Quadriceps m.
Urinary bladder

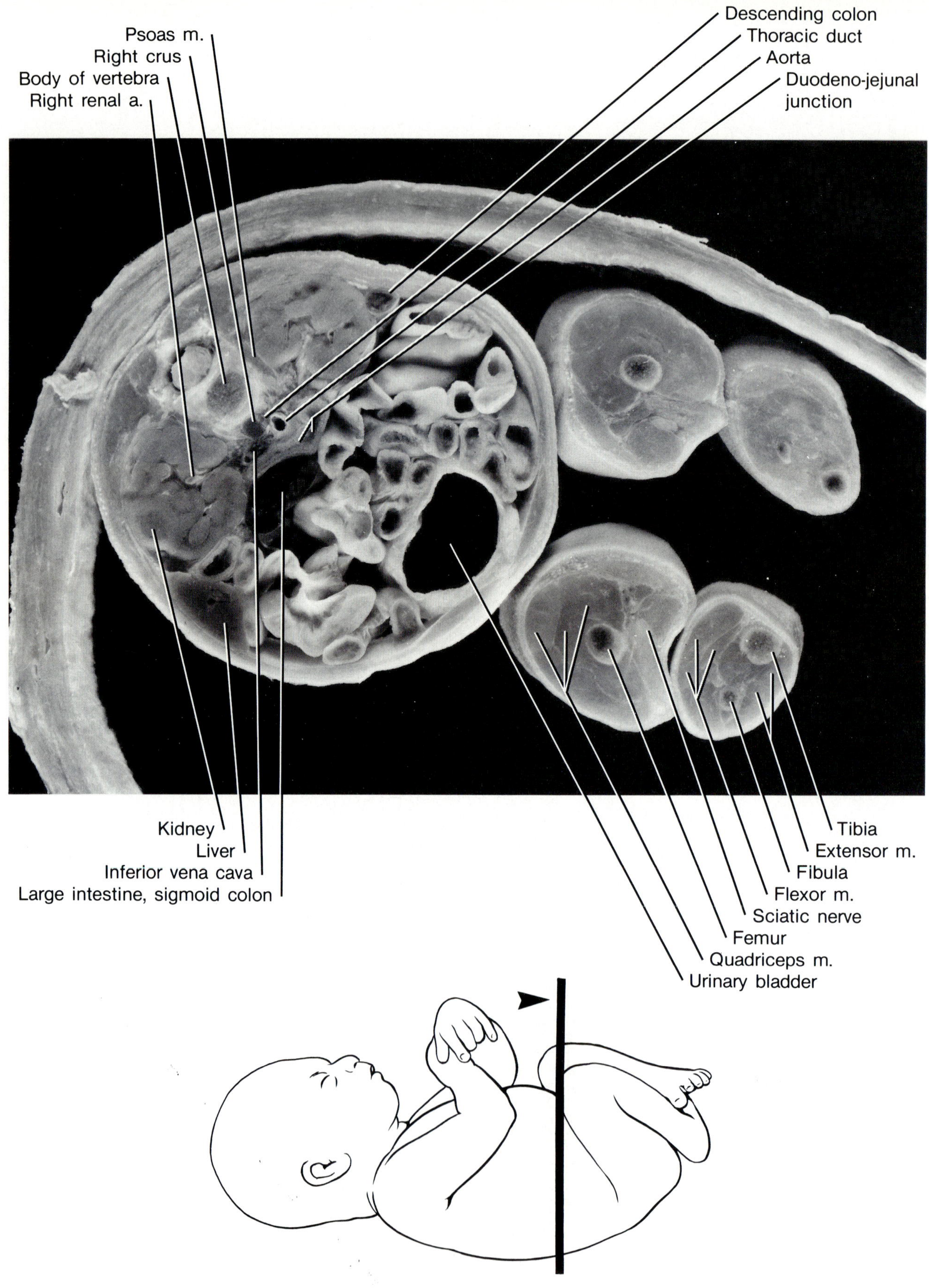

Figure 1.40

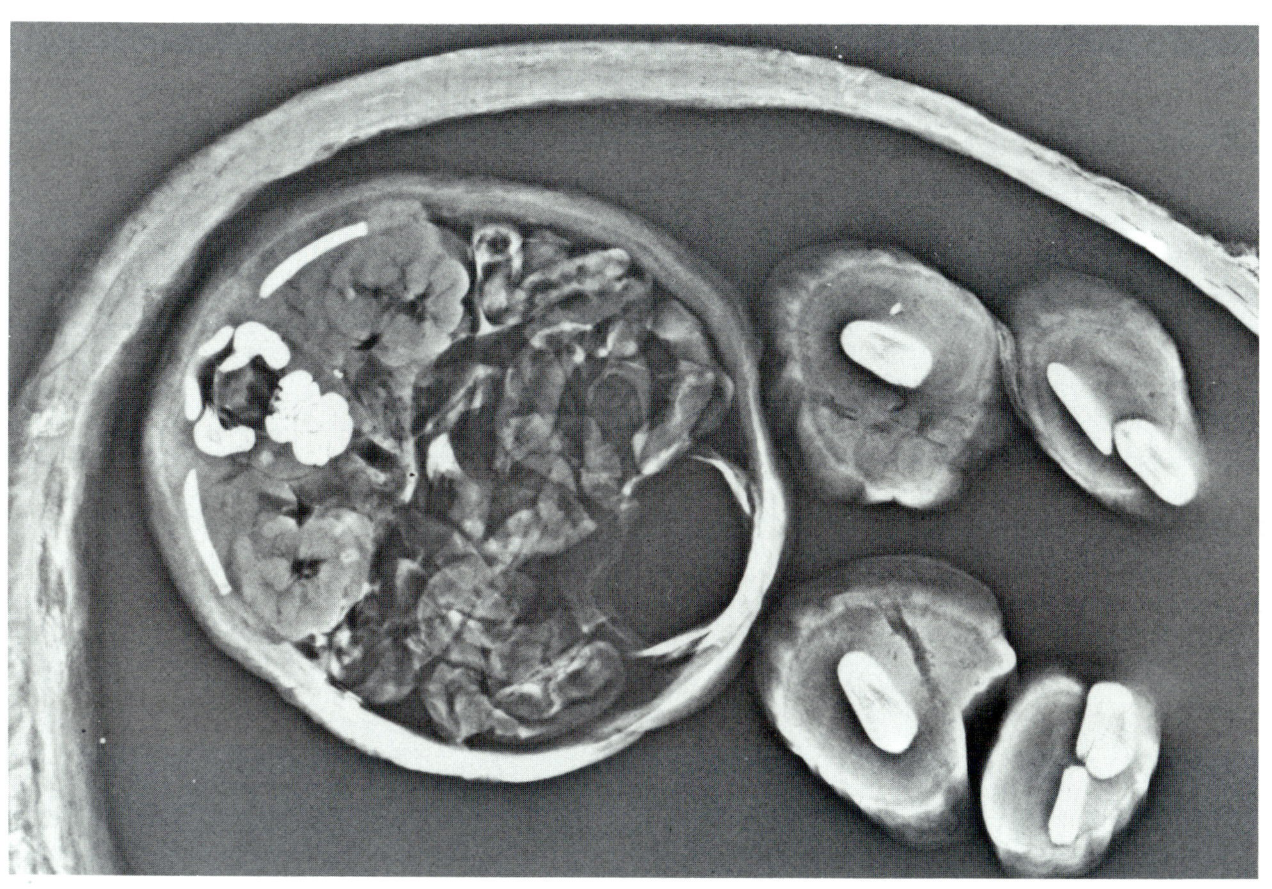

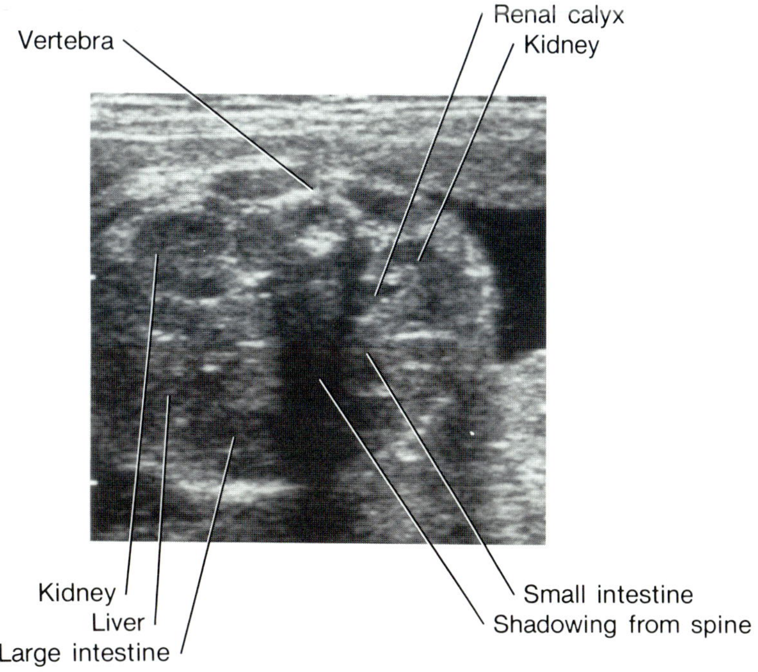

Vertebra
Renal calyx
Kidney
Kidney
Liver
Large intestine
Small intestine
Shadowing from spine

Descending colon
Kidney
Psoas m.
Aorta
Quadratus lumborum m.
Internal vertebral plexus of veins
Small intestine
Urinary bladder
Rectus abdominis m.
Quadriceps m.
Sigmoid colon
Renal papilla
Ascending colon
Inferior vena cava

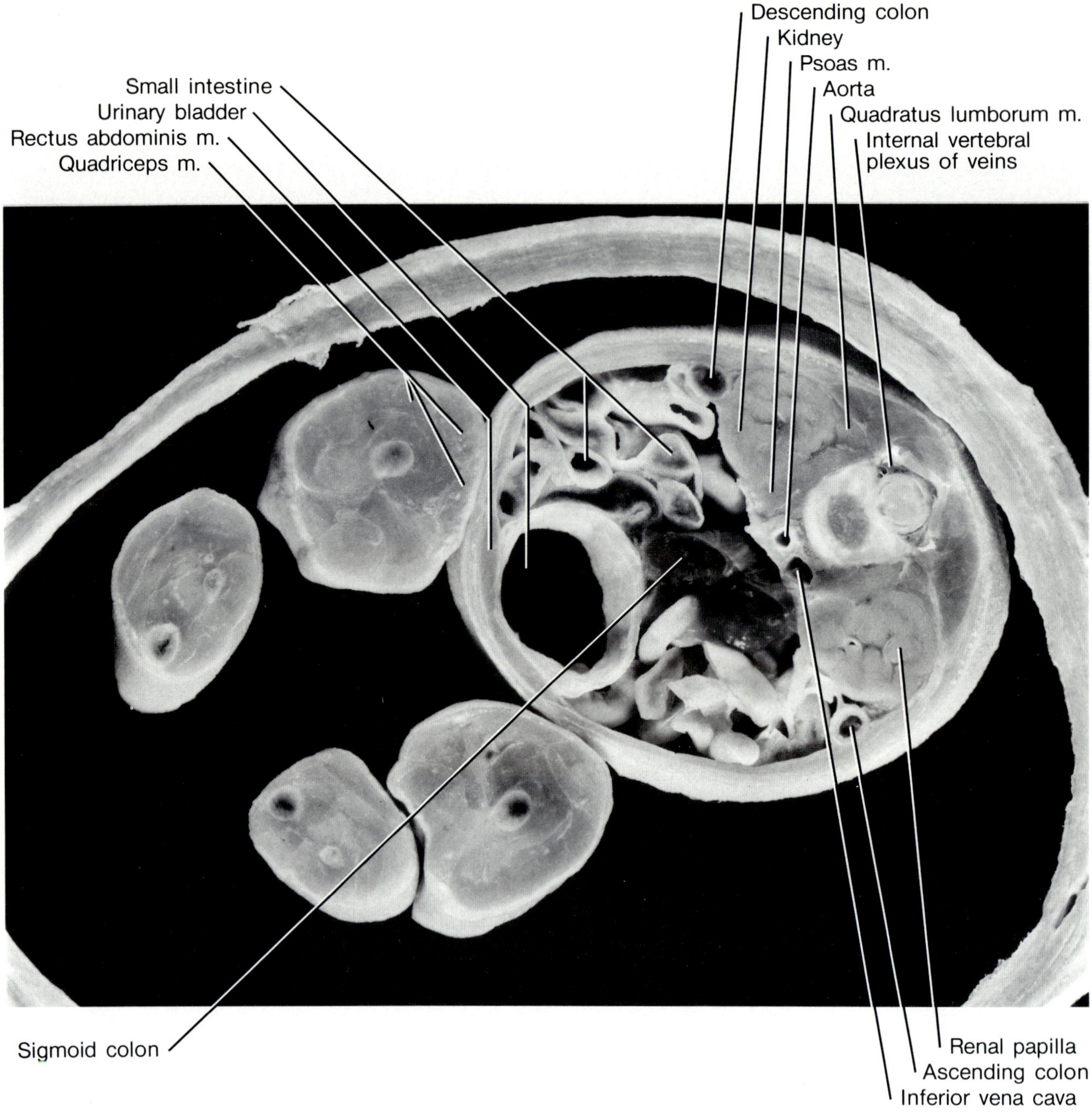

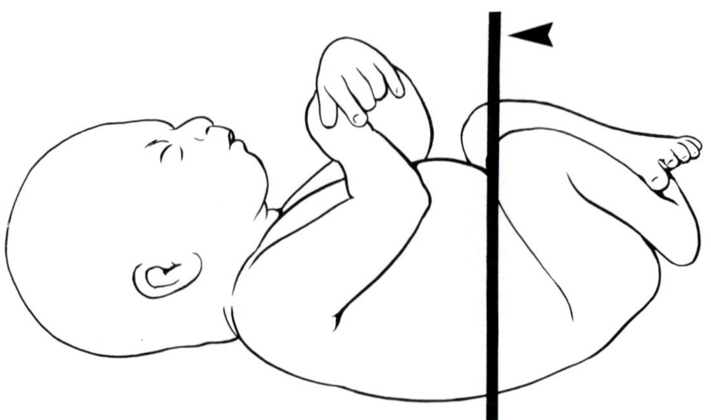

Figure 1.41

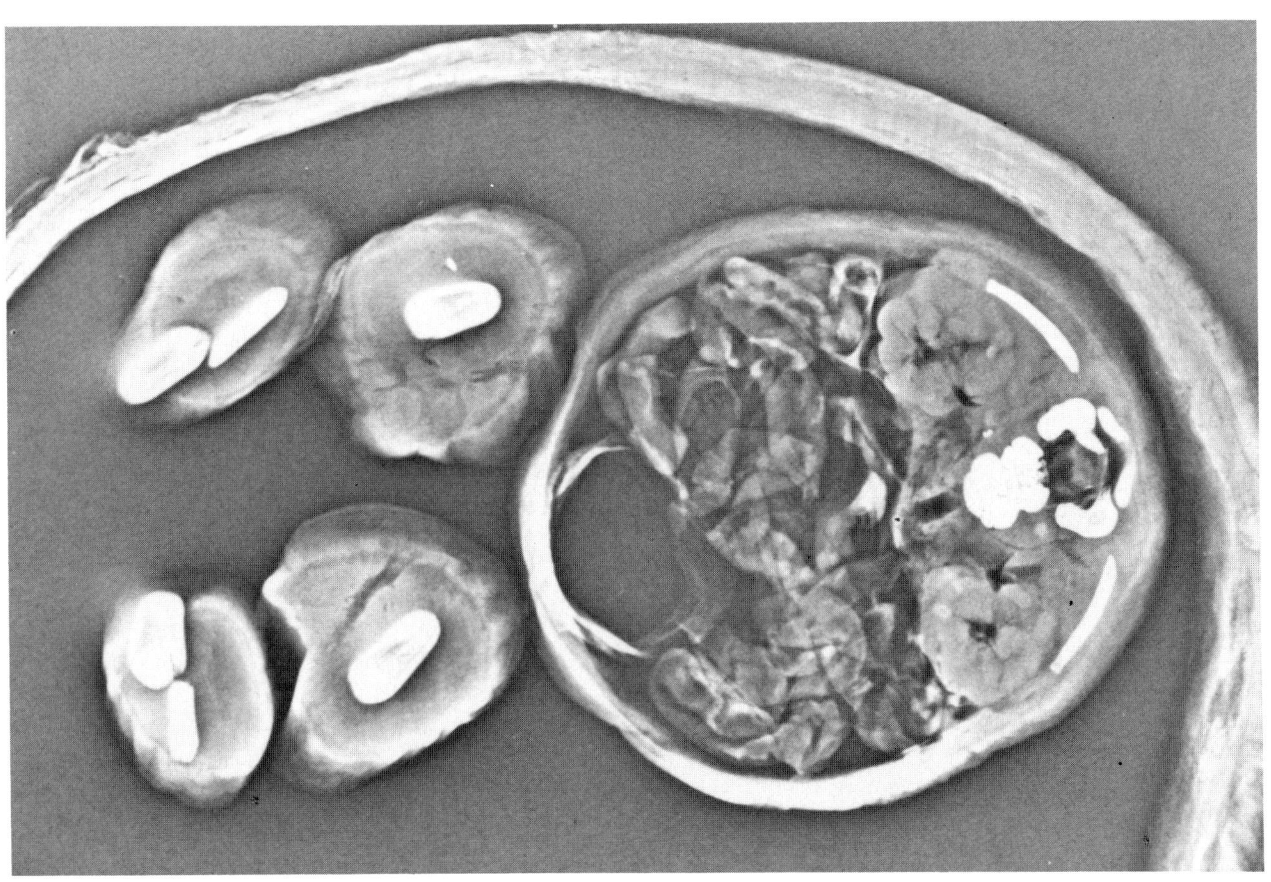

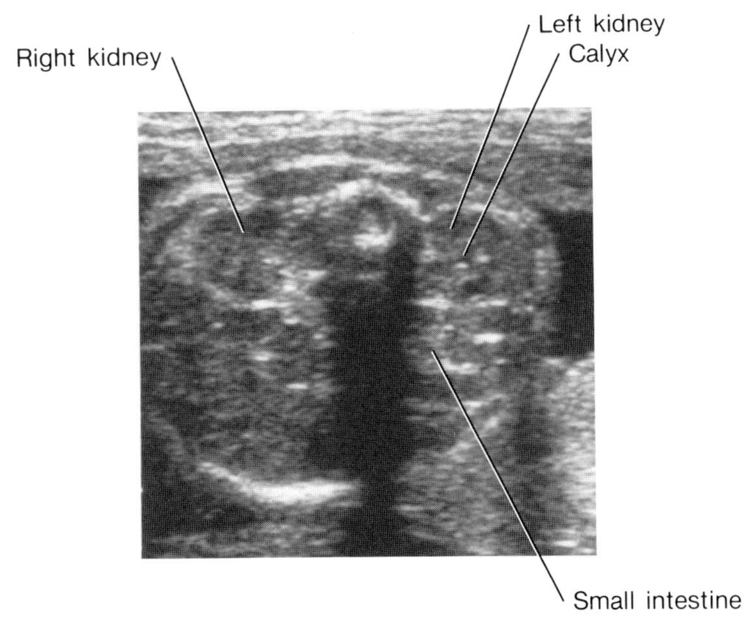

Right kidney
Left kidney
Calyx
Small intestine

Inferior vena cava
Psoas m.
Lamina of vertebra
Multifidus m.
Descending colon
Aorta
Sigmoid colon
Urinary bladder
Quadratus lumborum m.
Kidney
Ureter
Iliocecal junction
Tibia
Fibula
Femoral vessels
Femur

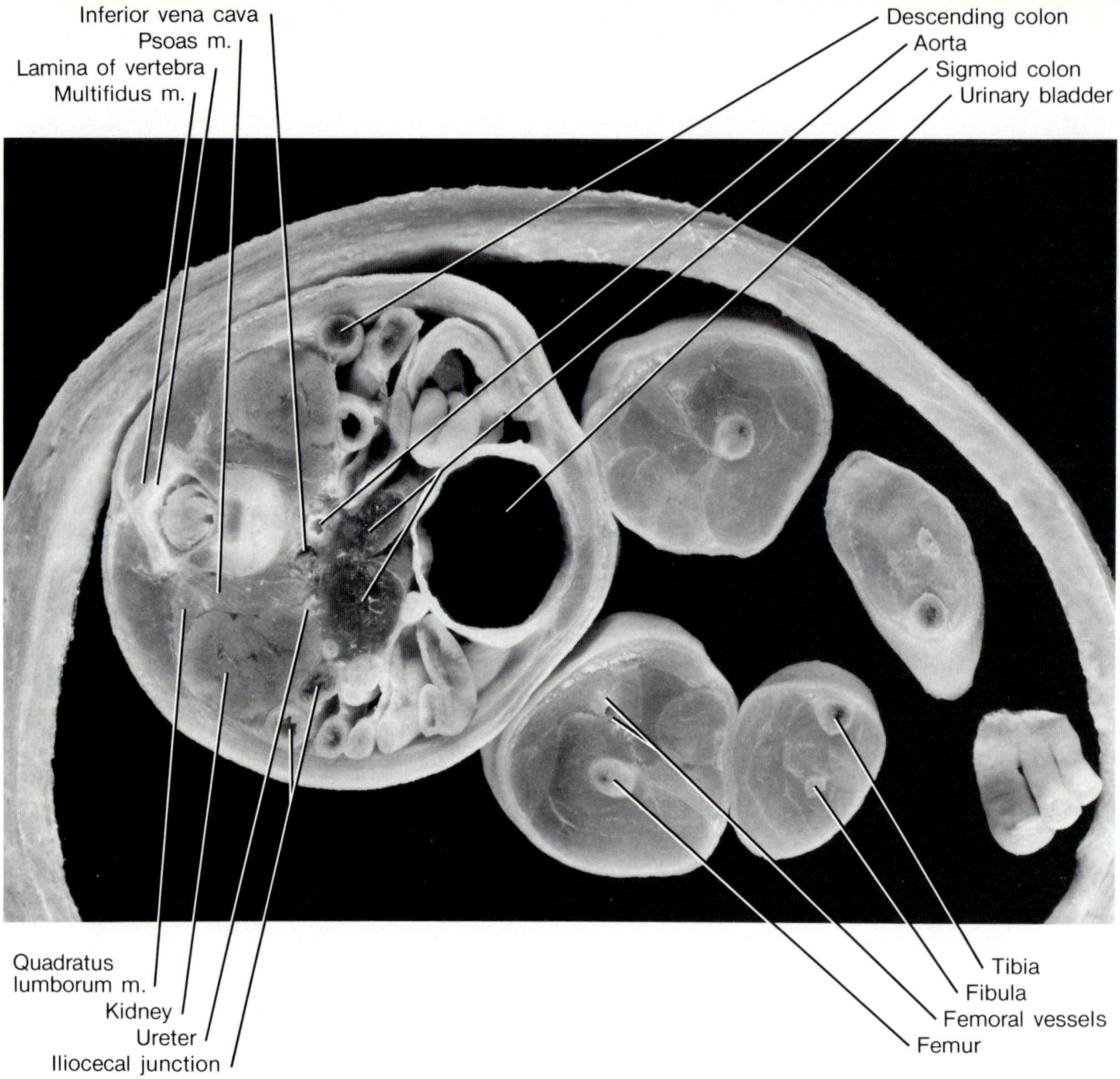

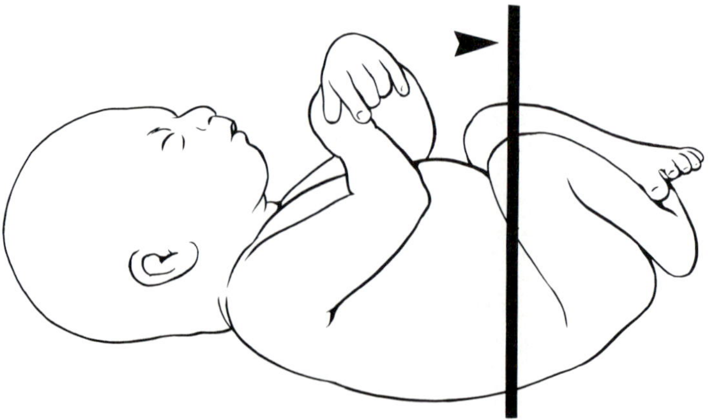

Figure 1.42

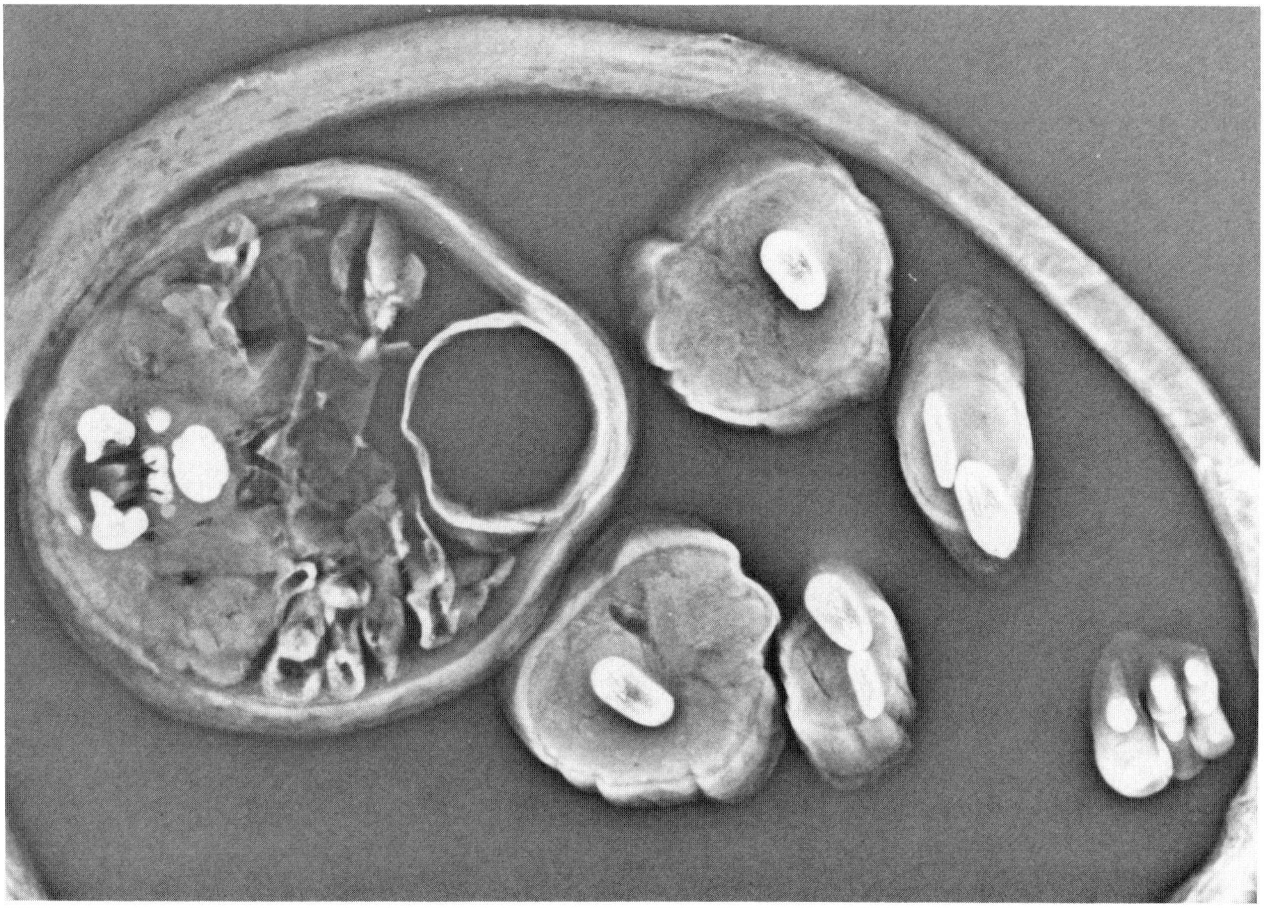

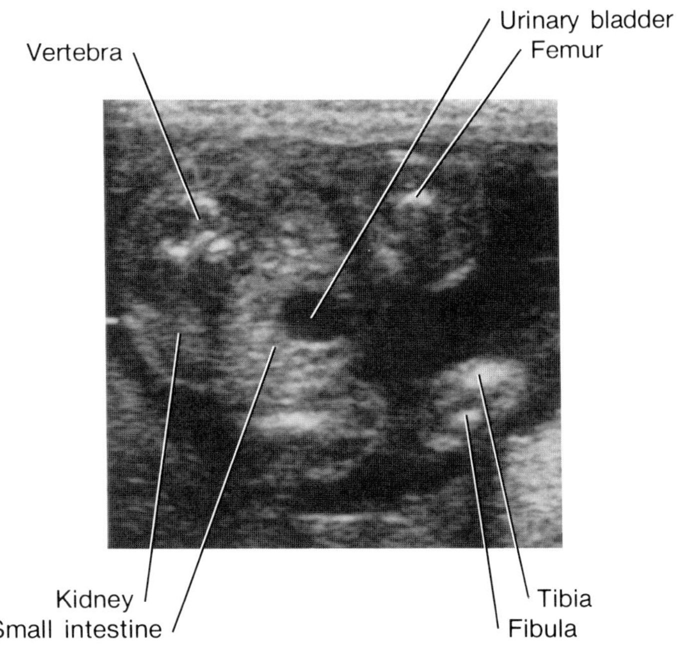

Vertebra
Urinary bladder
Femur
Kidney
Small intestine
Tibia
Fibula

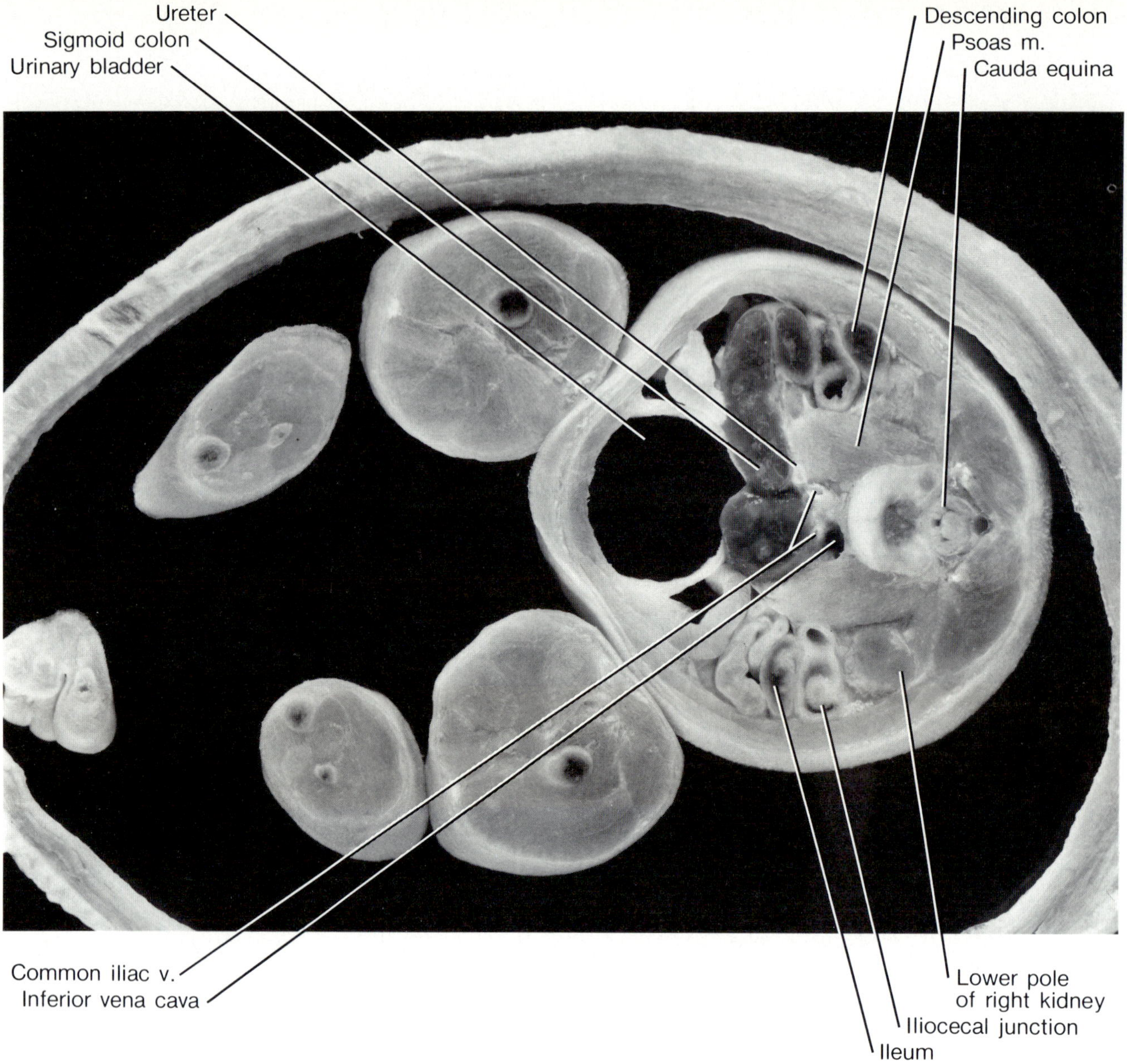

Ureter
Sigmoid colon
Urinary bladder
Descending colon
Psoas m.
Cauda equina
Common iliac v.
Inferior vena cava
Lower pole of right kidney
Iliocecal junction
Ileum

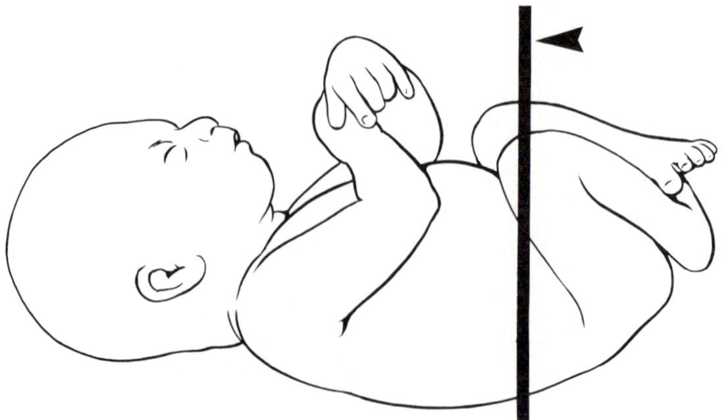

Figure 1.43

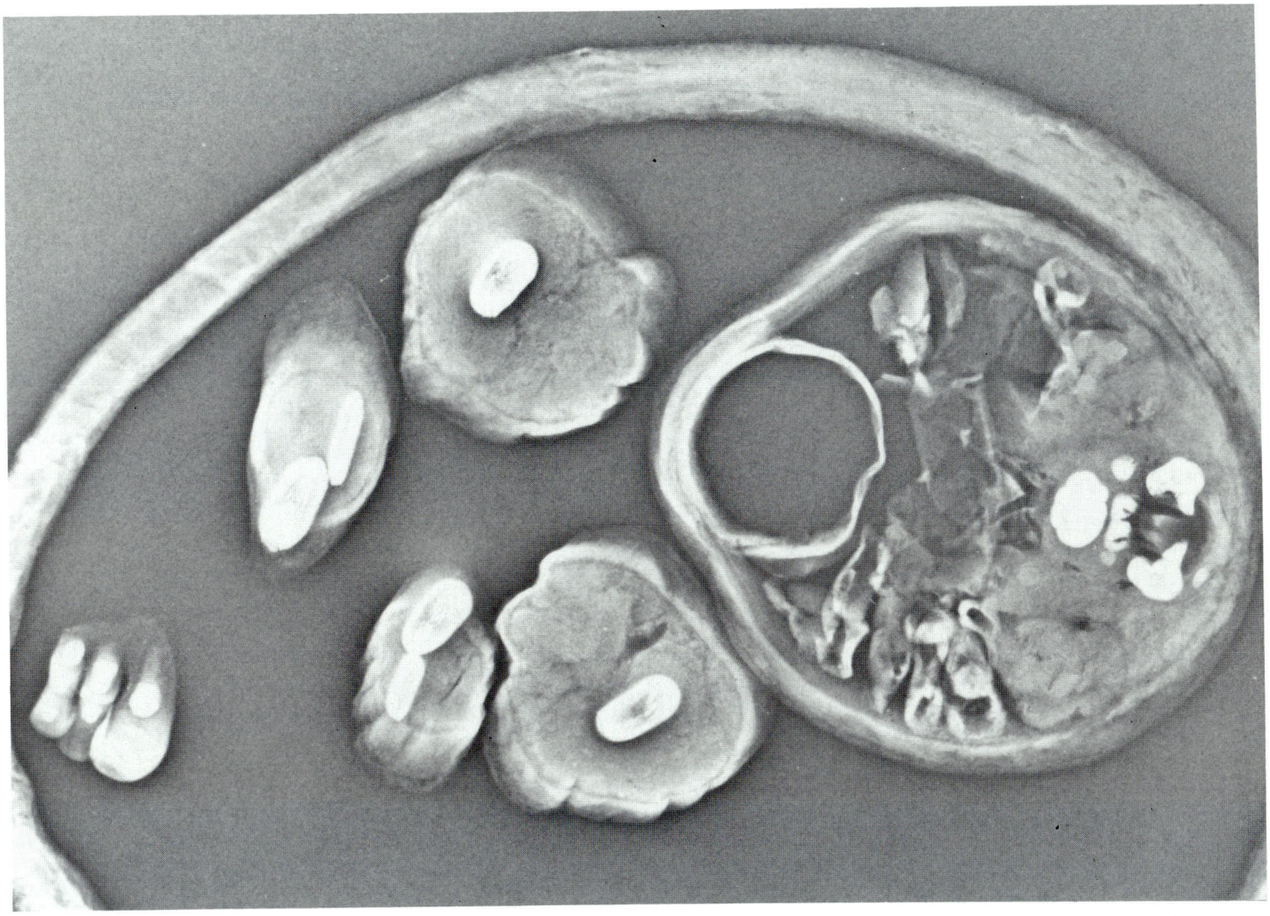

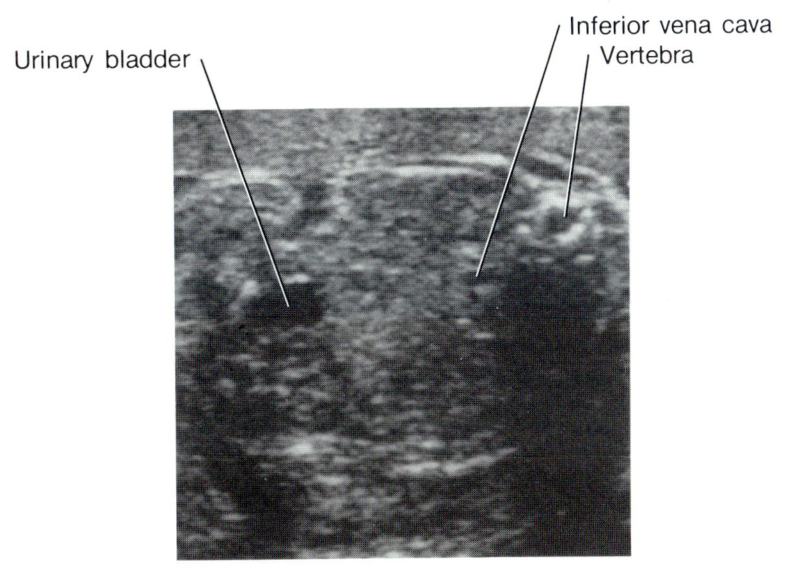

Urinary bladder
Inferior vena cava
Vertebra

Sigmoid colon
Psoas m.
Cauda equina
Dural sac
Ureter
Rectum
Testis
Urinary bladder
Cecum
Testis
Rectus femoris m.
Sartorius m.
Vastus intermedius m.
Vastus lateralis m.
Gracilis m.
Adductor magnus m.
Hamstring m.
Sciatic n.
Adductor longus m.
Femur

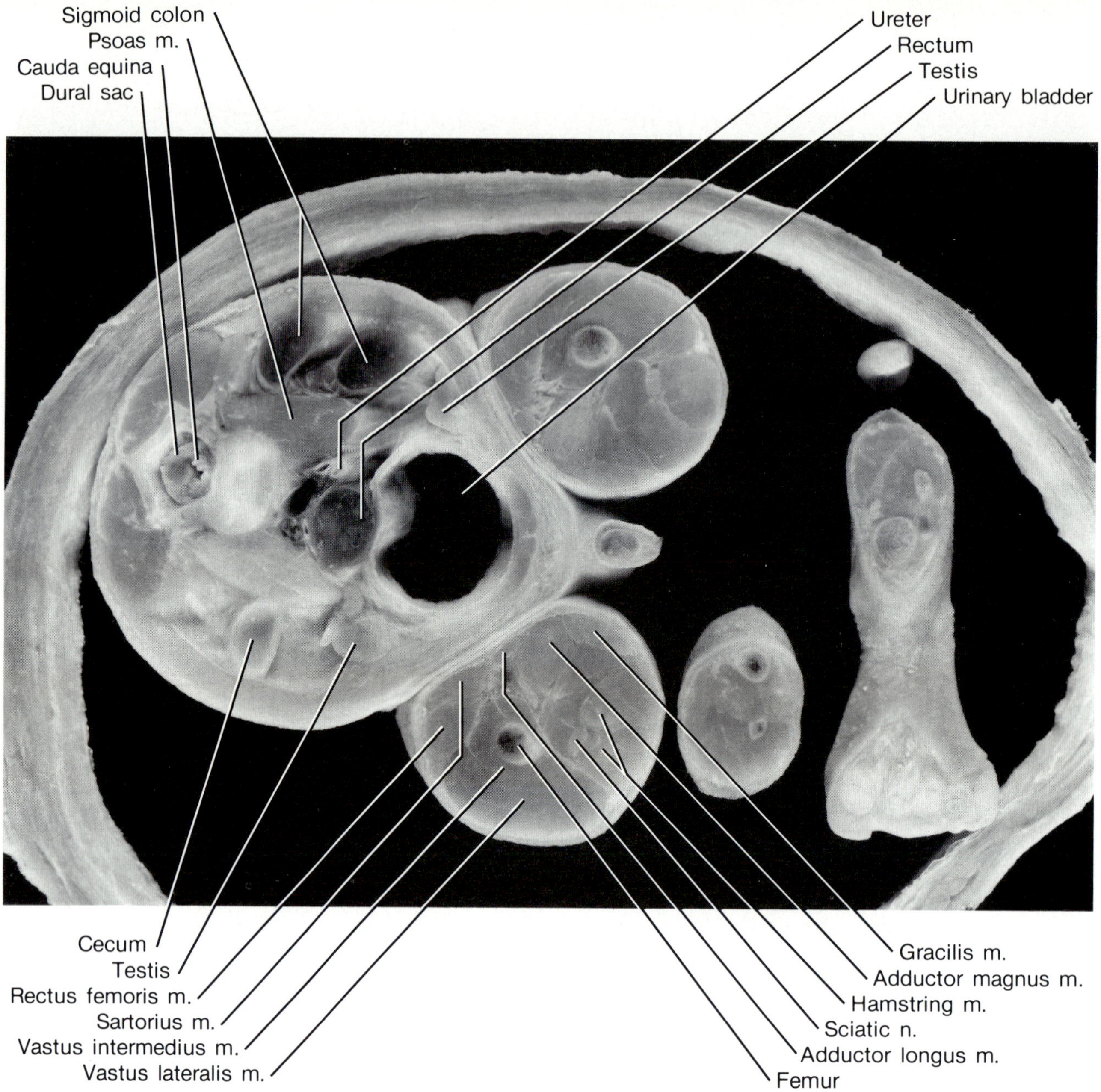

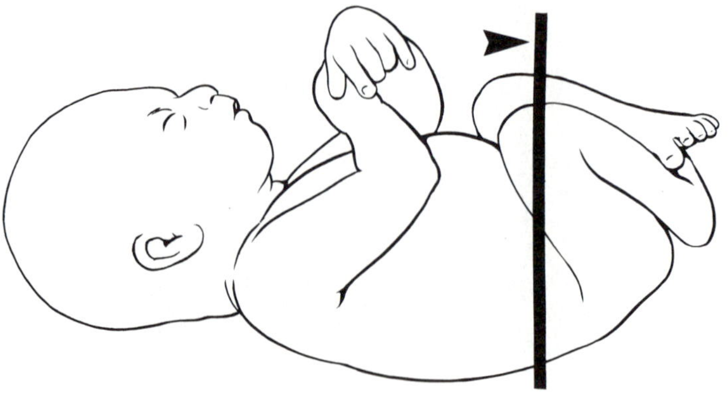

Figure 1.44

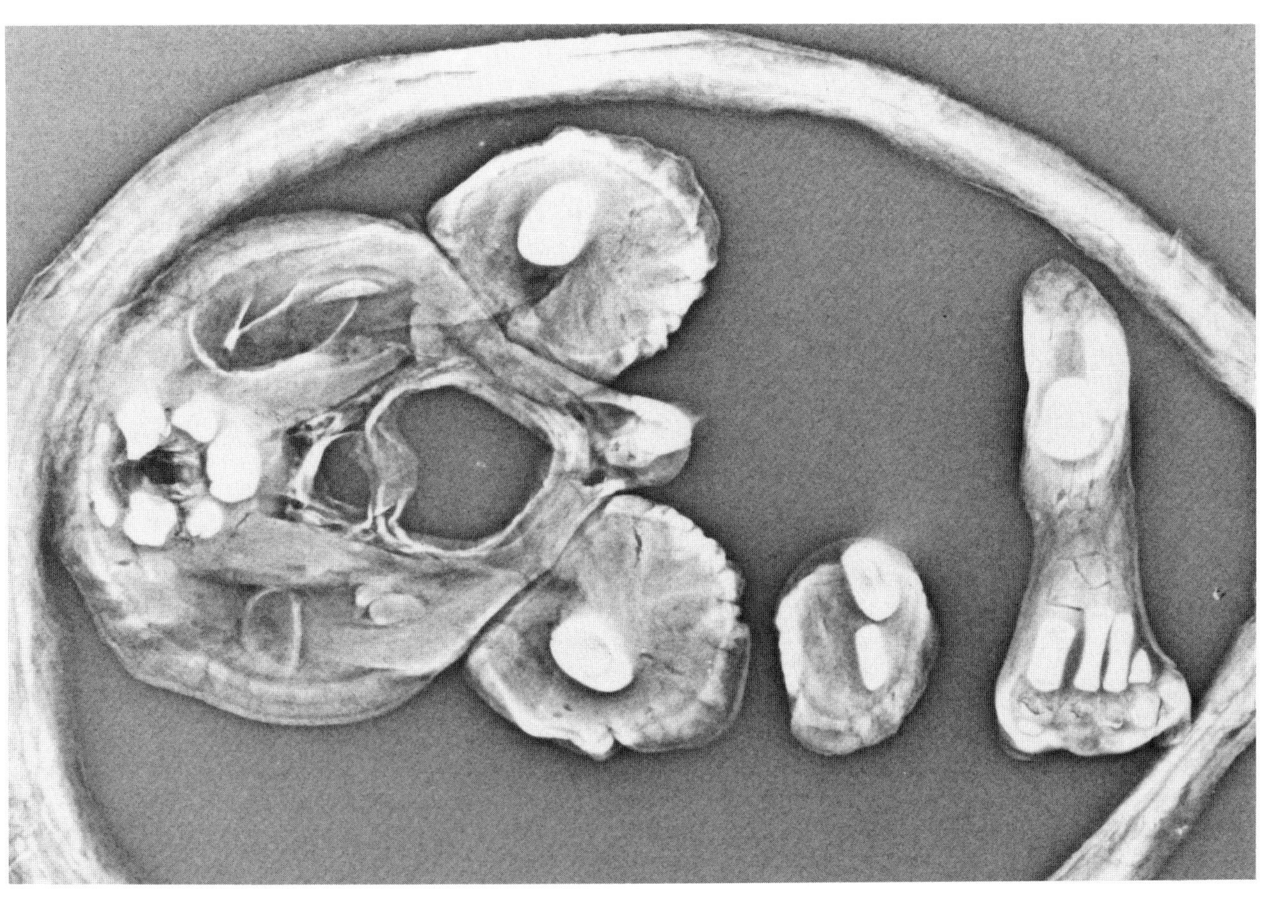

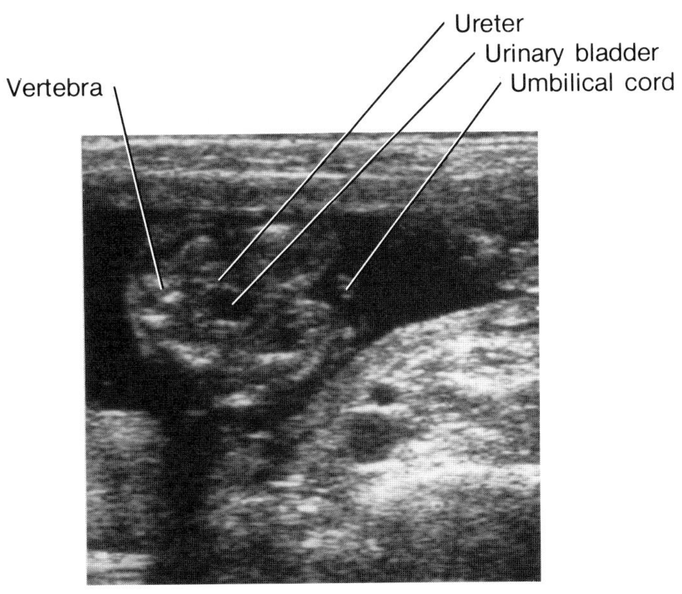

Ureter
Urinary bladder
Umbilical cord
Vertebra

Penis (3 bodies)
Urethra
Posterior crural m.
Tibia
Fibula
Anterior crural m.
Tibia
Fibula
Vesical a.
Ilium
Iliacus m.
Ureter
Iliac vessels
Quadratus lumborum m.
Dura mater
Multifidus m.
Tarsal bones or tarsus
Hamstring m.
Adductor m. group
Vastus lateralis m.
Shaft of femur
Femoral n.
Psoas m.
Rectum
Ureter
Urinary bladder
Rectus abdominis m.

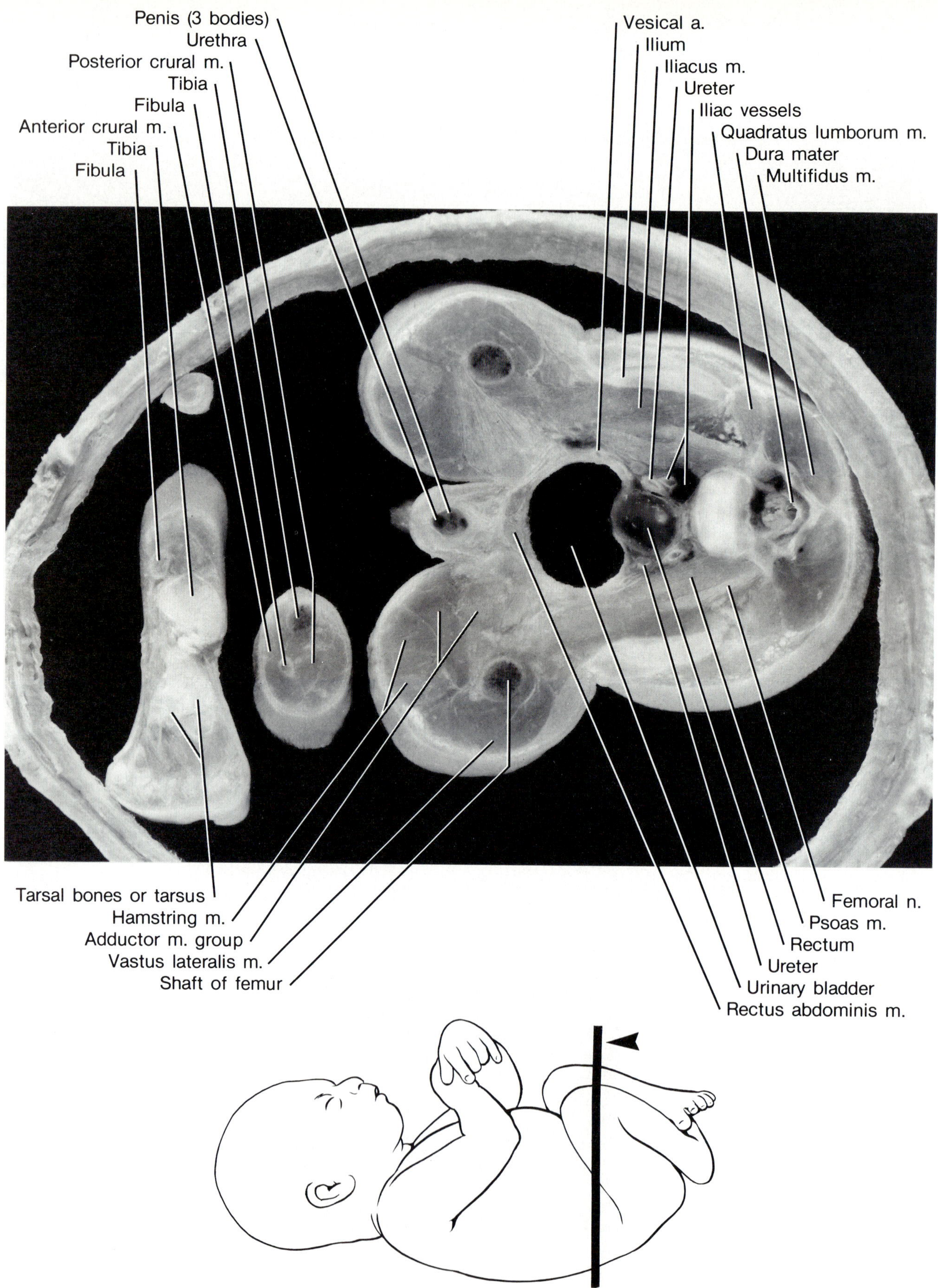

Figure 1.45

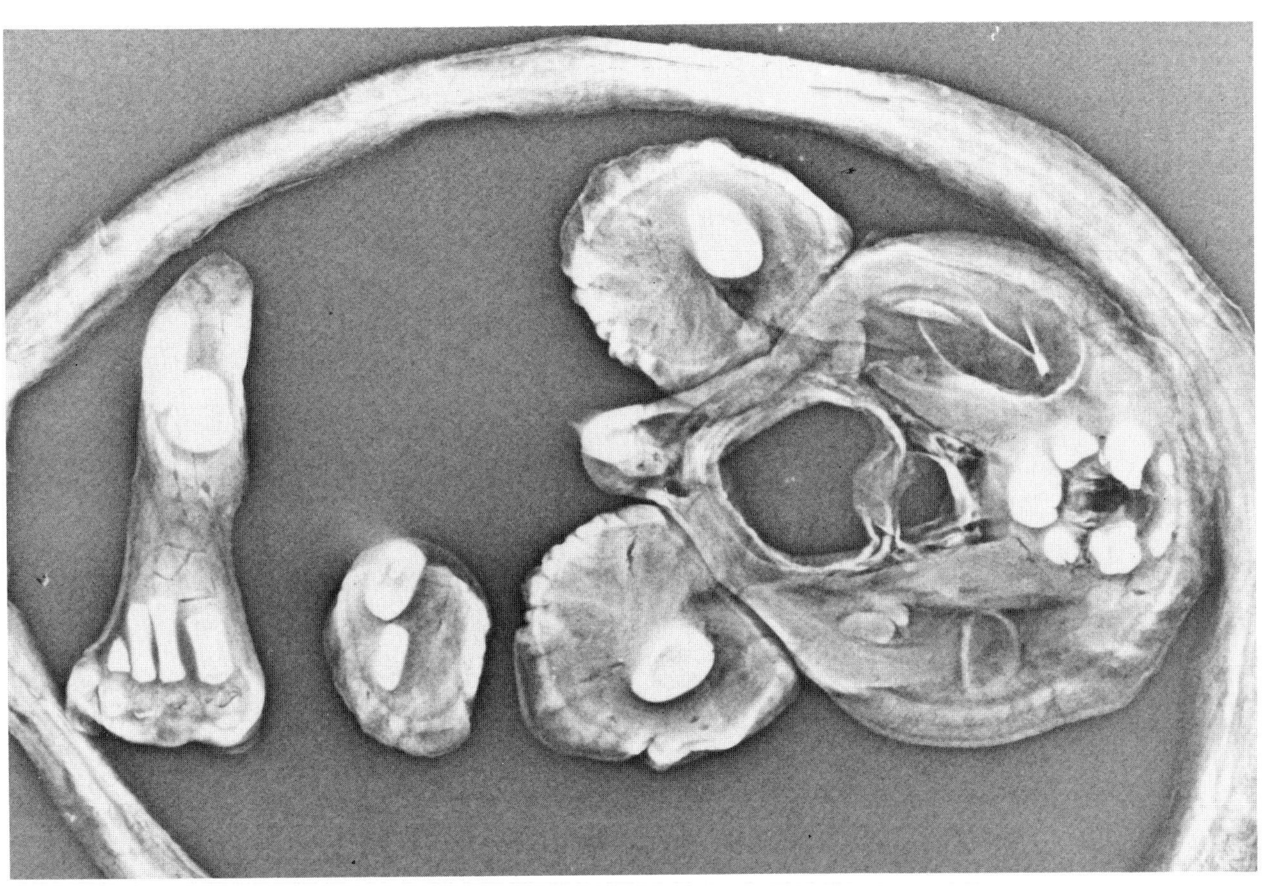

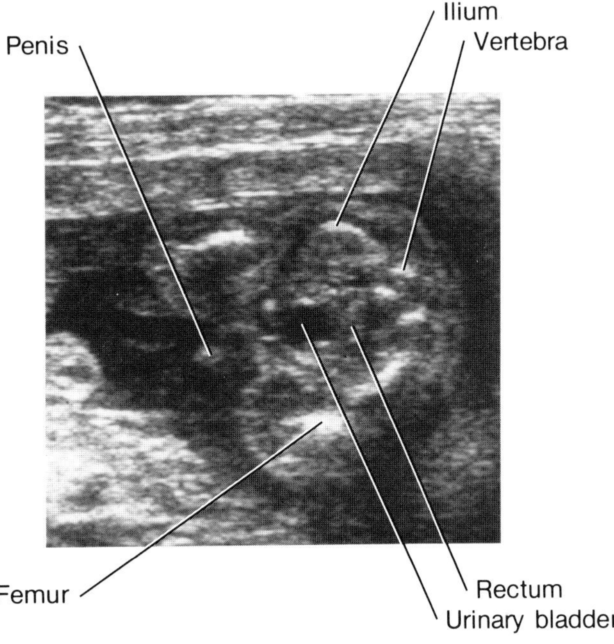

Penis
Ilium
Vertebra
Femur
Rectum
Urinary bladder

Opening of ureter
Ureter
Internal iliac vessels
Spinal nerves
Adductor m. group
Corpora of penis
Urethra
Dural sac
Iliacus m.
Psoas m.
Ureter
Ilium
Femur
Vastus lateralis m.

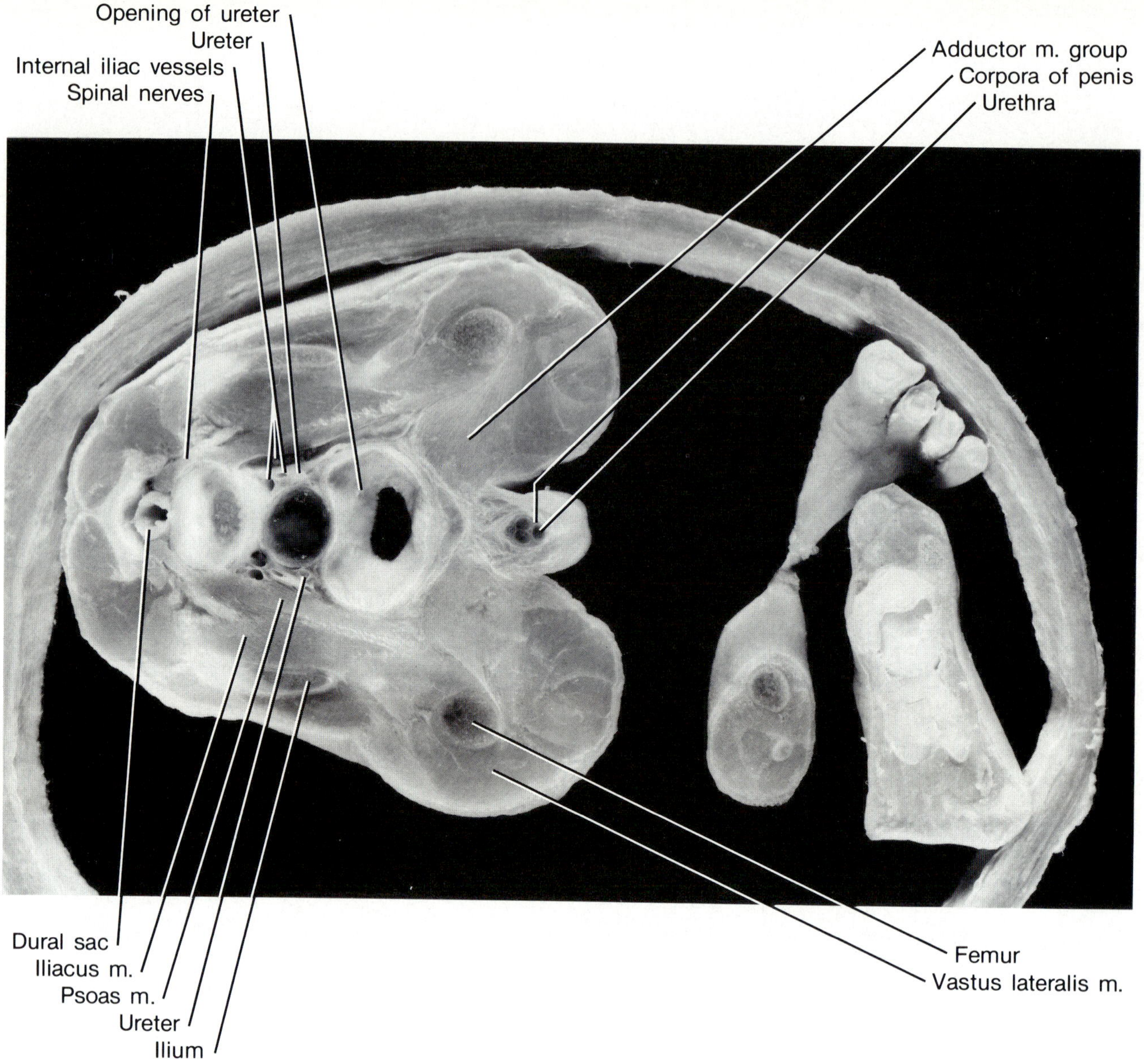

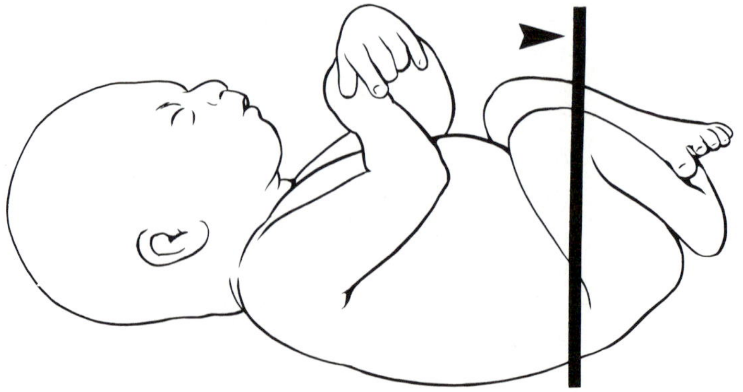

Figure 1.46

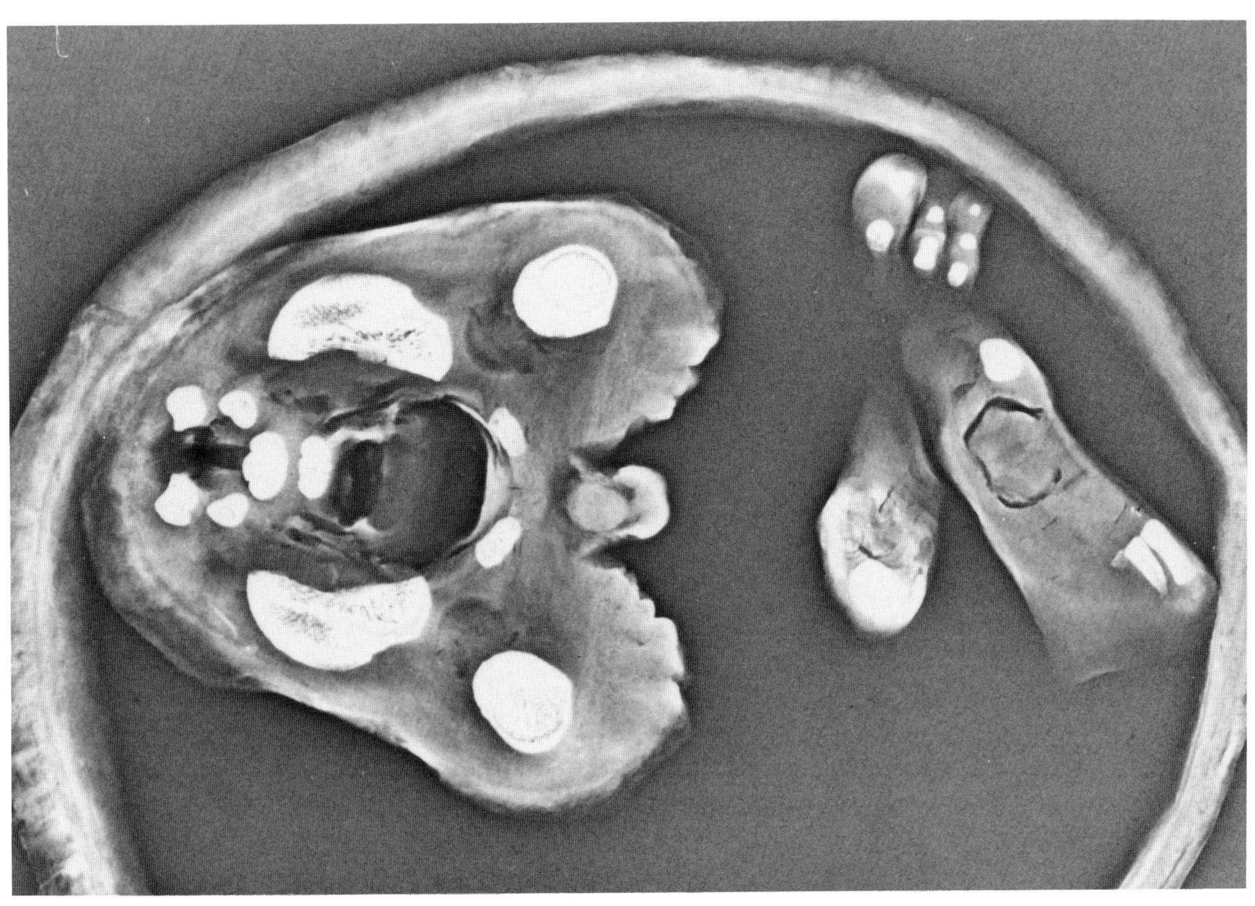

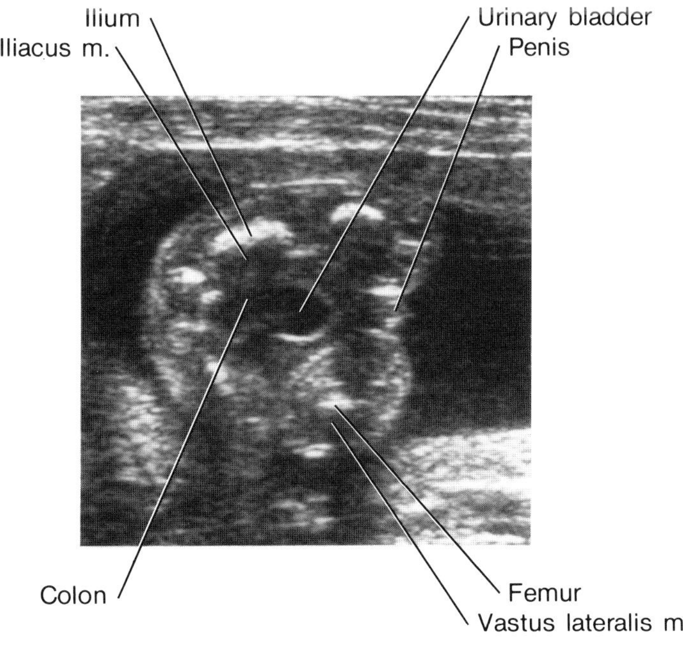

Ilium
Iliacus m.
Urinary bladder
Penis
Colon
Femur
Vastus lateralis m.

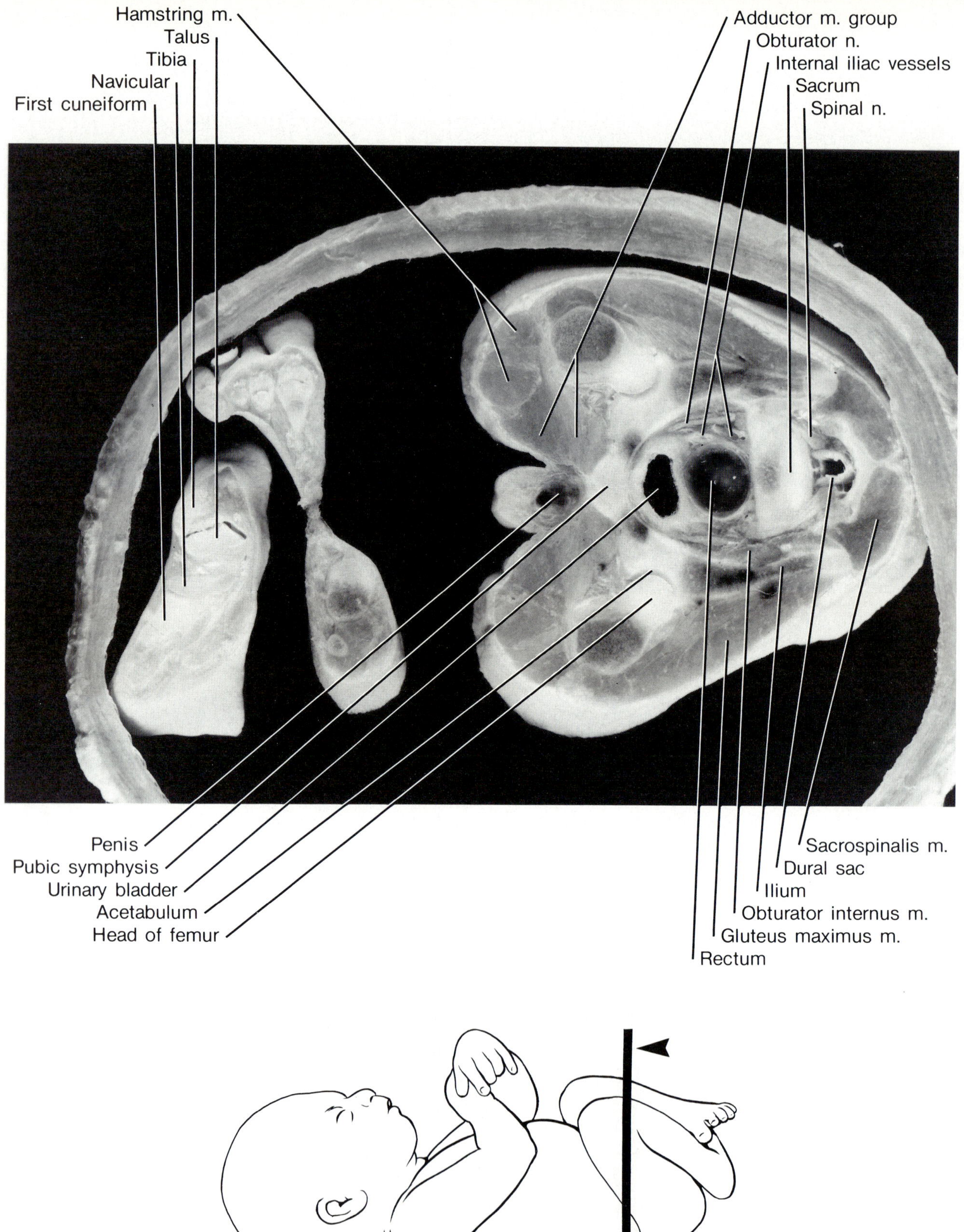

Figure 1.47

 FETAL SECTIONAL ANATOMY AND ULTRASONOGRAPHY

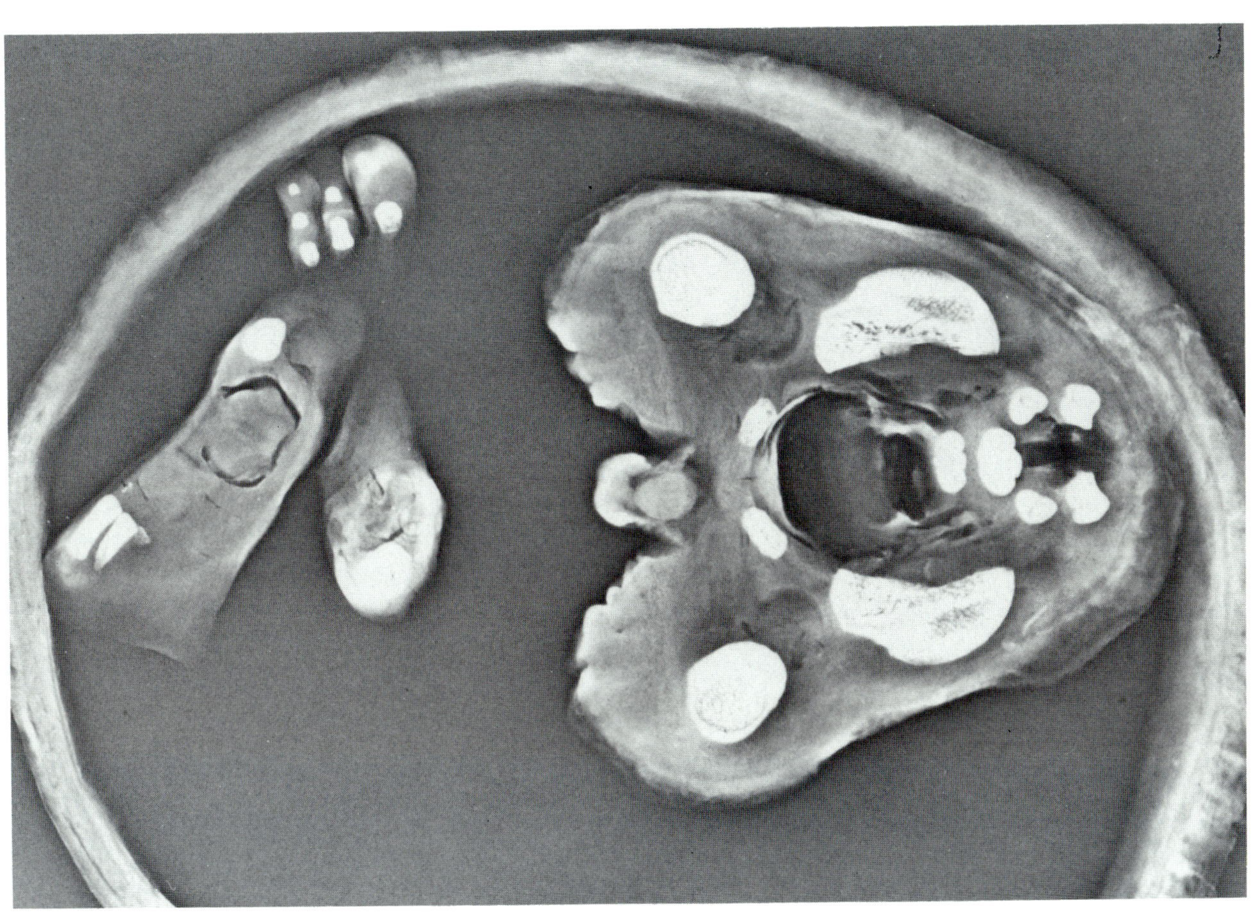

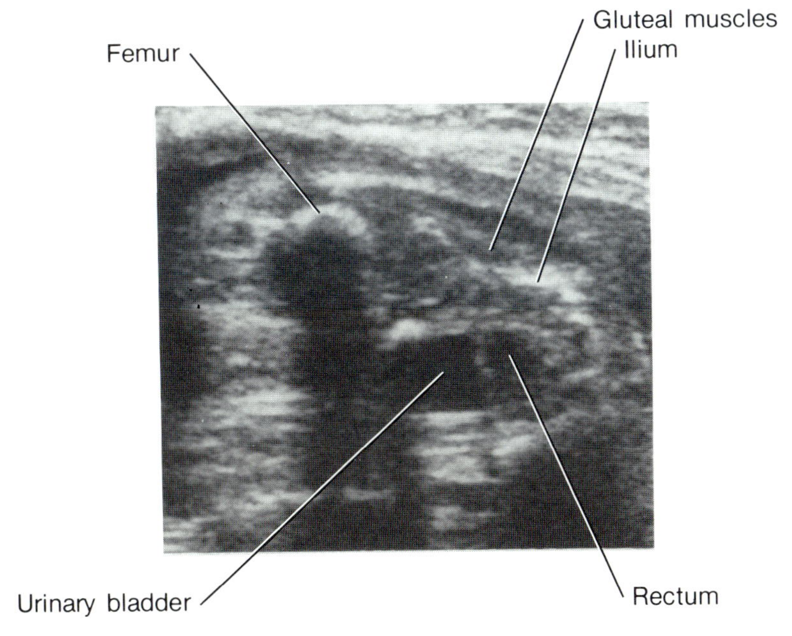

Femur
Gluteal muscles
Ilium
Urinary bladder
Rectum

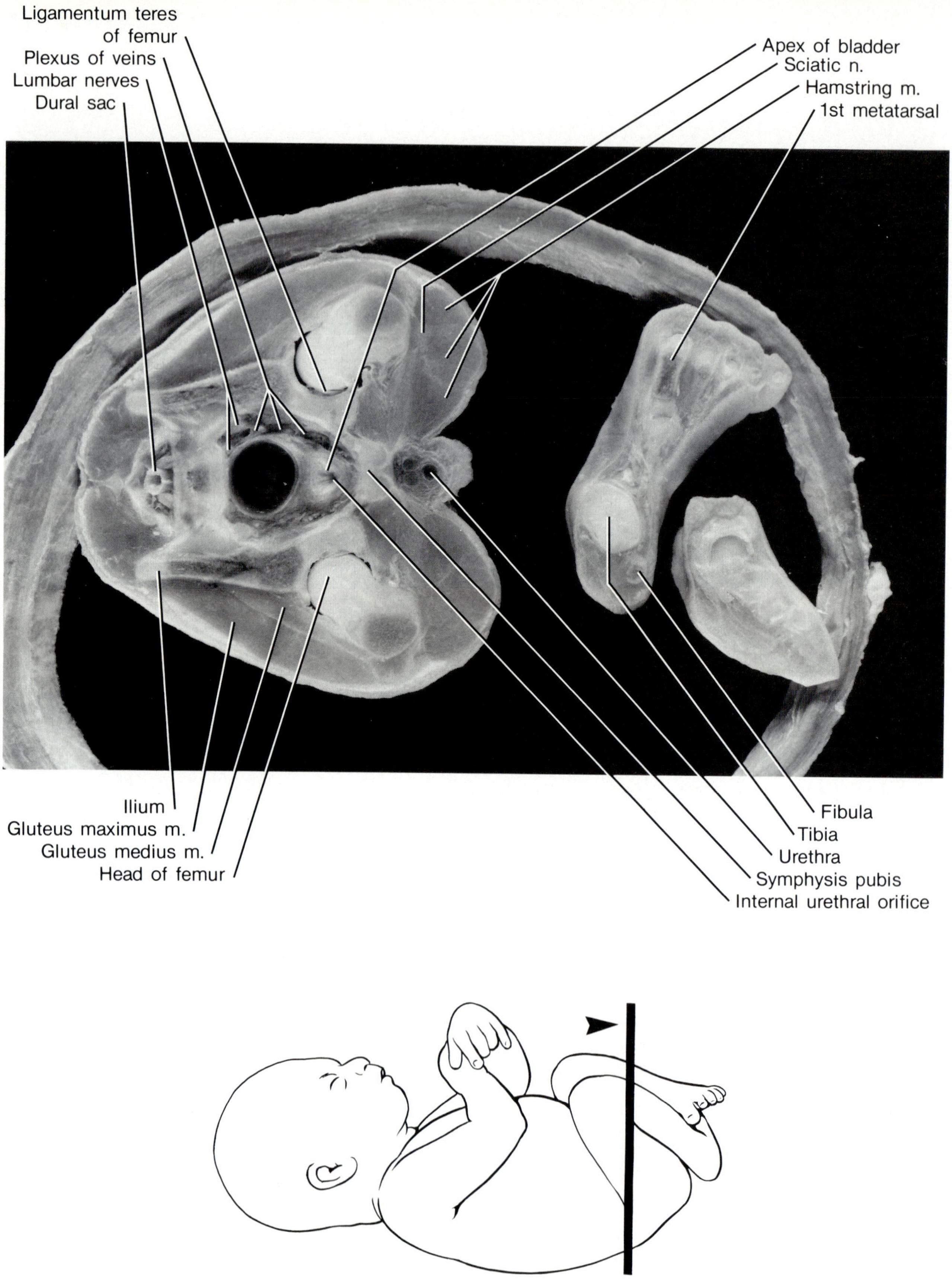

Ligamentum teres
of femur
Plexus of veins
Lumbar nerves
Dural sac

Apex of bladder
Sciatic n.
Hamstring m.
1st metatarsal

Ilium
Gluteus maximus m.
Gluteus medius m.
Head of femur

Fibula
Tibia
Urethra
Symphysis pubis
Internal urethral orifice

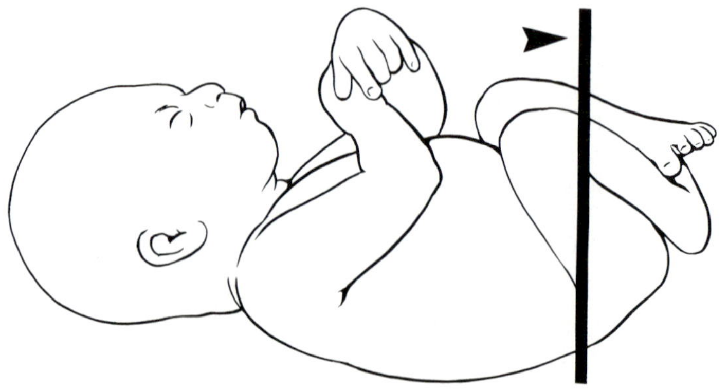

Figure 1.48

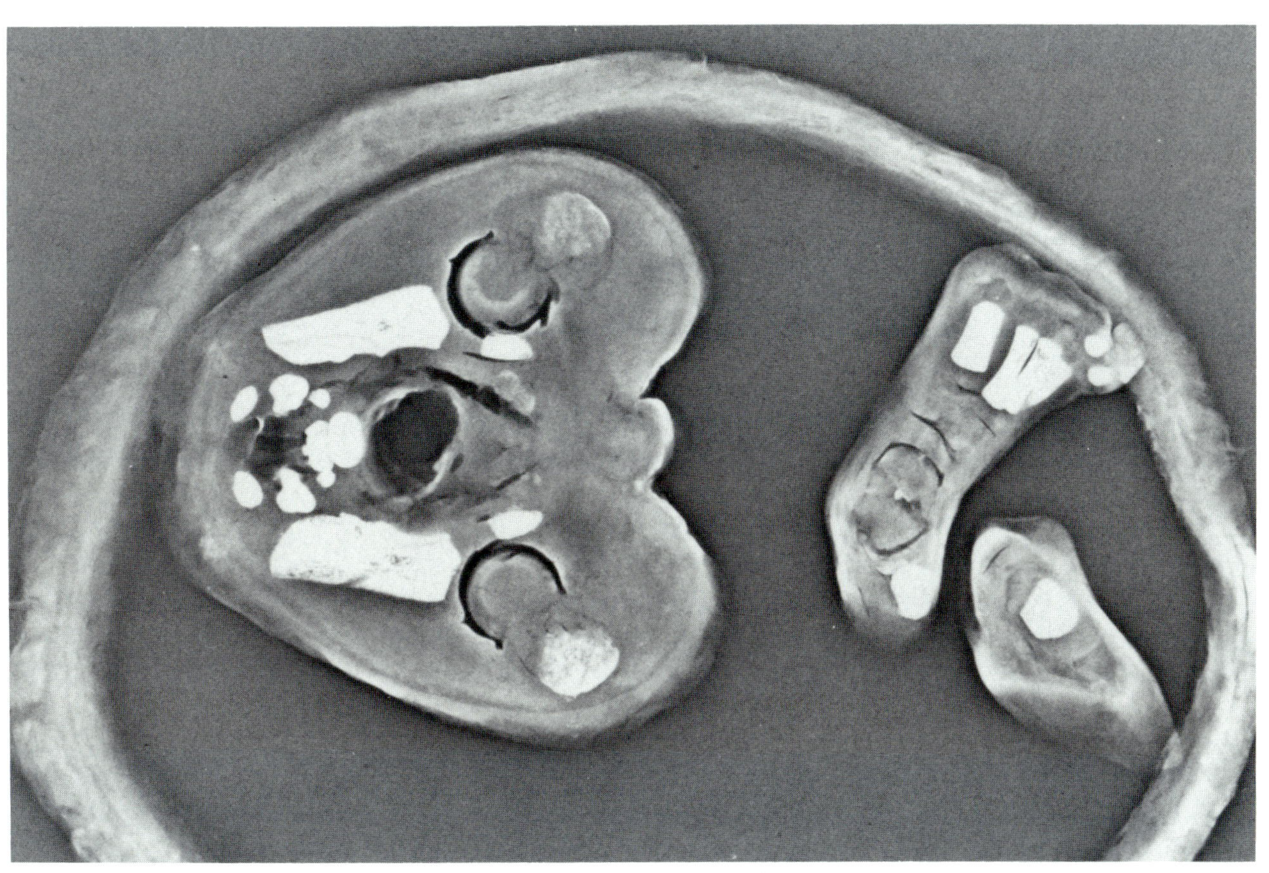

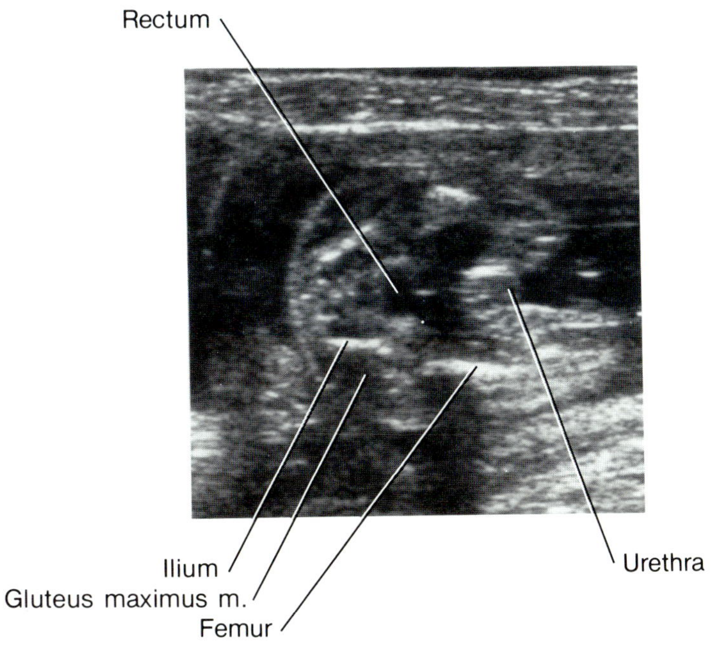

Rectum
Ilium
Gluteus maximus m.
Femur
Urethra

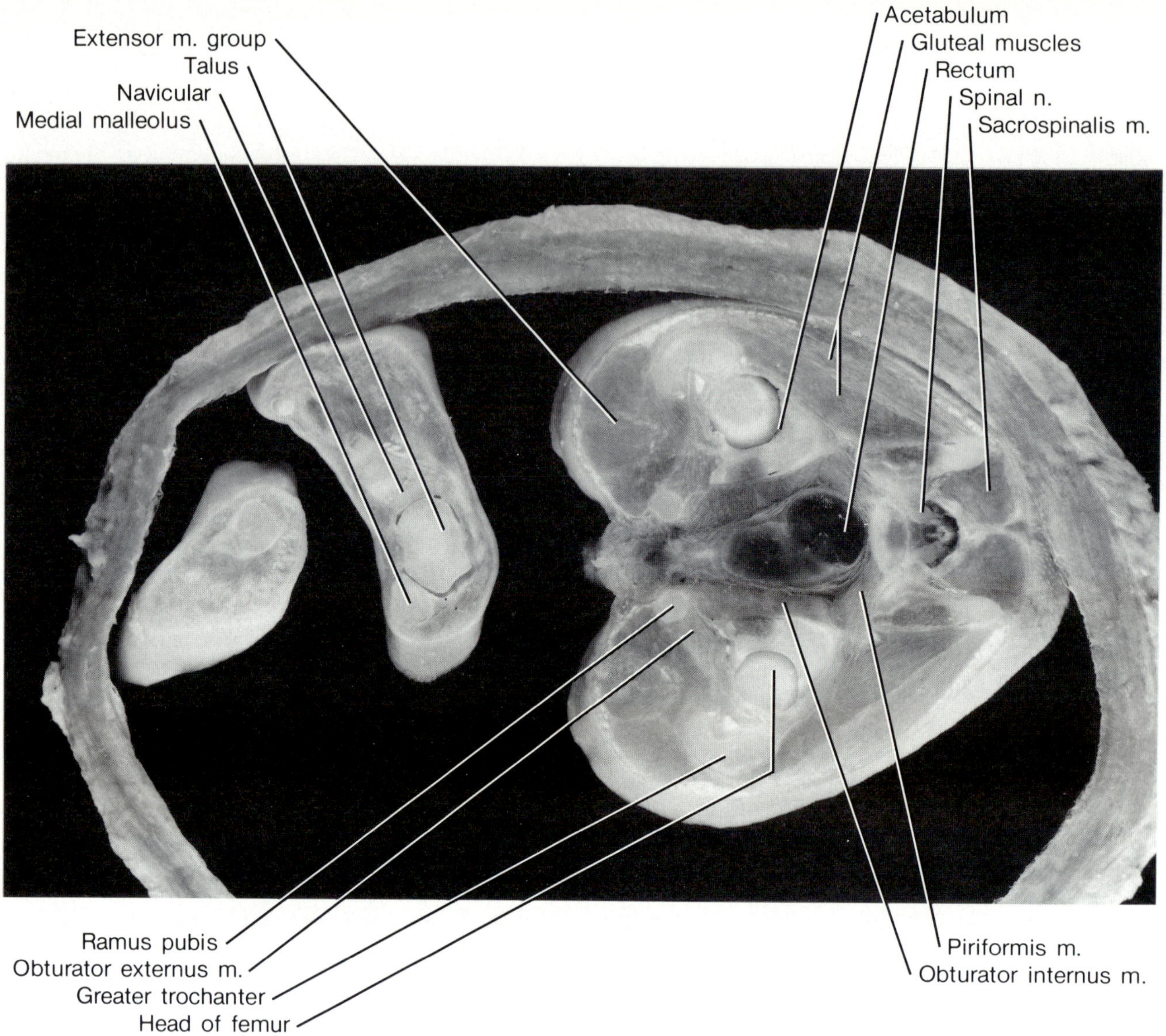

Extensor m. group
Talus
Navicular
Medial malleolus
Acetabulum
Gluteal muscles
Rectum
Spinal n.
Sacrospinalis m.
Ramus pubis
Obturator externus m.
Greater trochanter
Head of femur
Piriformis m.
Obturator internus m.

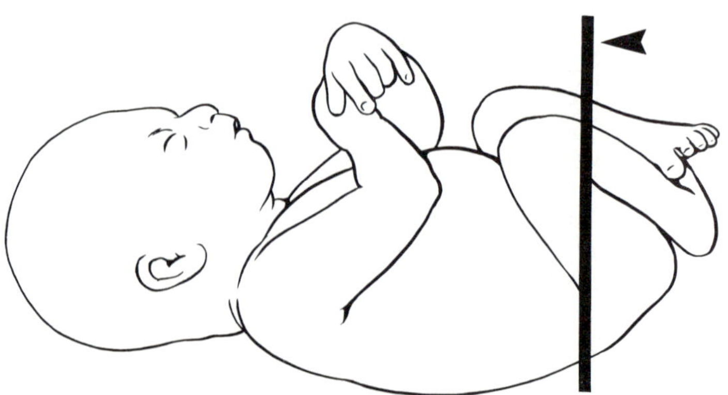

Figure 1.49

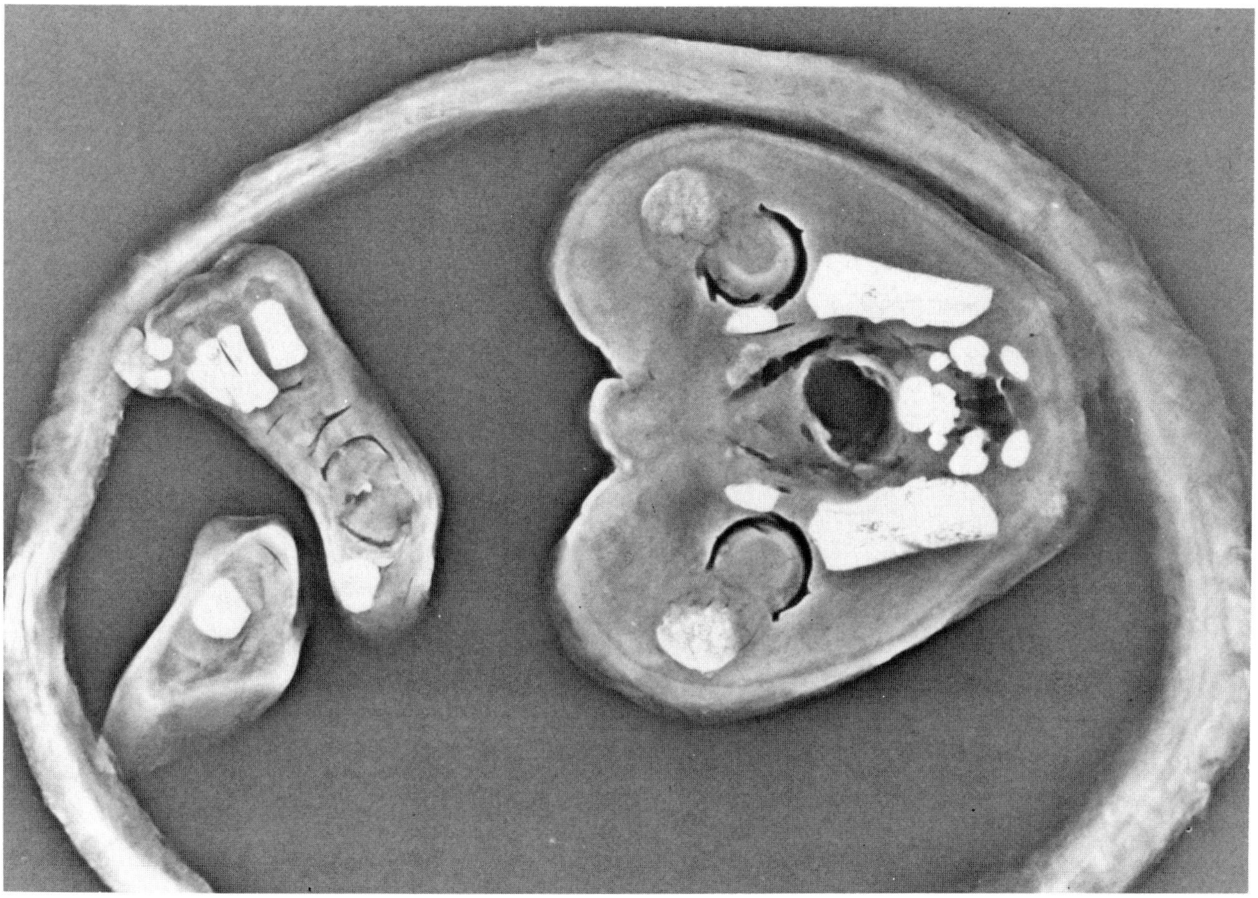

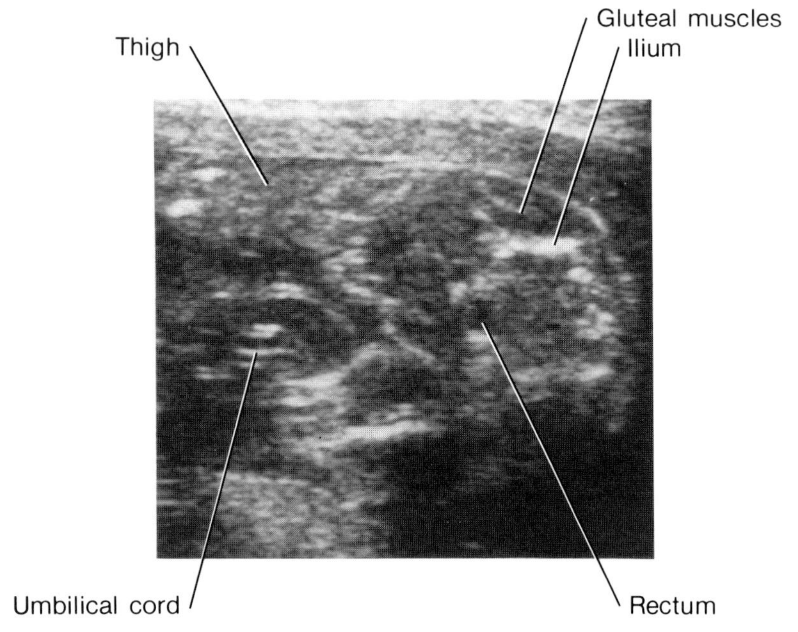

Thigh
Gluteal muscles
Ilium
Umbilical cord
Rectum

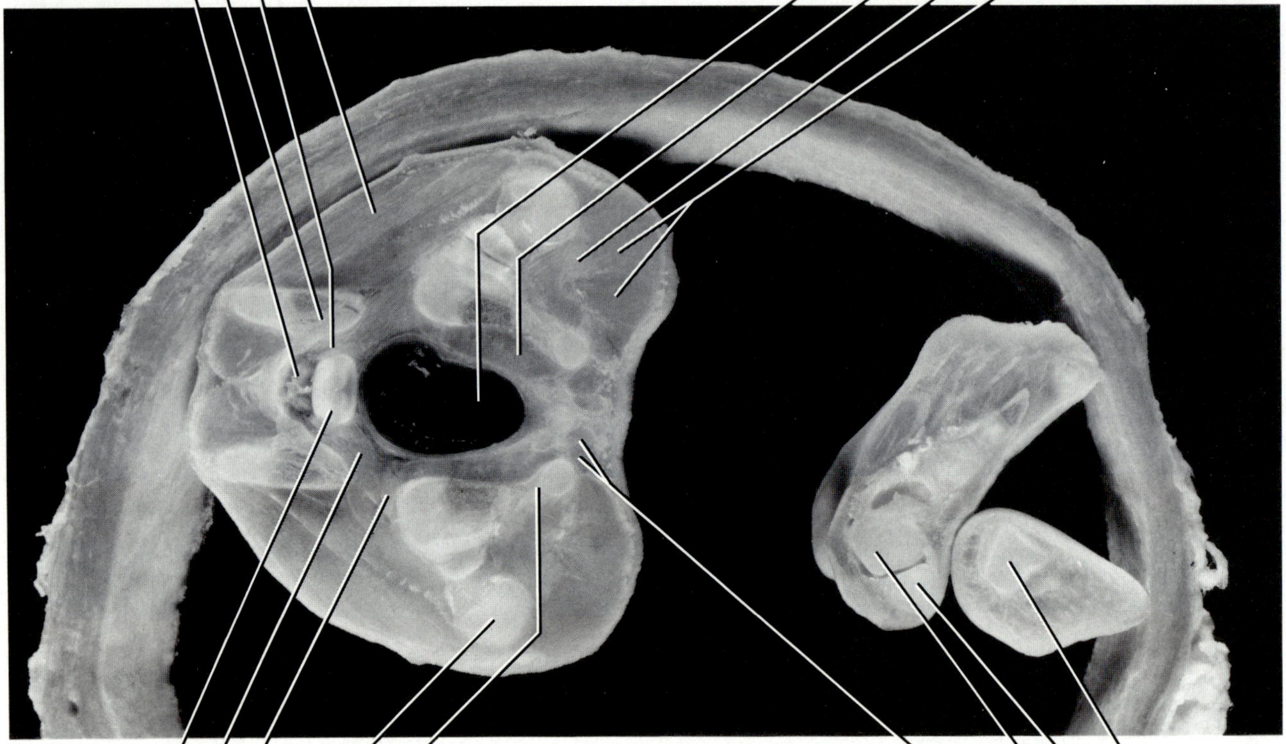

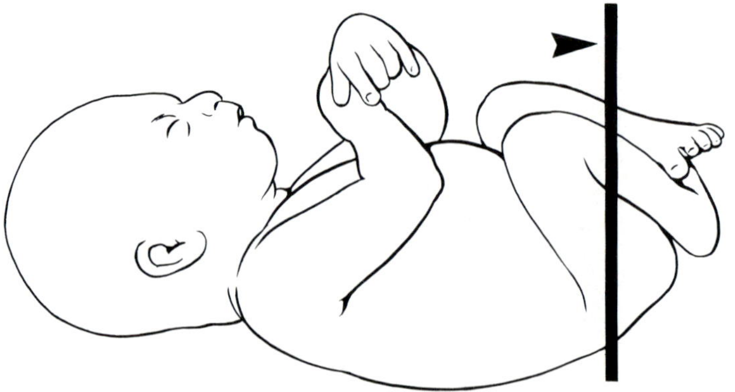

Figure 1.50

  FETAL SECTIONAL ANATOMY AND ULTRASONOGRAPHY

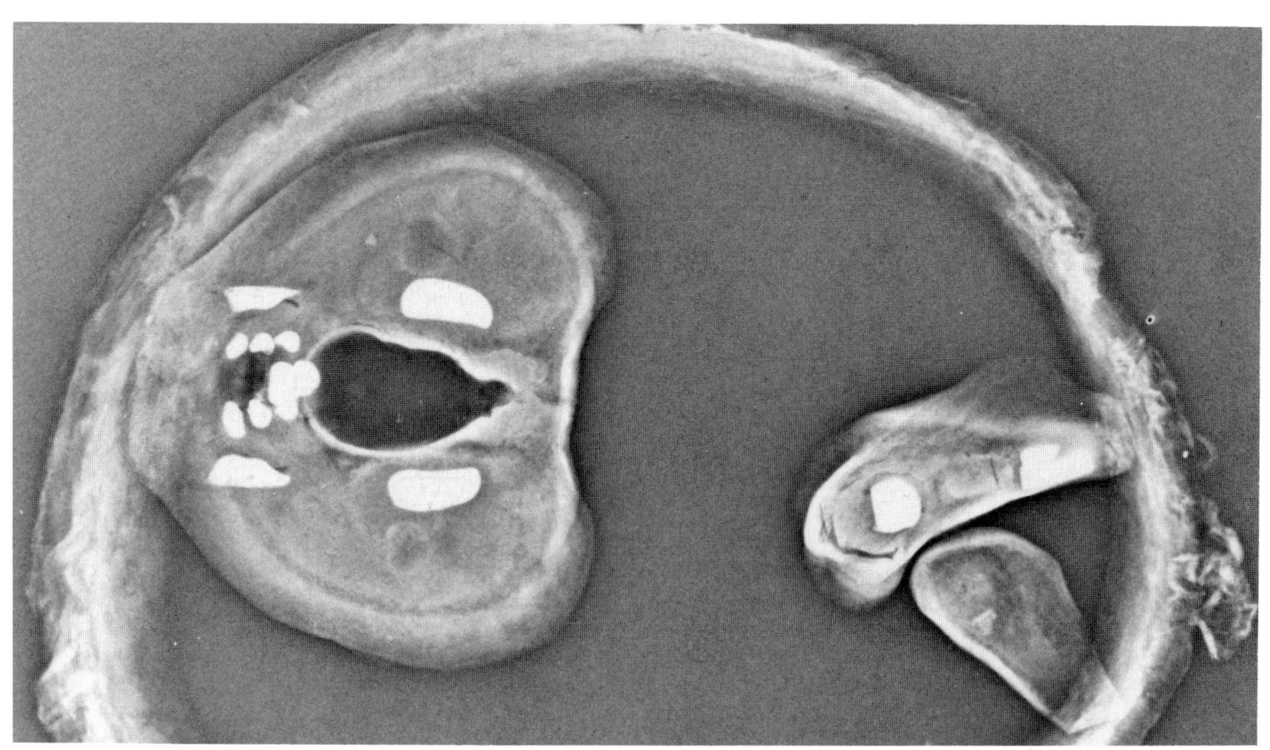

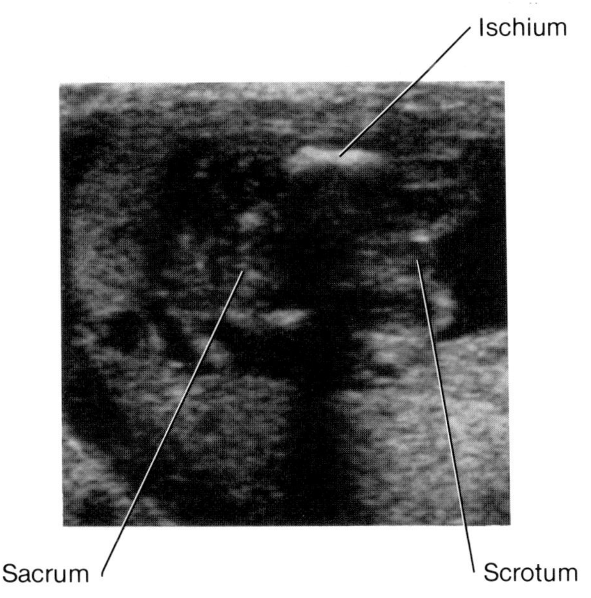

Ischium
Sacrum
Scrotum

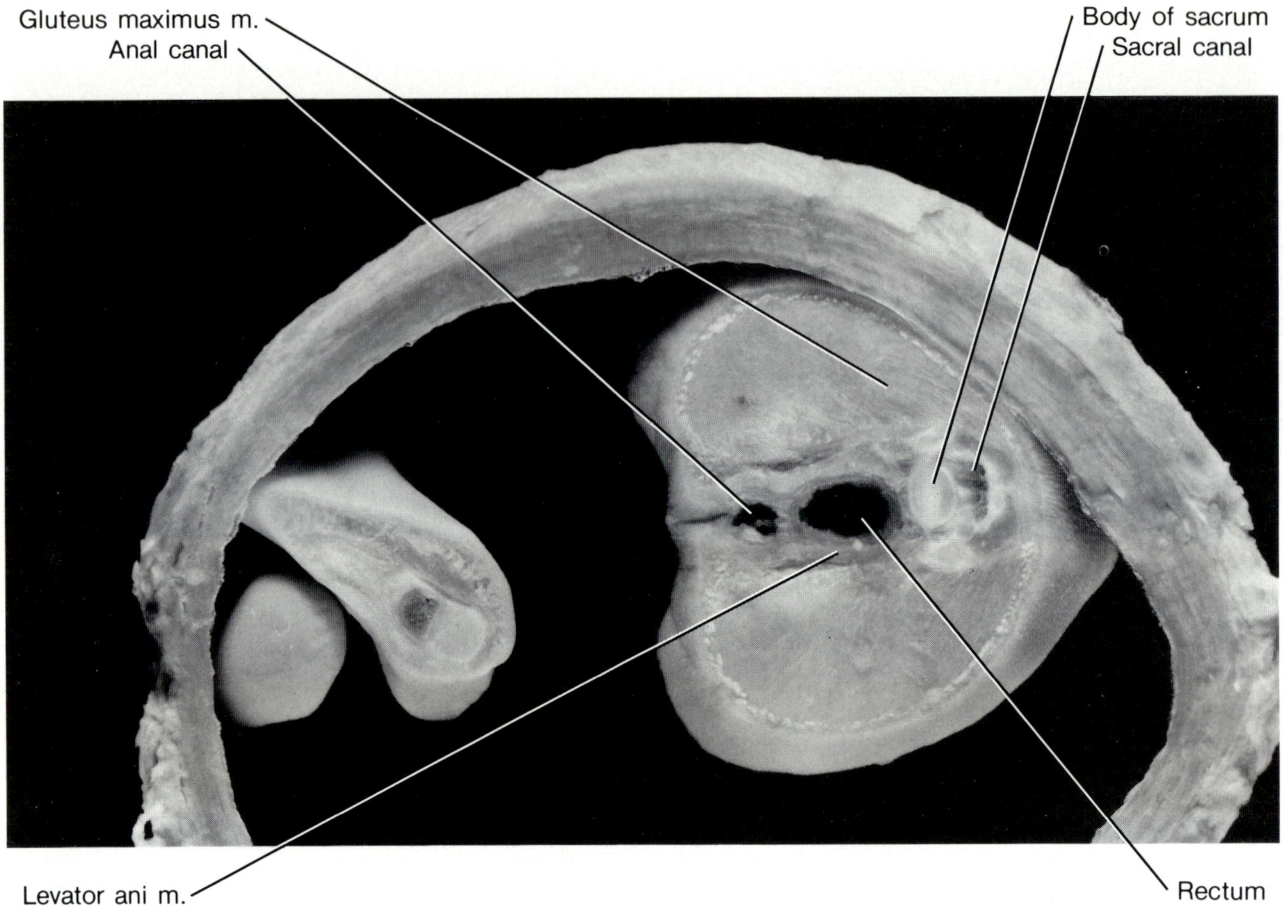
Gluteus maximus m.
Anal canal
Body of sacrum
Sacral canal
Levator ani m.
Rectum

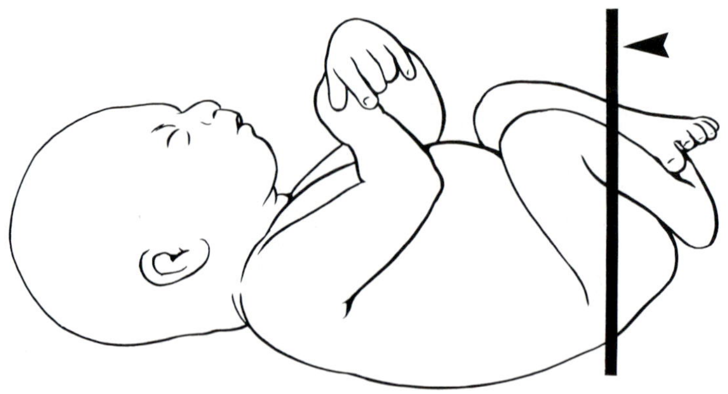

Figure 1.51

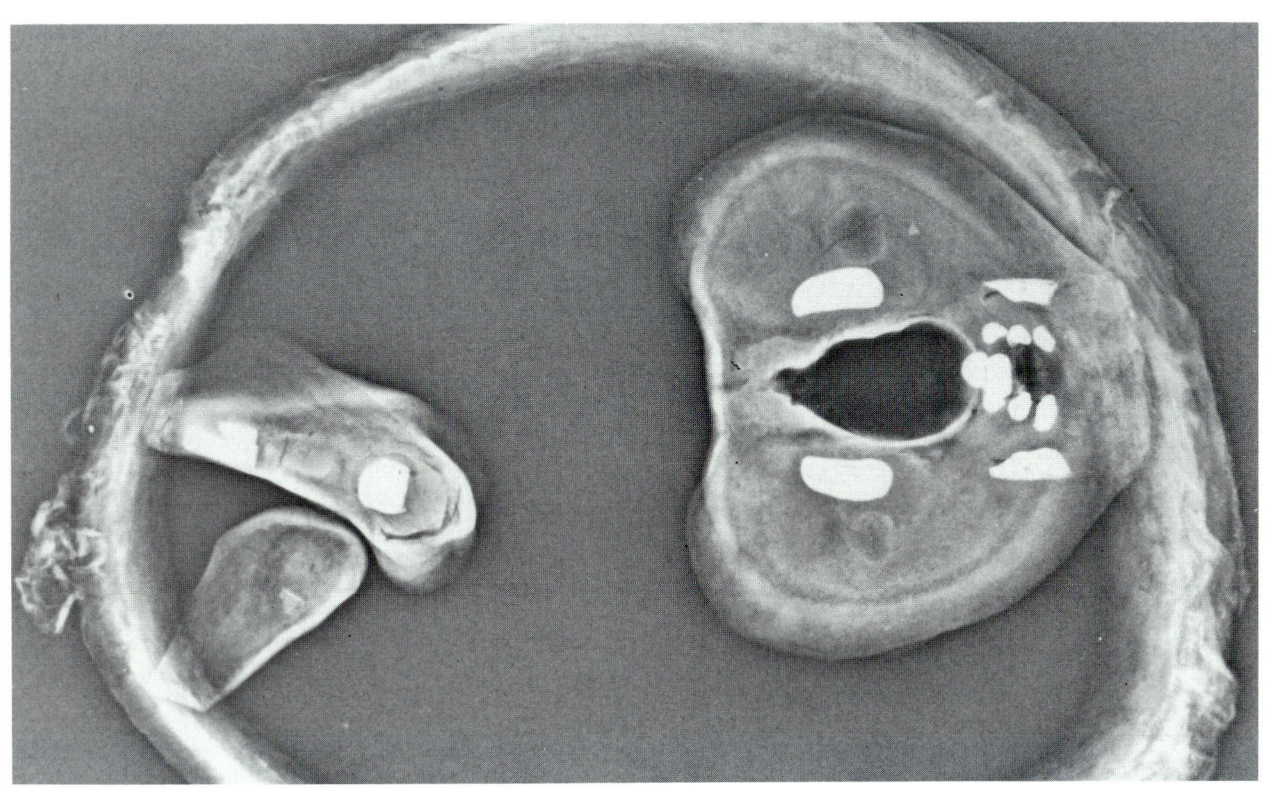

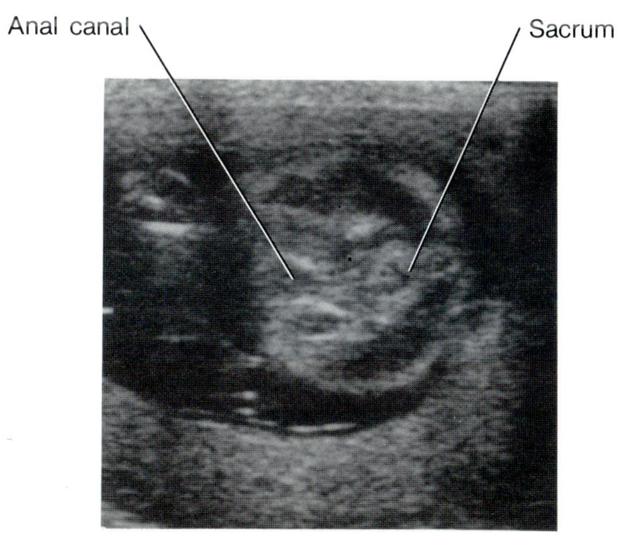

Anal canal
Sacrum

2

CROSS SECTIONS

heart of a
20-week fetus

Pleural cavity
Pericardial cavity
Arch of aorta
Thymus
Oblique fissure
Rib
Dura mater
Lamina
Superior vena cava
Primary bronchi
Intervertebral disc
Body of vertebra
Esophagus

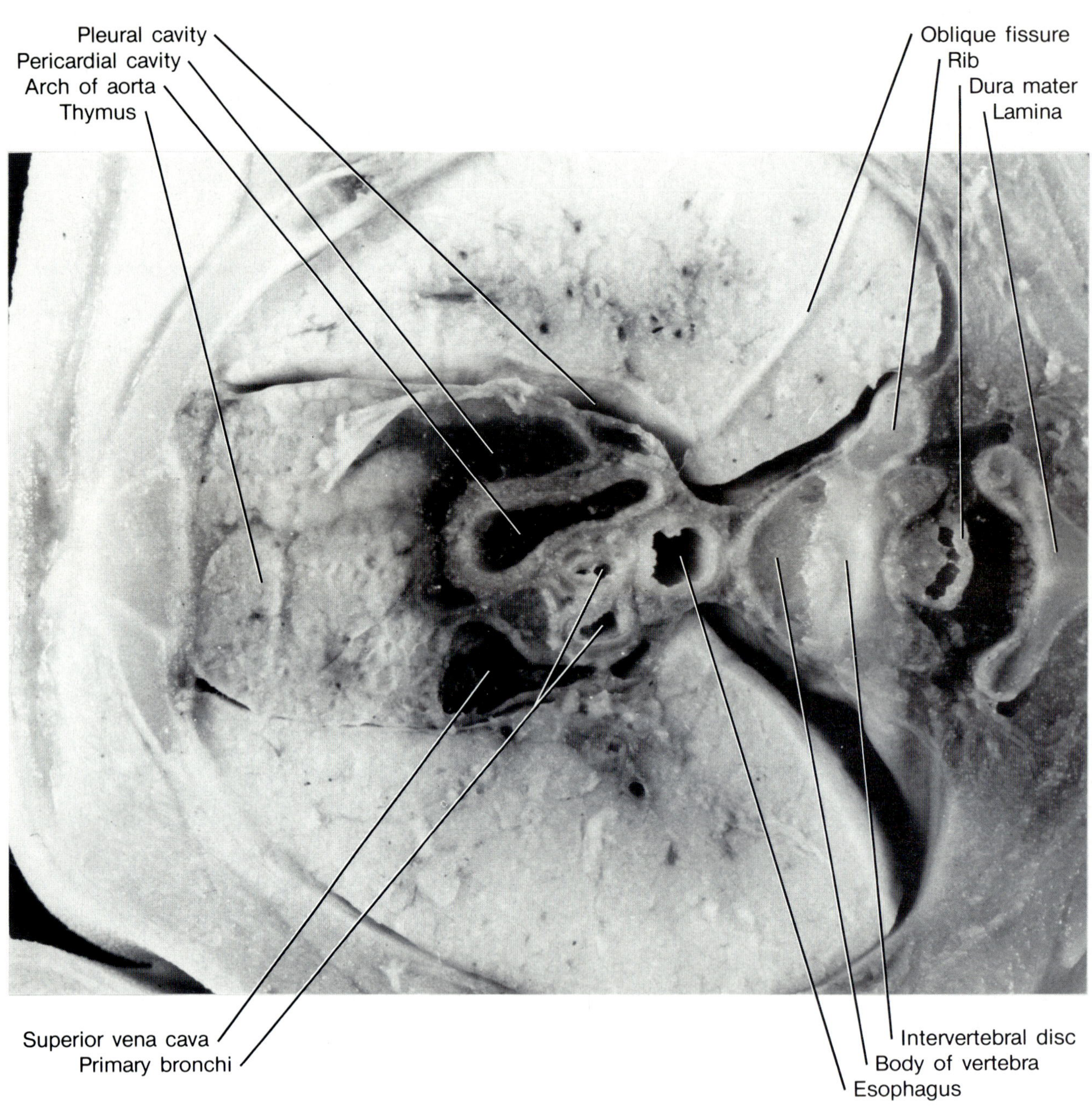

Figure 2.1

Descending aorta
Oblique fissure
Esophagus
Dura mater
Pulmonary trunk
Primary bronchi
Ascending aorta
Right auricle
Thymus
Pleural cavity
Lower lobe
of right lung
Oblique fissure
Pericardium
Superior vena cava
Right pulmonary v.
Azygos v.

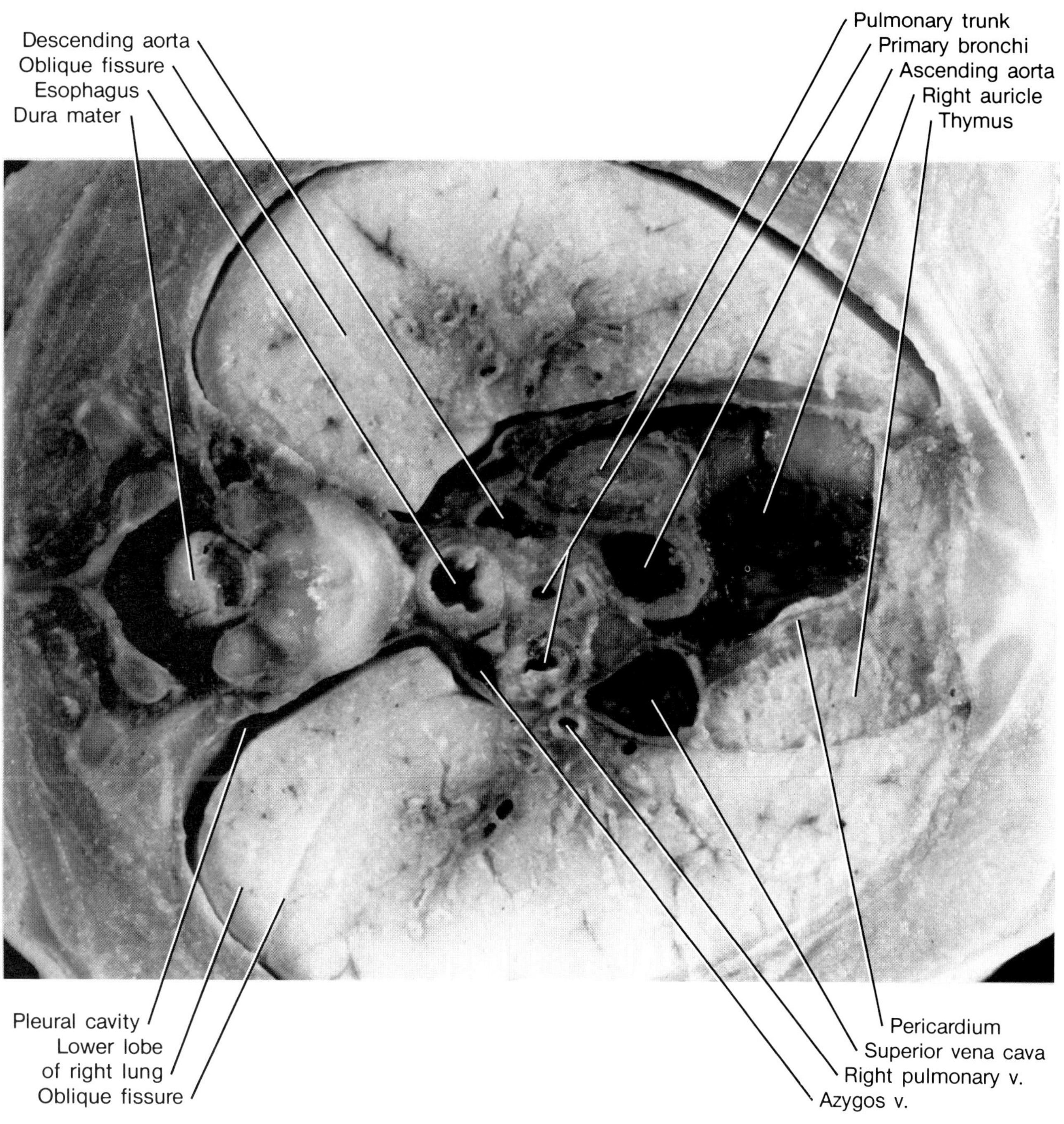

Figure 2.2

Left ventricle
Ascending aorta
Cusps of aortic valve
Right ventricle
Pericardial cavity
Left auricle
Pulmonary a.
Aorta
Intervertebral disc
Dura mater
Right atrium
Interatrial septum
Left atrium
Azygos v.
Esophagus
Secondary bronchus
Pulmonary a.

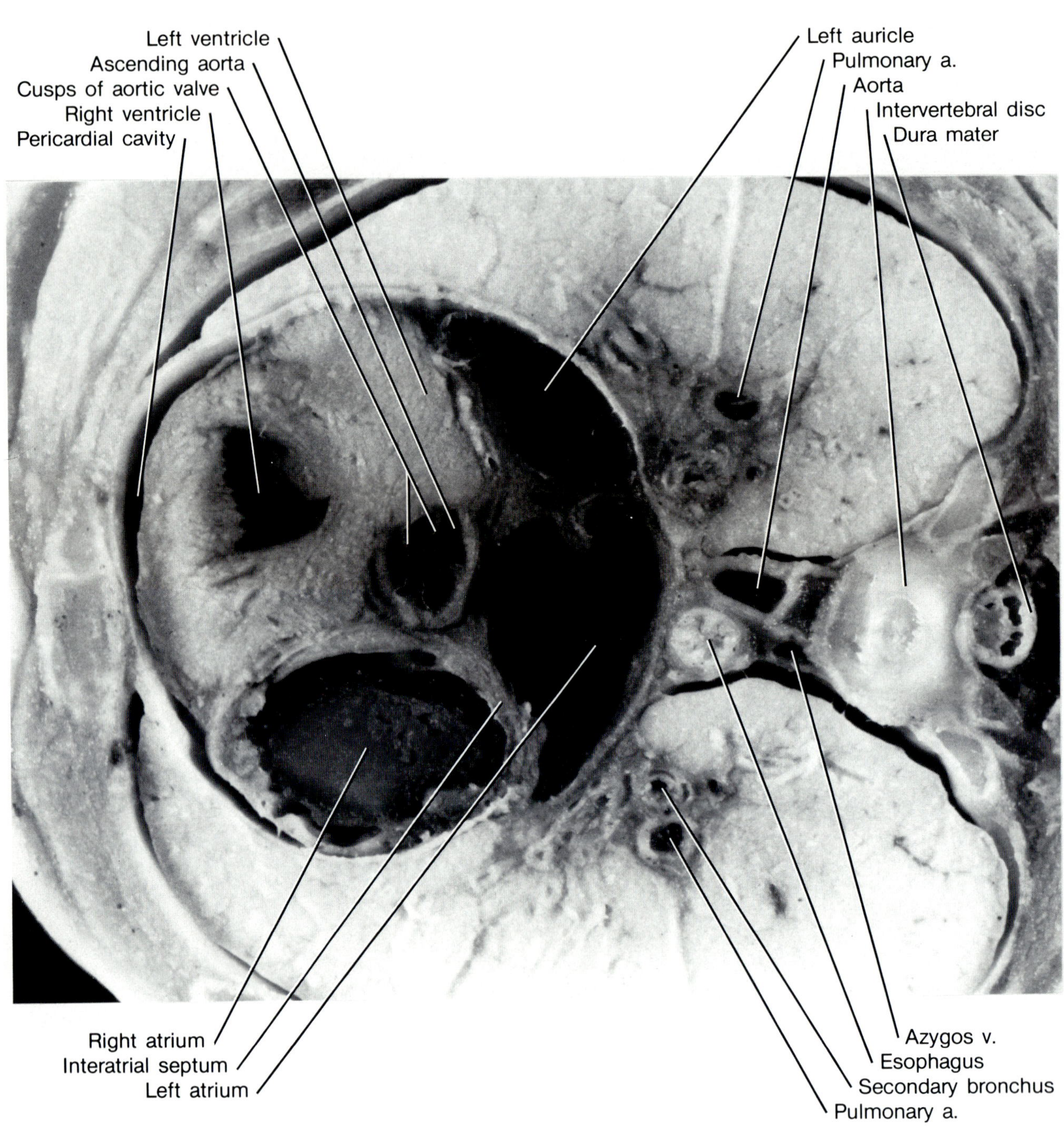

Figure 2.3

Pulmonary arteries
Pulmonary v.
Aorta
Secondary bronchus
Left auricle
Left ventricle
Ascending aorta
Azygos v.
Esophagus
Left atrium
Pericardium
Right ventricle
Right atrium

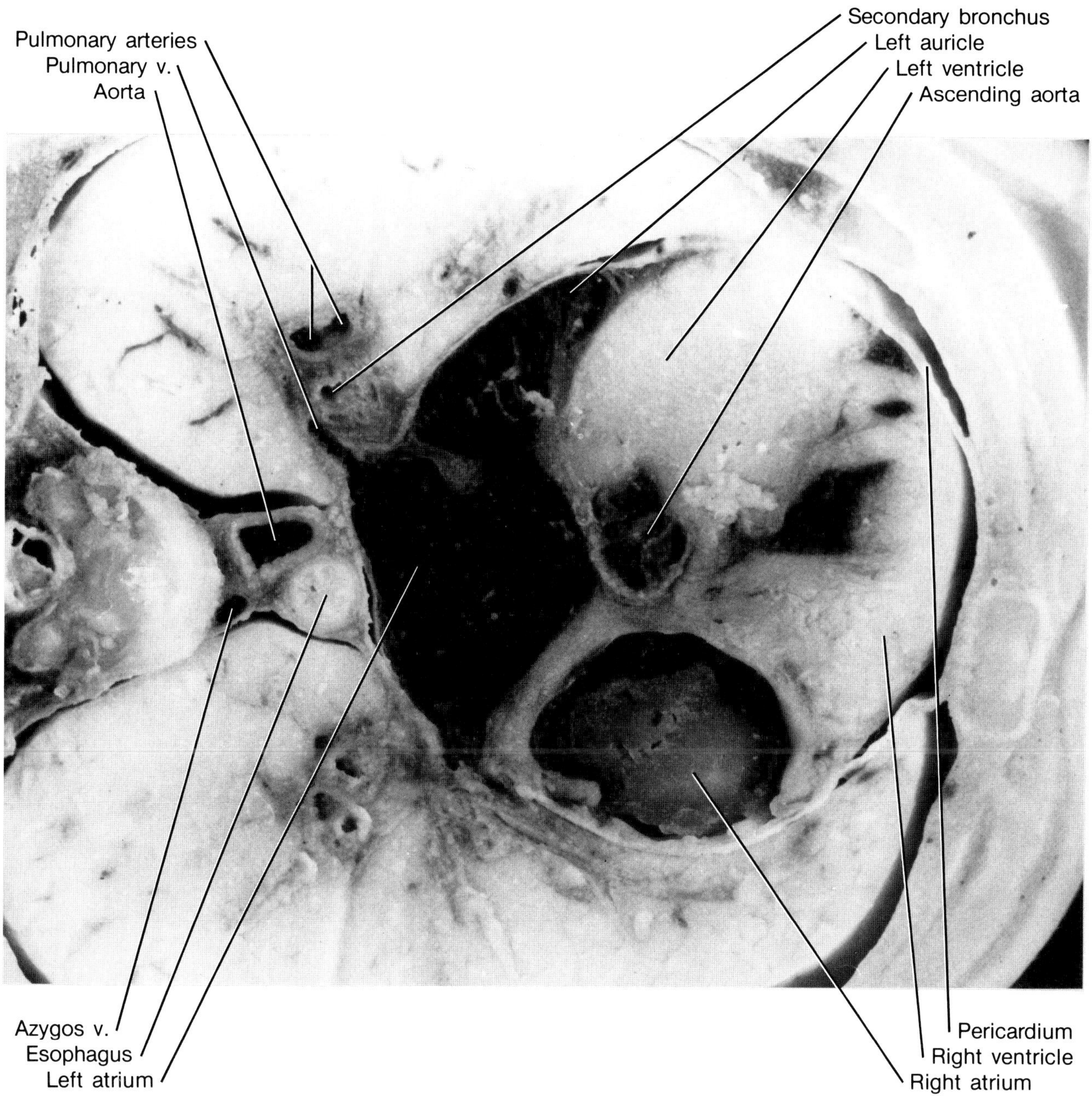

Figure 2.4

Oblique fissure
Pericardium
Papillary m.
Left ventricle
Pleural cavity
Esophagus
Aorta
Intervertebral disc
Right ventricle
Right atrium
Azygos v.
Left atrium
Interatrial septum

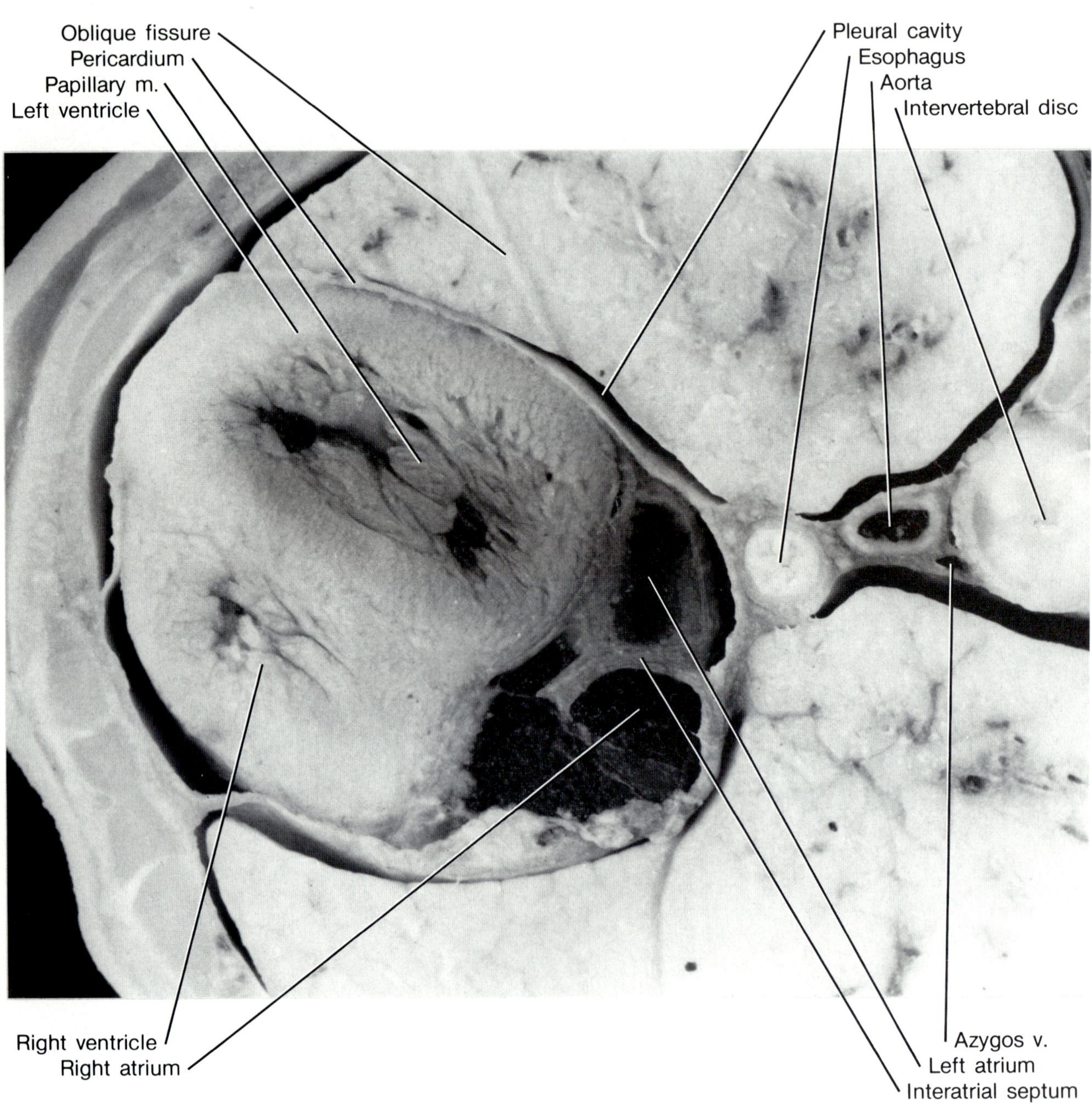

Figure 2.5

Coronary sinus
Left auricle
Aorta
Oblique fissure
Pericardium
Left ventricle
Azygos v.
Esophagus
Diaphragm
Right ventricle
Inferior vena cava
Liver

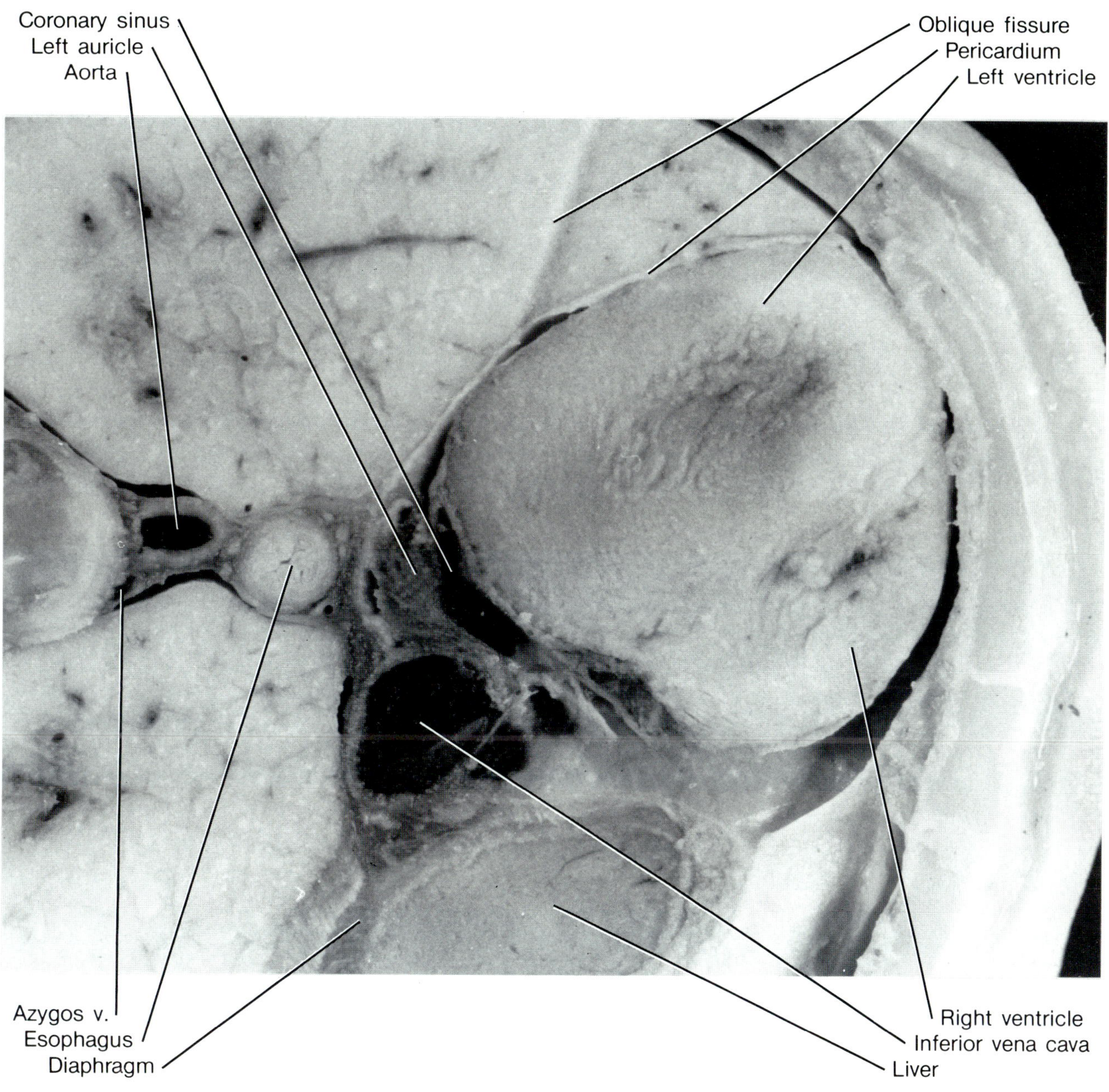

Figure 2.6

3

SAGITTAL SECTIONS

20-week fetus

Epiphyseal plate
Triceps m.
Liver
Humerus
External auditory canal
Dura mater
Latissimus dorsi m.
Diaphragm
Serratus anterior m.
Scapula
Clavicle
Scapula
Supraspinatus m.
Subscapularis m.

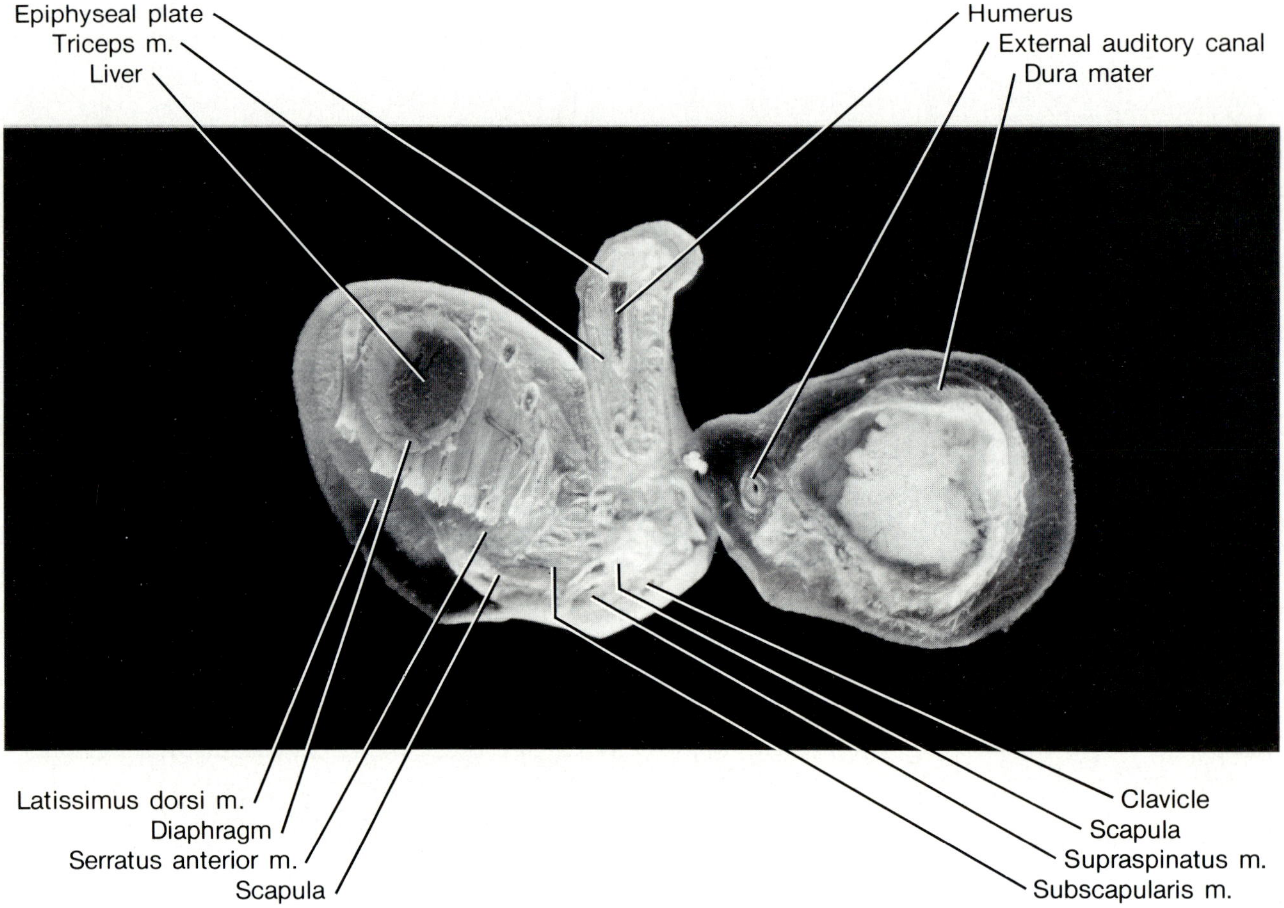

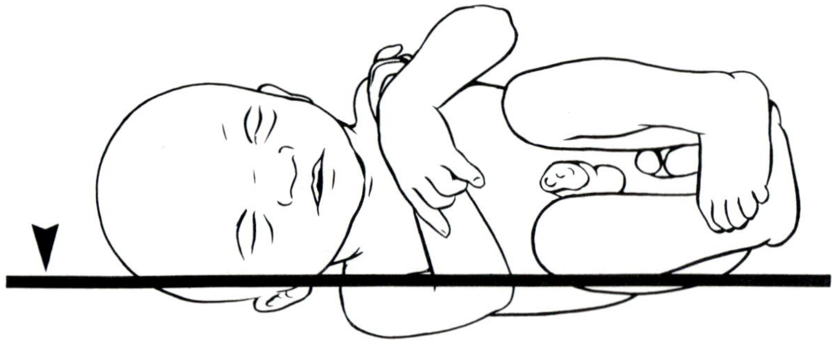

Figure 3.1

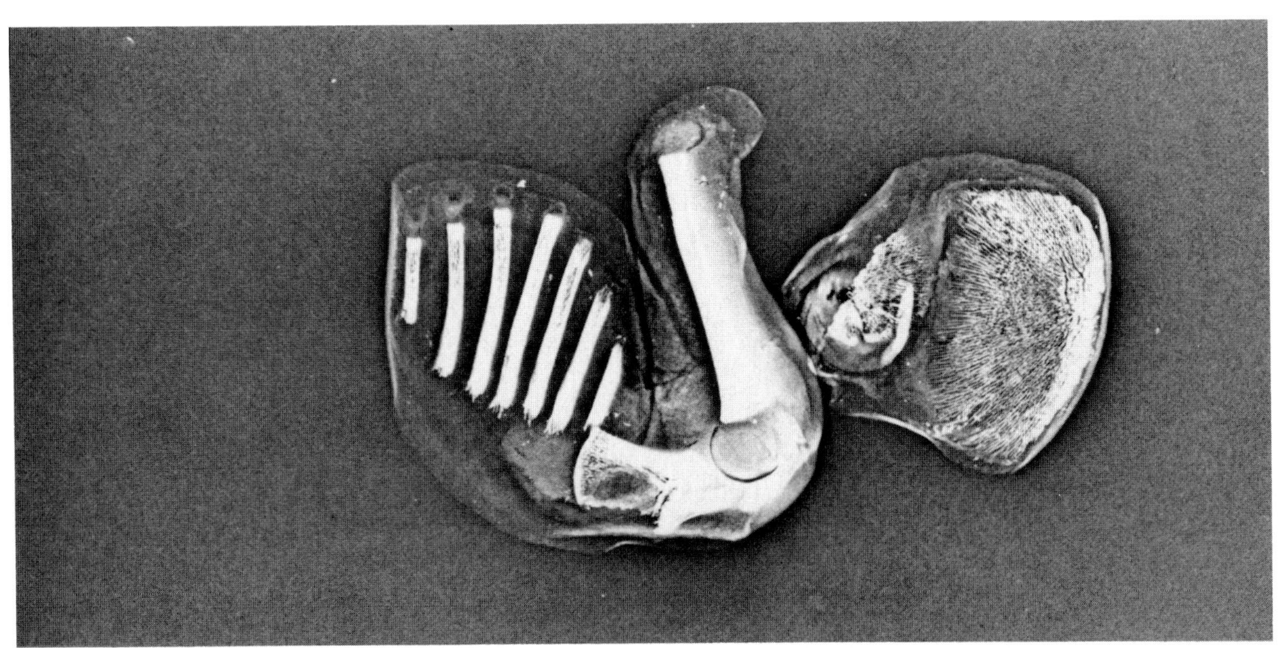

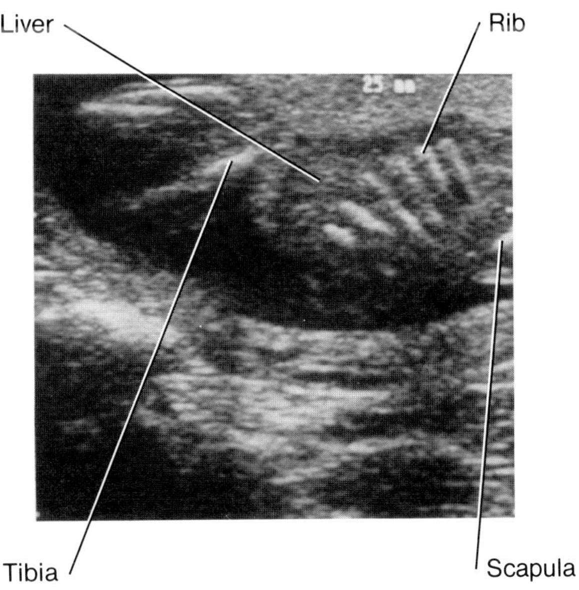
Liver
Rib
Tibia
Scapula

Brachialis m.
Biceps brachii m.
Temporalis m.
Dura mater
Radius
Humerus
Liver
Middle ear
External auditory meatus
Masseter m.
Diaphragm
Right lung
Acromion

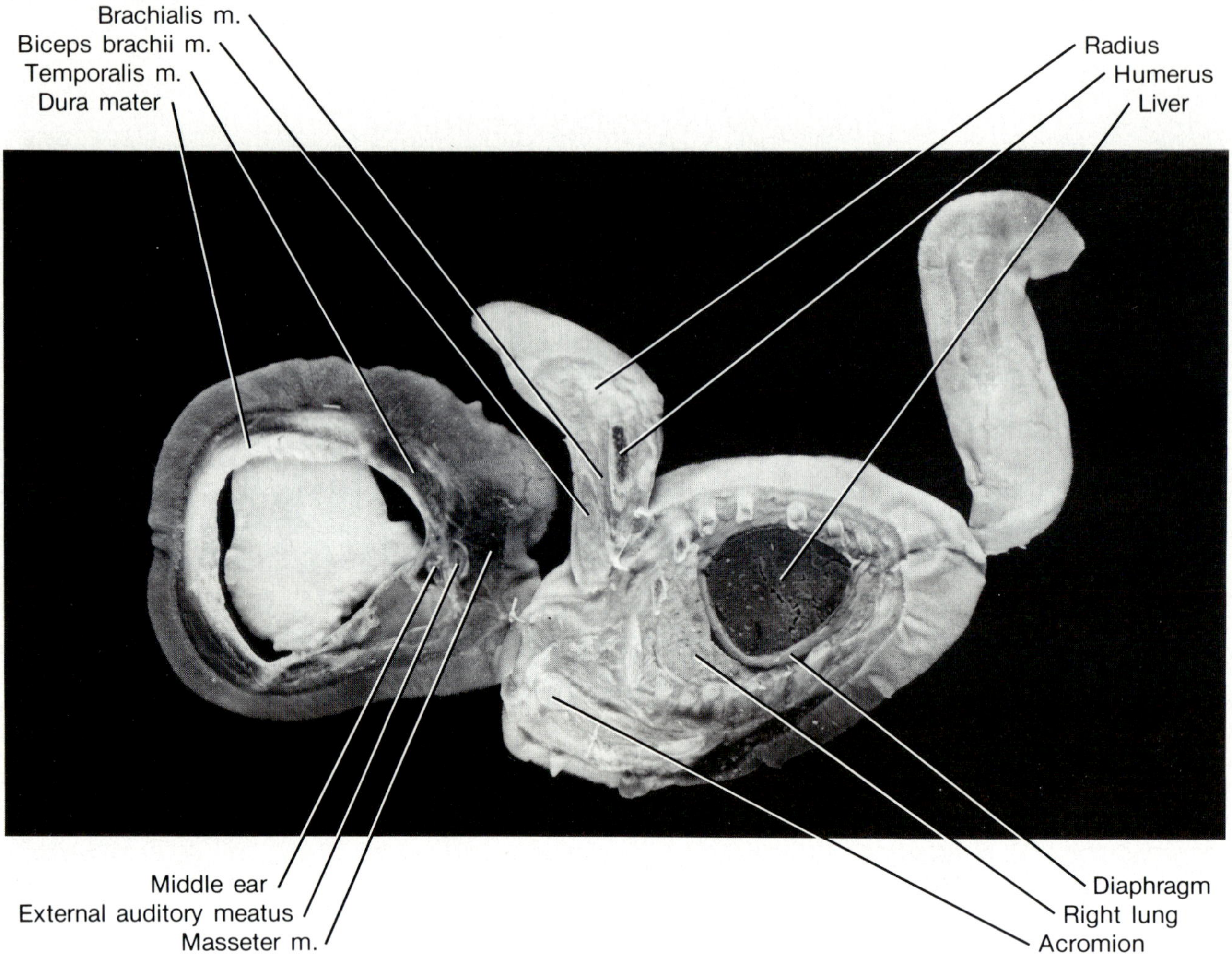

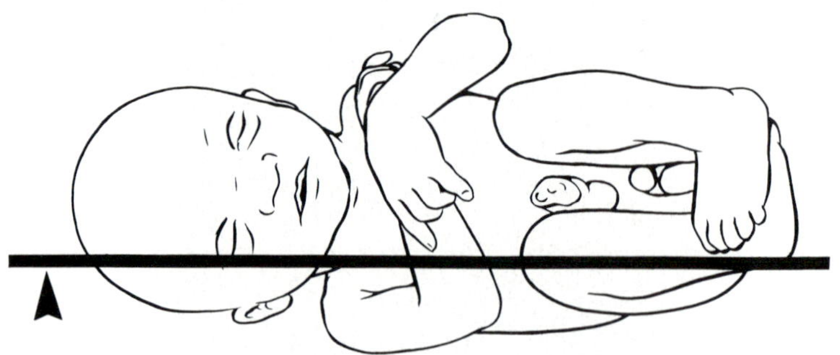

Figure 3.2

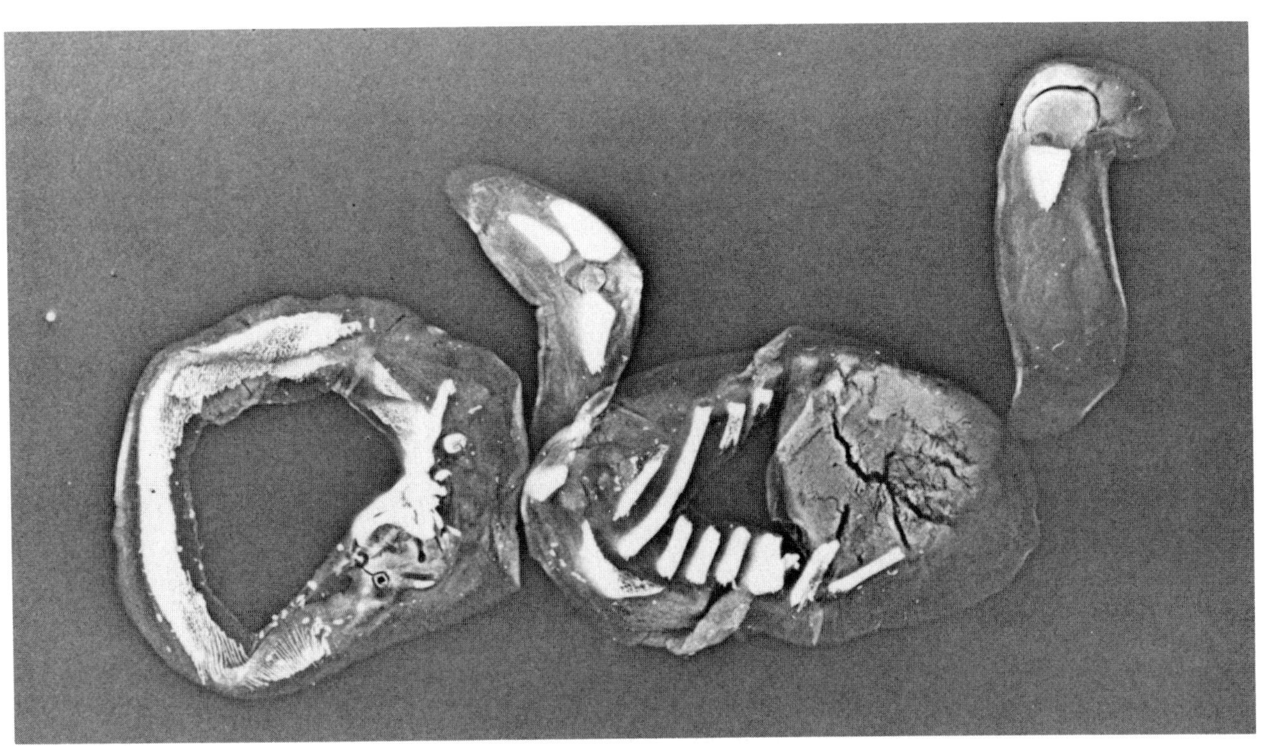

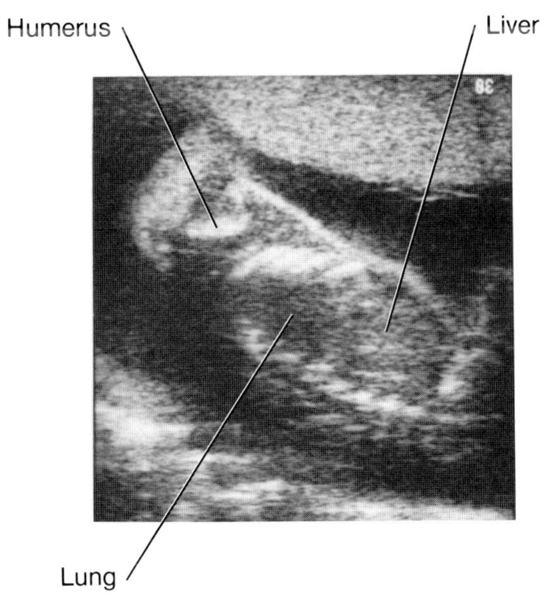

Humerus
Liver
Lung

Radius
Humerus
Pectoralis minor m.
Liver
Patella
Ulna
Pectoralis major m.
Condyle of mandible
Temporomandibular joint
Temporal lobe
Fibula
Tibia
Femur
Diaphragm
Upper, middle, and lower lobes of lung
First rib
Dura mater
Incus
Malleus
Tympanic membrane
Coracoid process
Brachial plexus and subclavian vessels

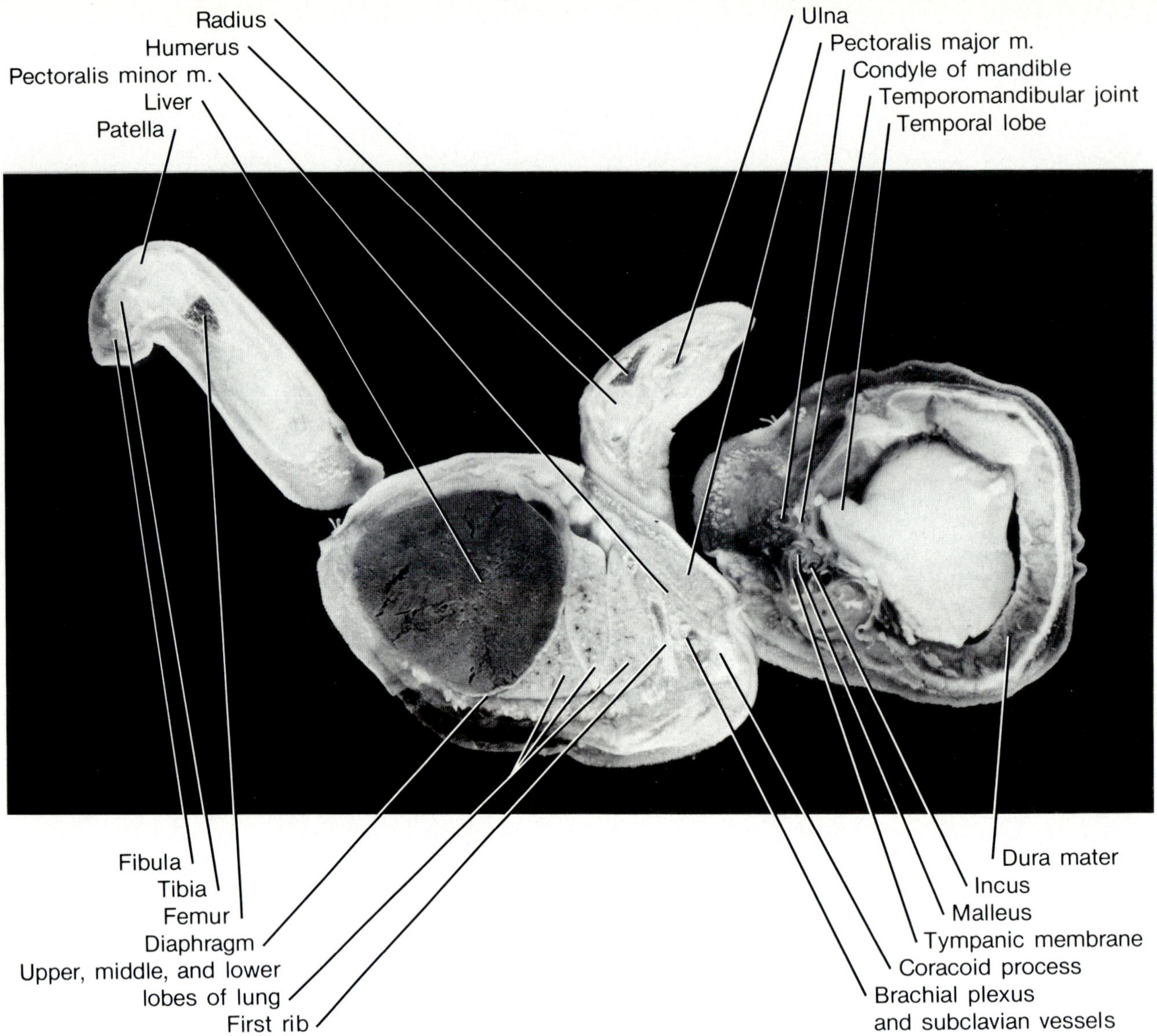

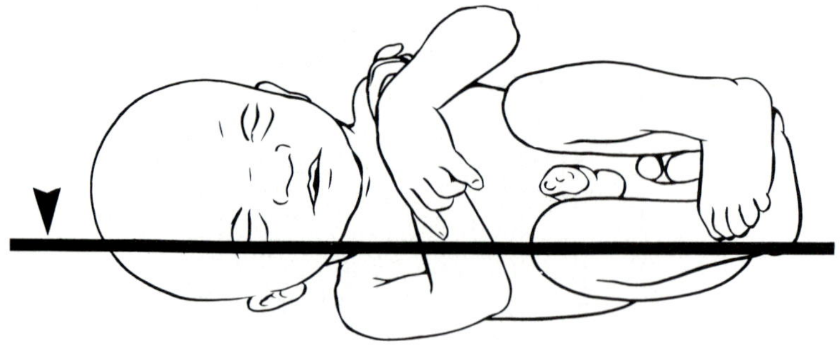

Figure 3.3

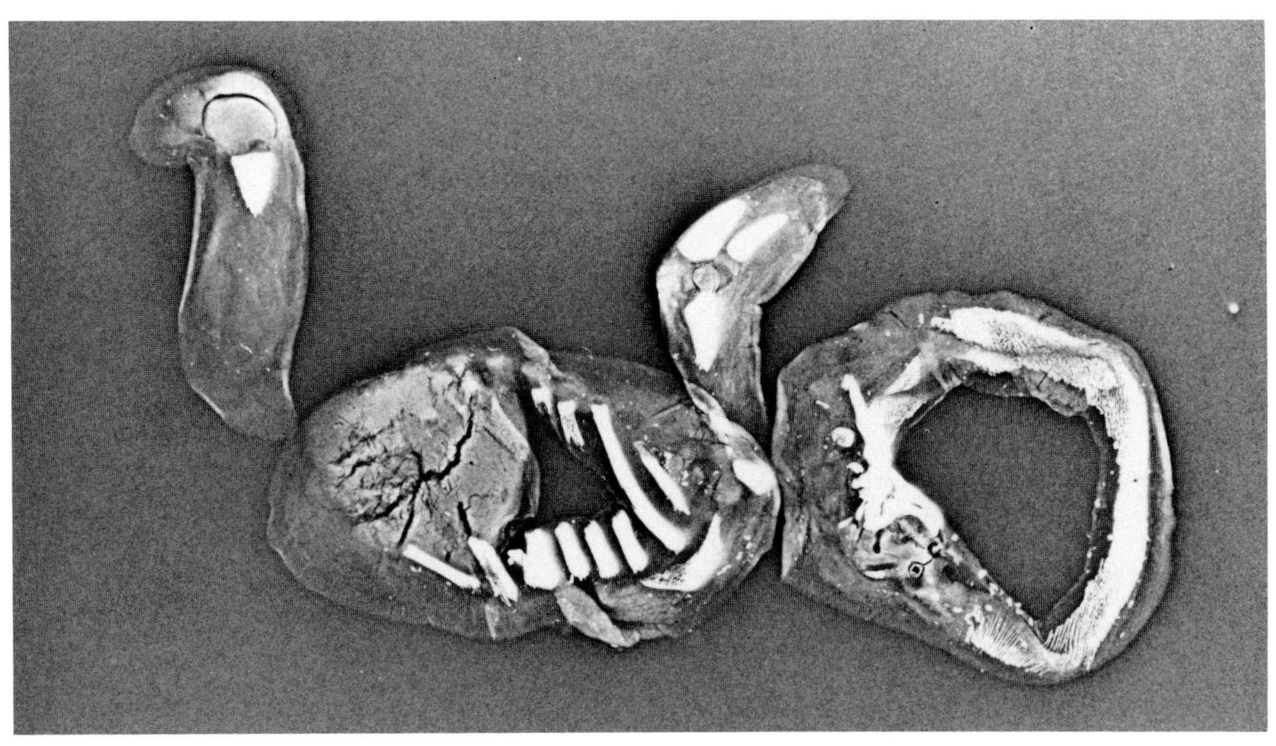

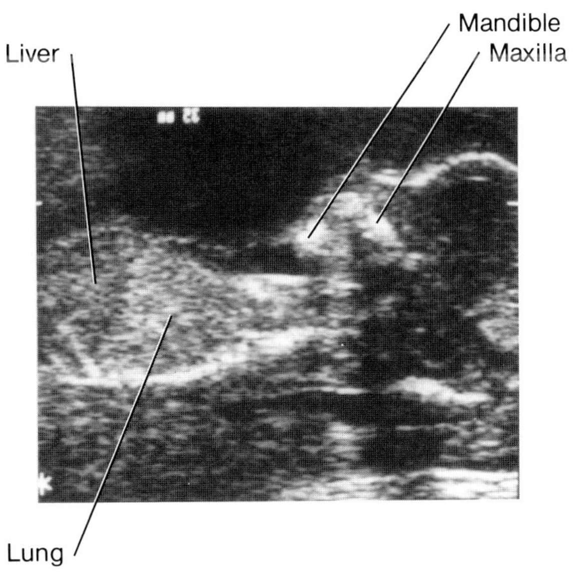

Liver
Mandible
Maxilla
Lung

Middle lobe of lung
Ulna
Radius
Masseter m.
Lateral pterygoid m.
Temporalis m.
Lesser wing of sphenoid
Diaphragm
Liver
Lateral condyle of femur
Patella
Quadriceps femoris m.
Tibia
Fibula
Hamstring m.
Sigmoid sinus
Inner ear
Stapes
Parotid gland
Condyle of mandible
Clavicle
Lower lobe of lung
Upper lobe of lung
Scapula
Pectoralis major m.
Brachial plexus and subclavian vessels

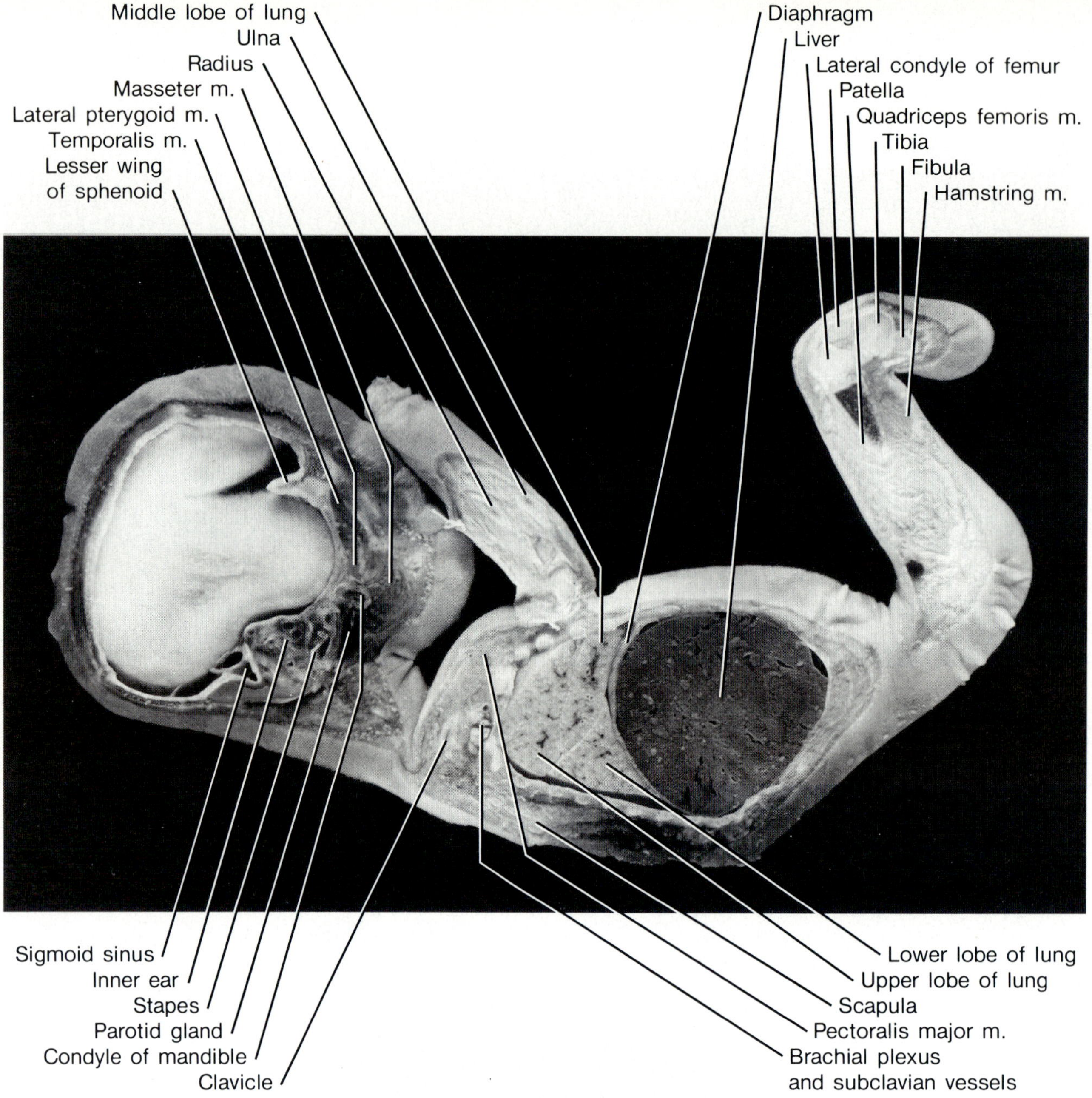

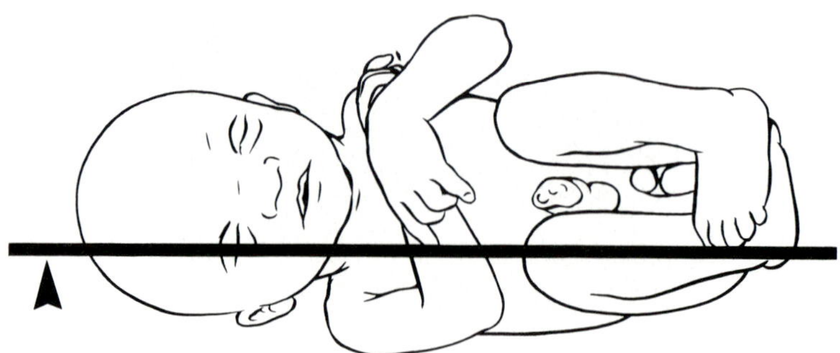

Figure 3.4

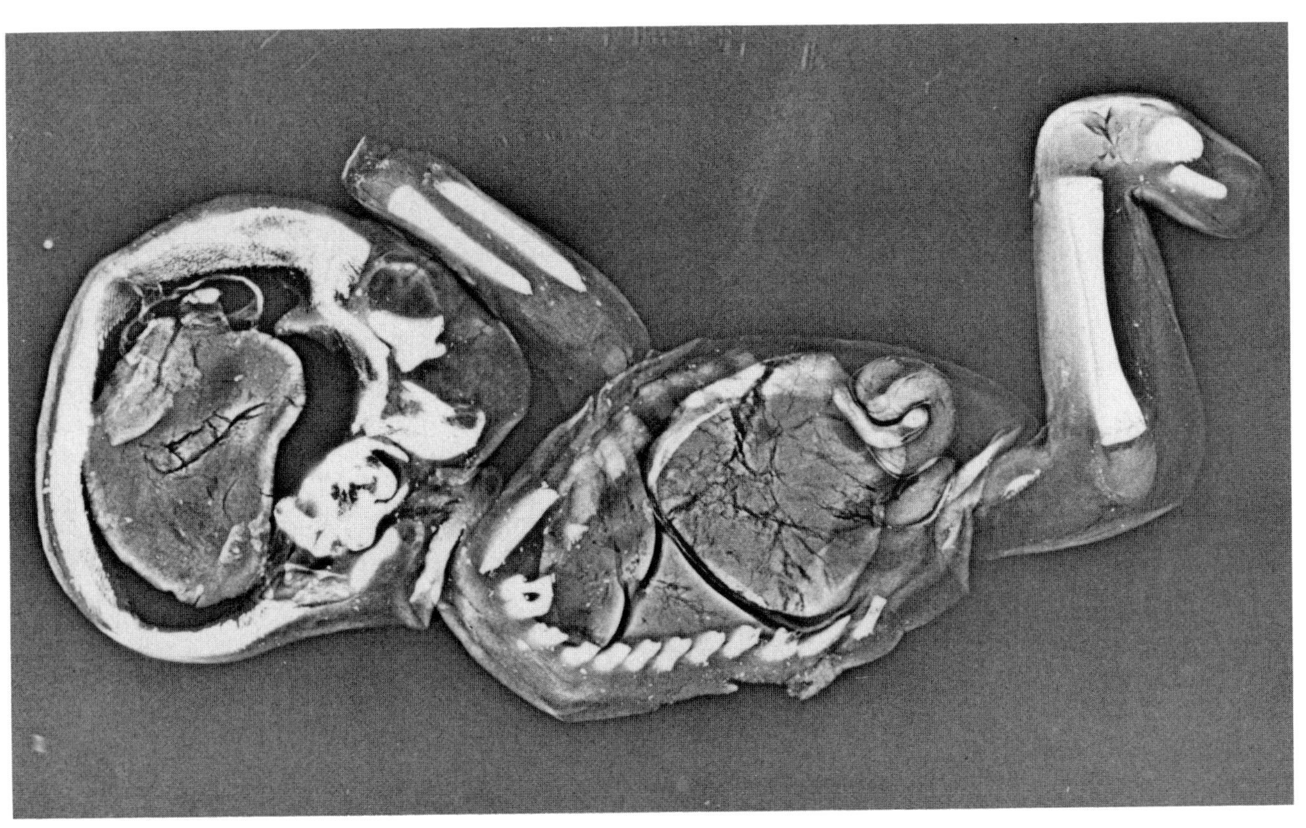

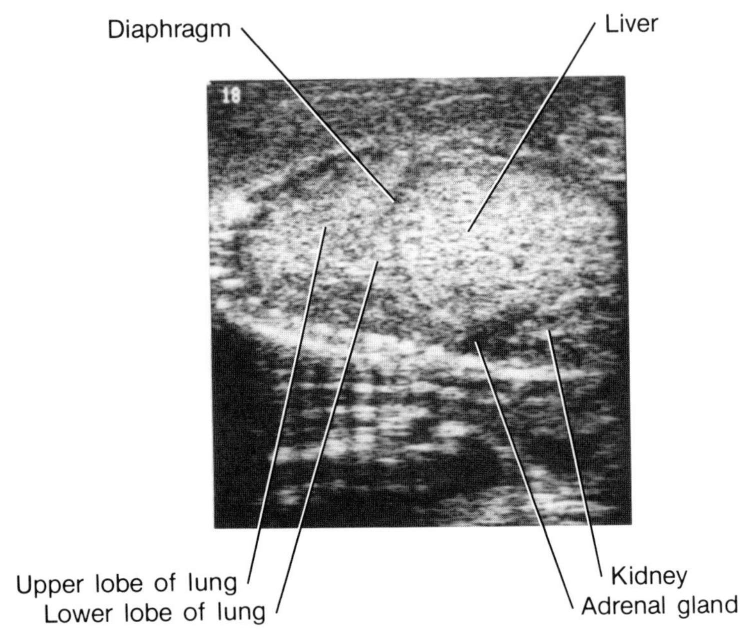

Diaphragm
Liver
18
Upper lobe of lung
Lower lobe of lung
Kidney
Adrenal gland

Lateral pterygoid m.
Right atrium
Liver
Ileum
Sclera
Orbital plate of frontal bone
Dura mater
Ascending colon
Pyramid of kidney
Cortex of kidney
Lower lobe of lung
Oblique fissure
Tentorium cerebelli
Cerebellum
Sigmoid sinus
Inner ear
Internal jugular v.

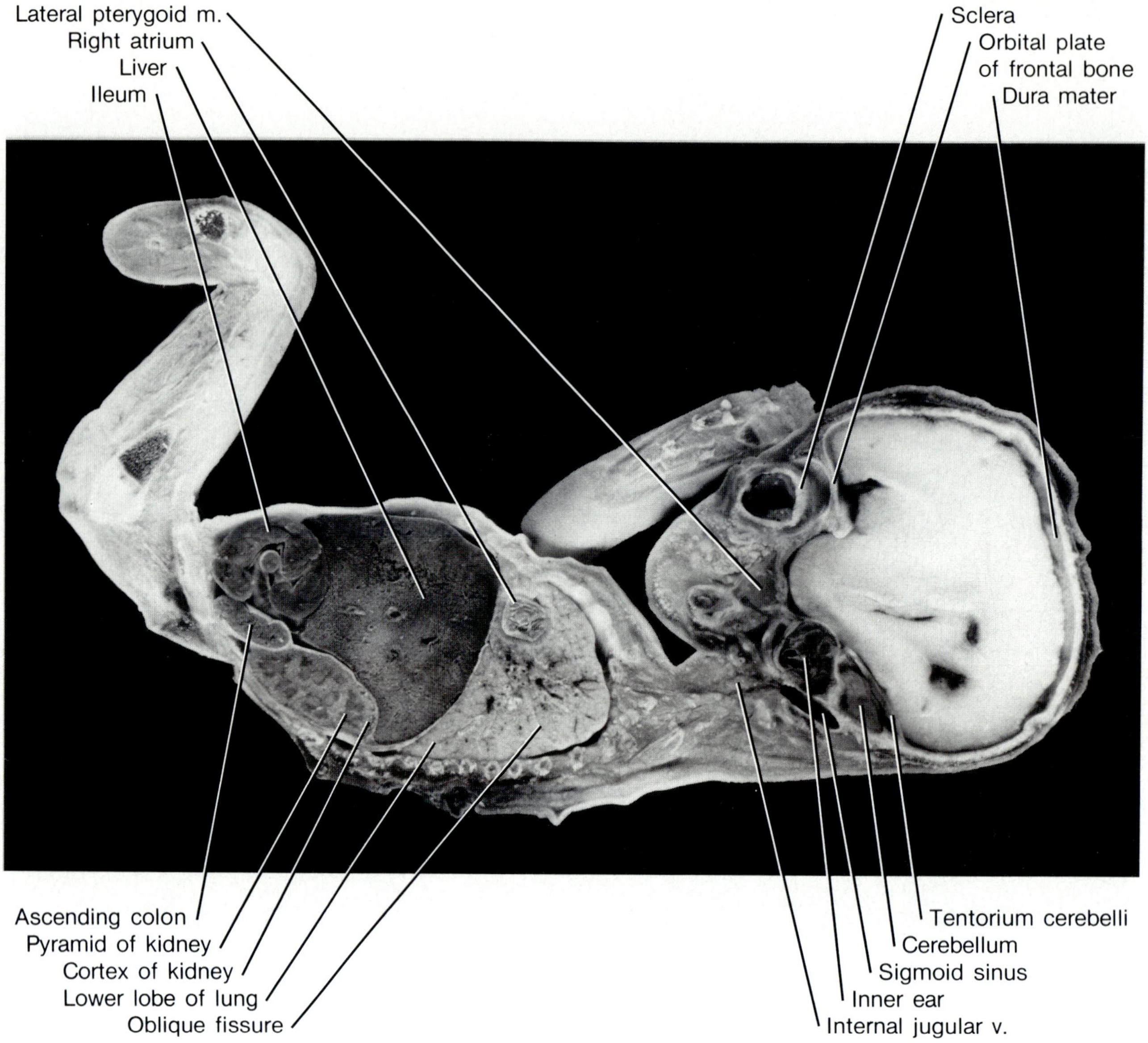

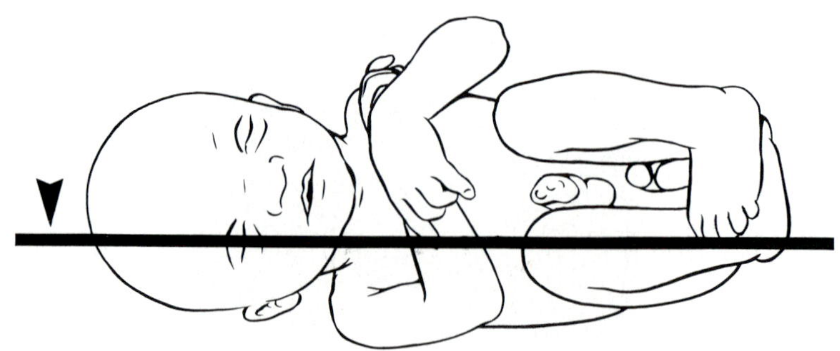

Figure 3.5

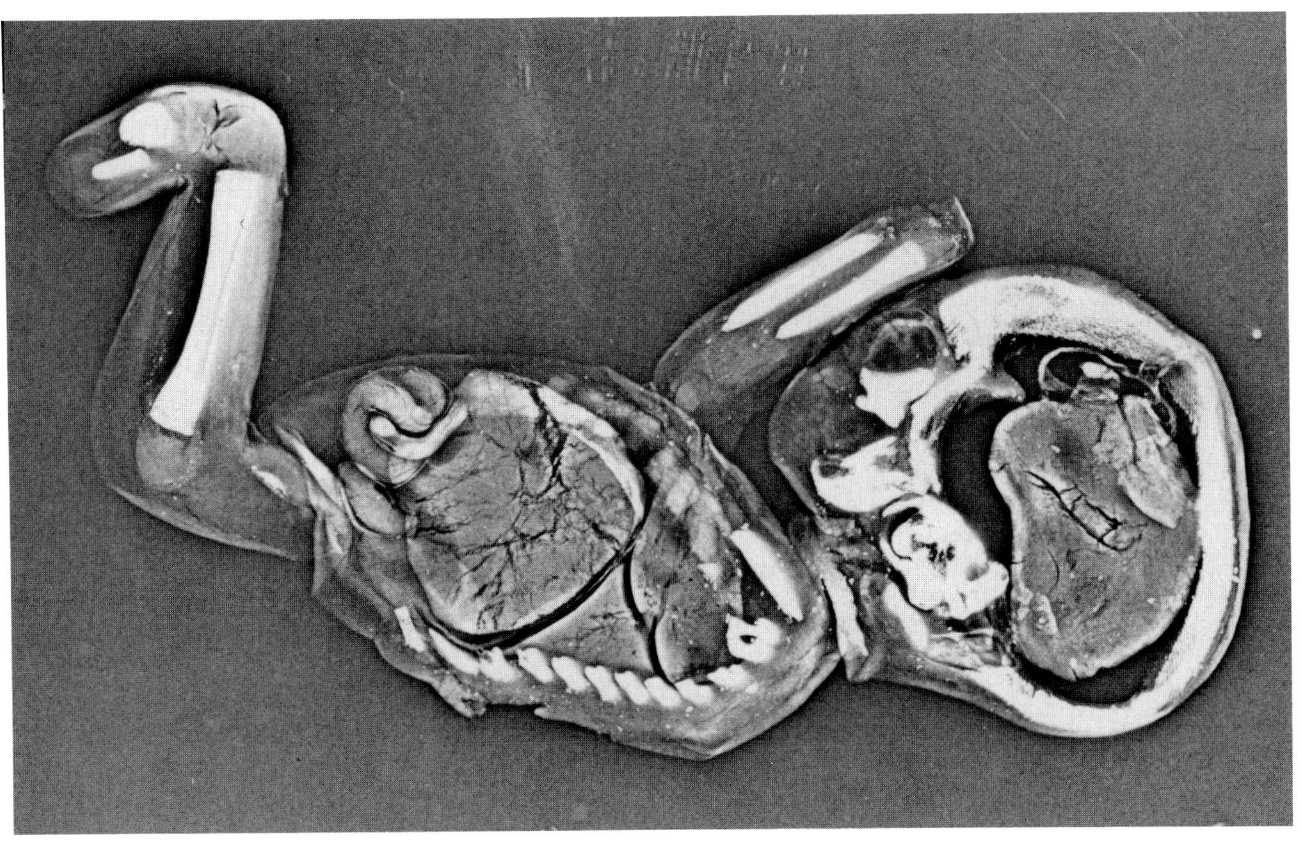

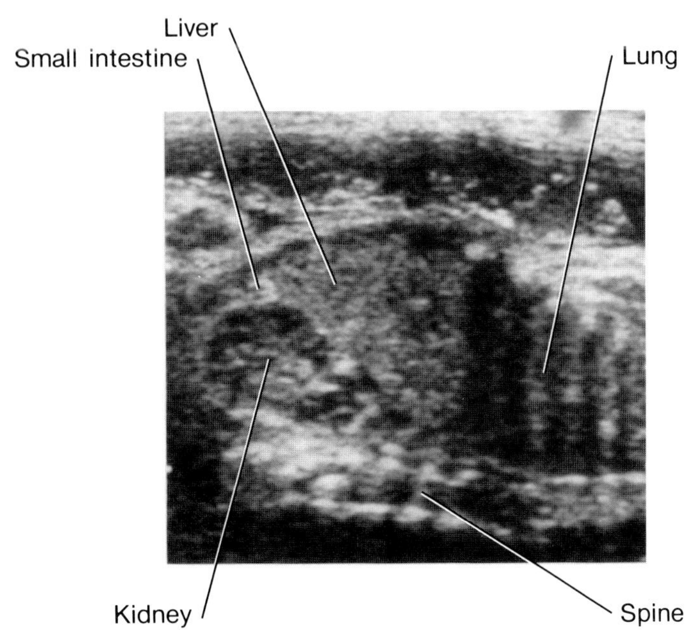
Liver
Small intestine
Lung
Kidney
Spine

Mandible
Buccinator m.
Internal carotid a.
Zygoma
Cornea
Lens
Sphenoid bone
Sclera
Orbital plate
of frontal bone
Parotid gland
Clavicle
Pericardium
Pectinate m.
Hepatic triad
Tibia
Fibula
Large intestine
Hamstring m.
Gluteus maximus m.
Frontal lobe
Occipital lobe
Temporal lobe
Inner ear
Lateral pterygoid m.
Medial pterygoid m.
Vagus n.
Trapezius m.
Superior vena cava
Sacrum
Ileum
Cecum
Ascending colon
Renal pyramid
Renal cortex
Hyparterial bronchus
Pulmonary vessels
Eparterial bronchus
Oblique fissure

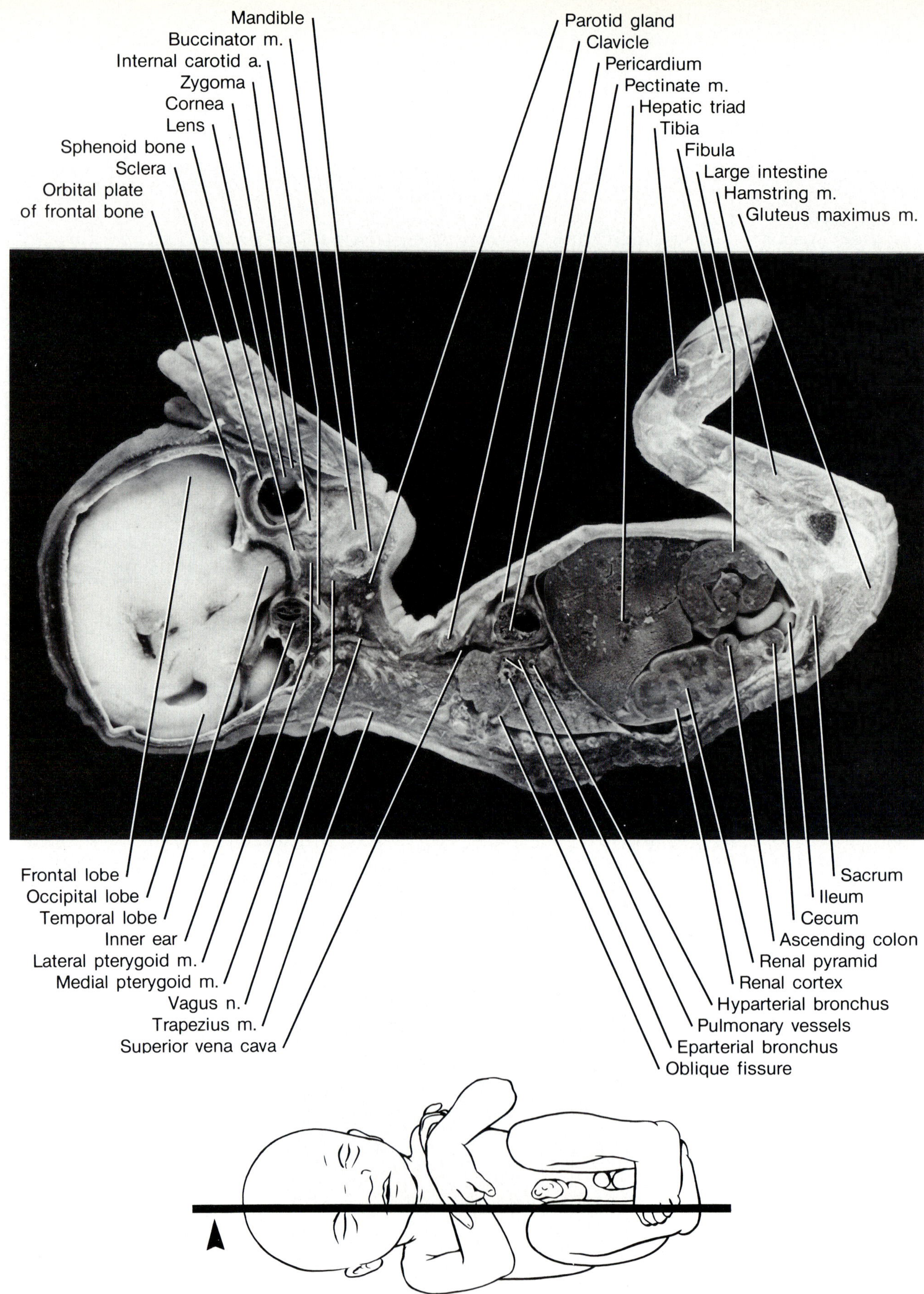

Figure 3.6

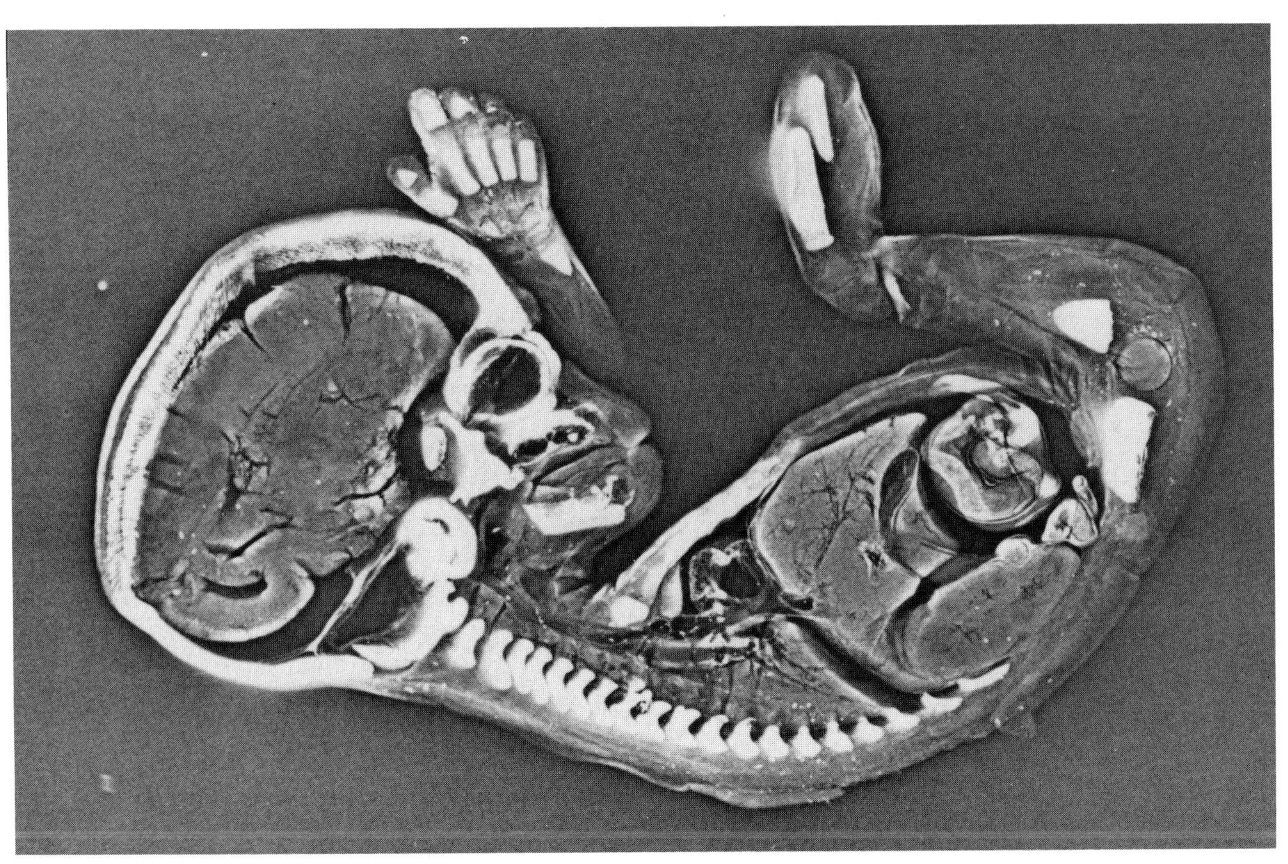

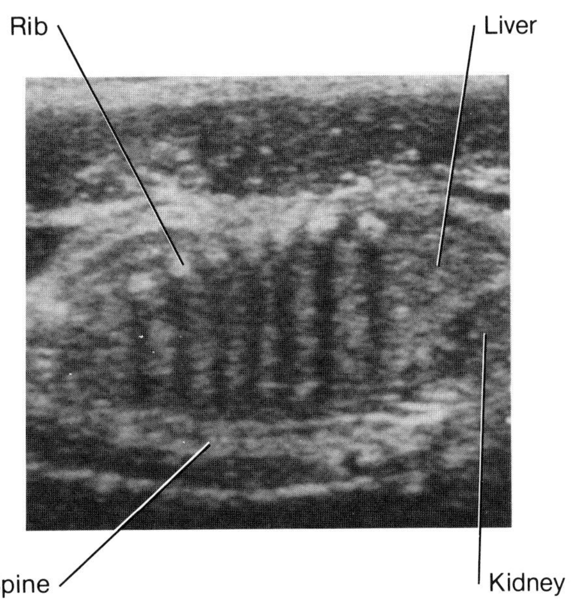
Rib
Liver
Spine
Kidney

Sternal angle
Right auricle
Arch of aorta
Diaphragm
Right atrium
Liver
Tooth bud
Maxilla
Inferior rectus m.
Optic n.
Superior rectus m.
Head of femur
Testis
Gall bladder
Suprarenal gland
Inferior vena cava
Trachea
Dura mater
Tentorium cerebelli
Cerebellum
Foramen magnum
Tongue
Vertebral canal
Left brachiocephalic v.

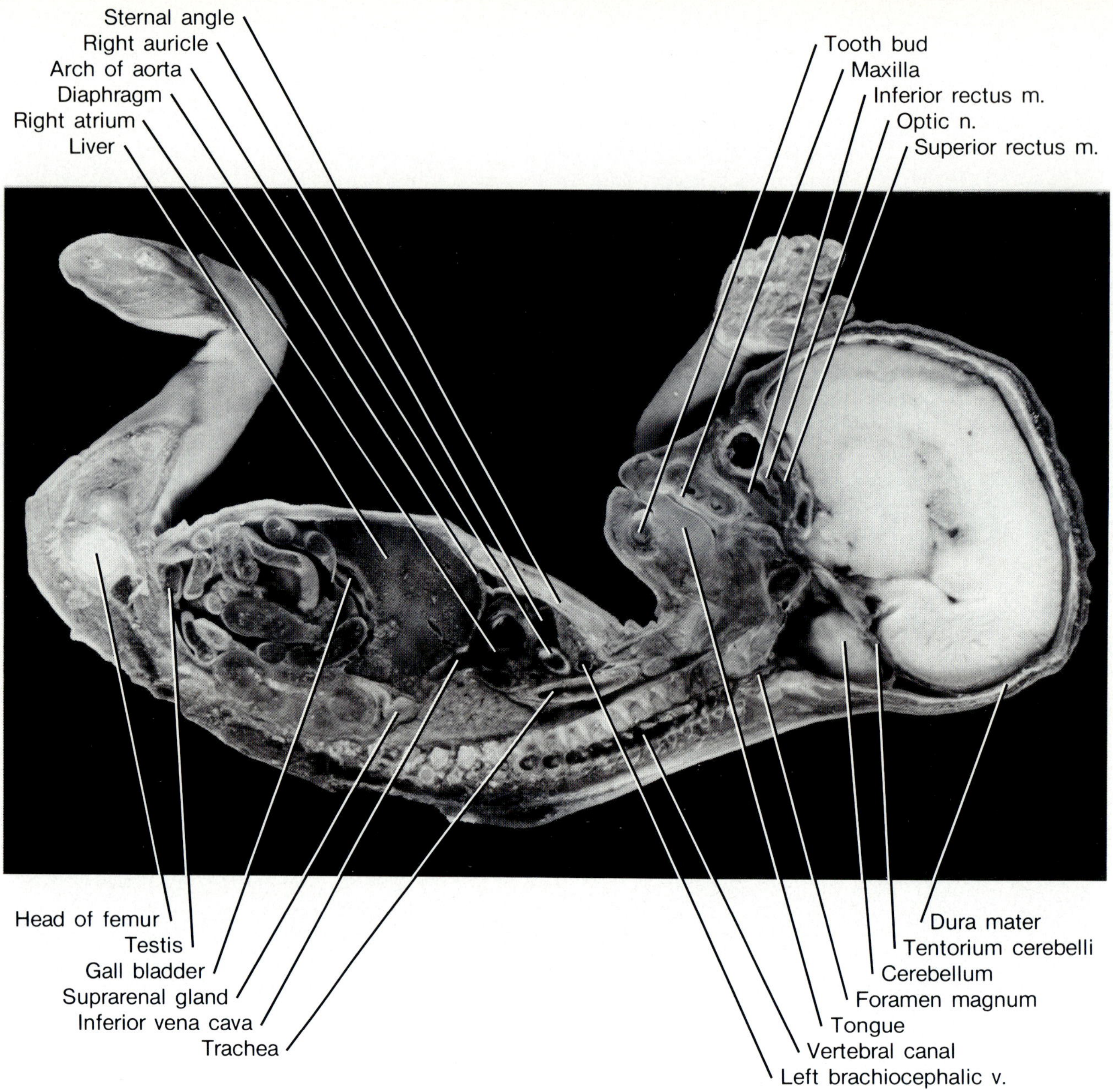

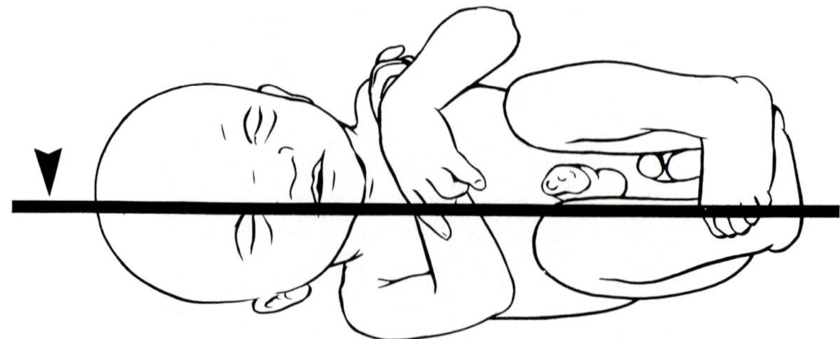

Figure 3.7

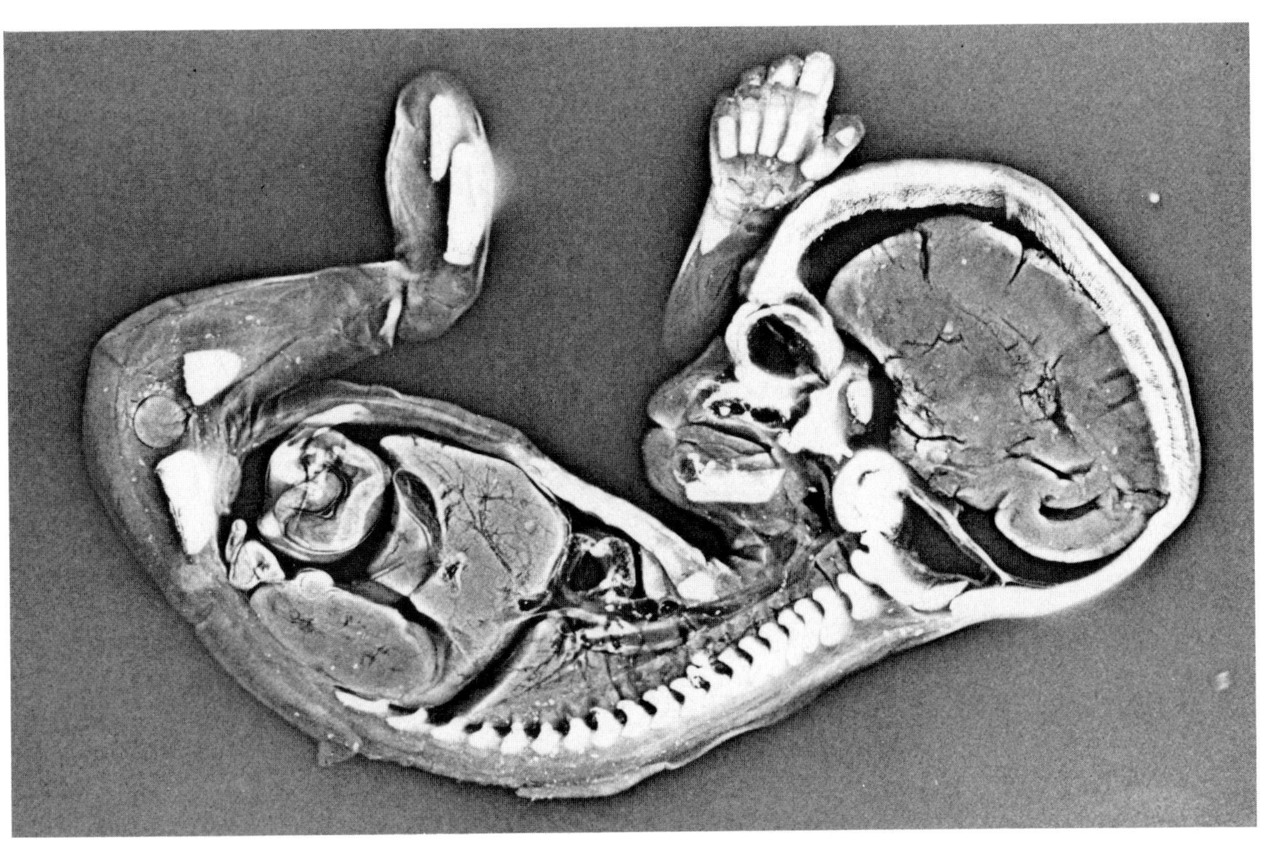

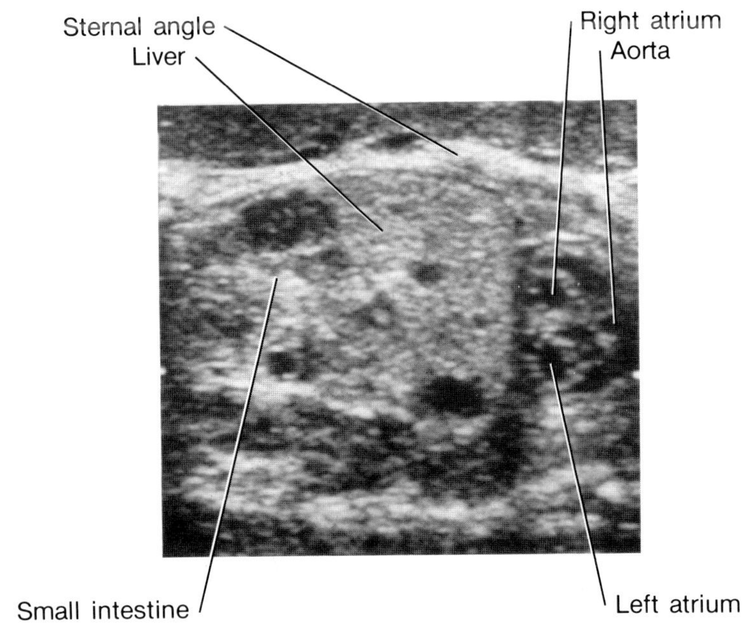

Sternal angle
Liver
Right atrium
Aorta
Small intestine
Left atrium

Thymus
Body of mandible
Tongue
Sclera
Inferior rectus m.
Orbital plate
of frontal bone
Dura mater
Right ventricle
Right atrium
Interatrial septum
Diaphragm
Hepatic v.
Liver
Ileum
Tentorium cerebelli
Cerebellum
Superior rectus m.
Anterior wall of pharynx
Spinal cord
Trachea
Left brachiocephalic v.
Aortic arch
Ascending colon
Kidney
Suprarenal gland
Inferior vena cava
Valve of inferior vena cava
Left atrium
Esophagus
Right pulmonary a.

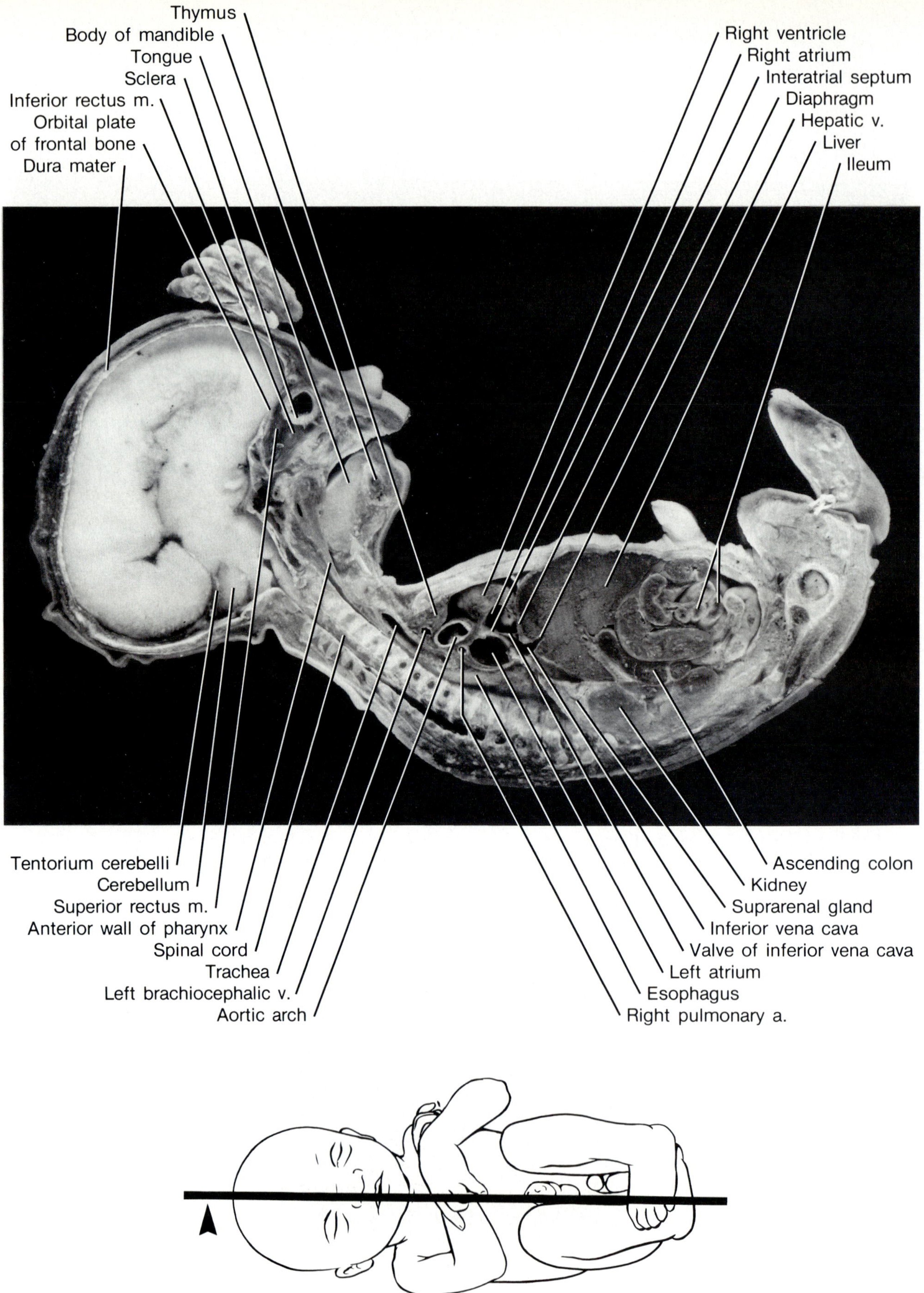

Figure 3.8

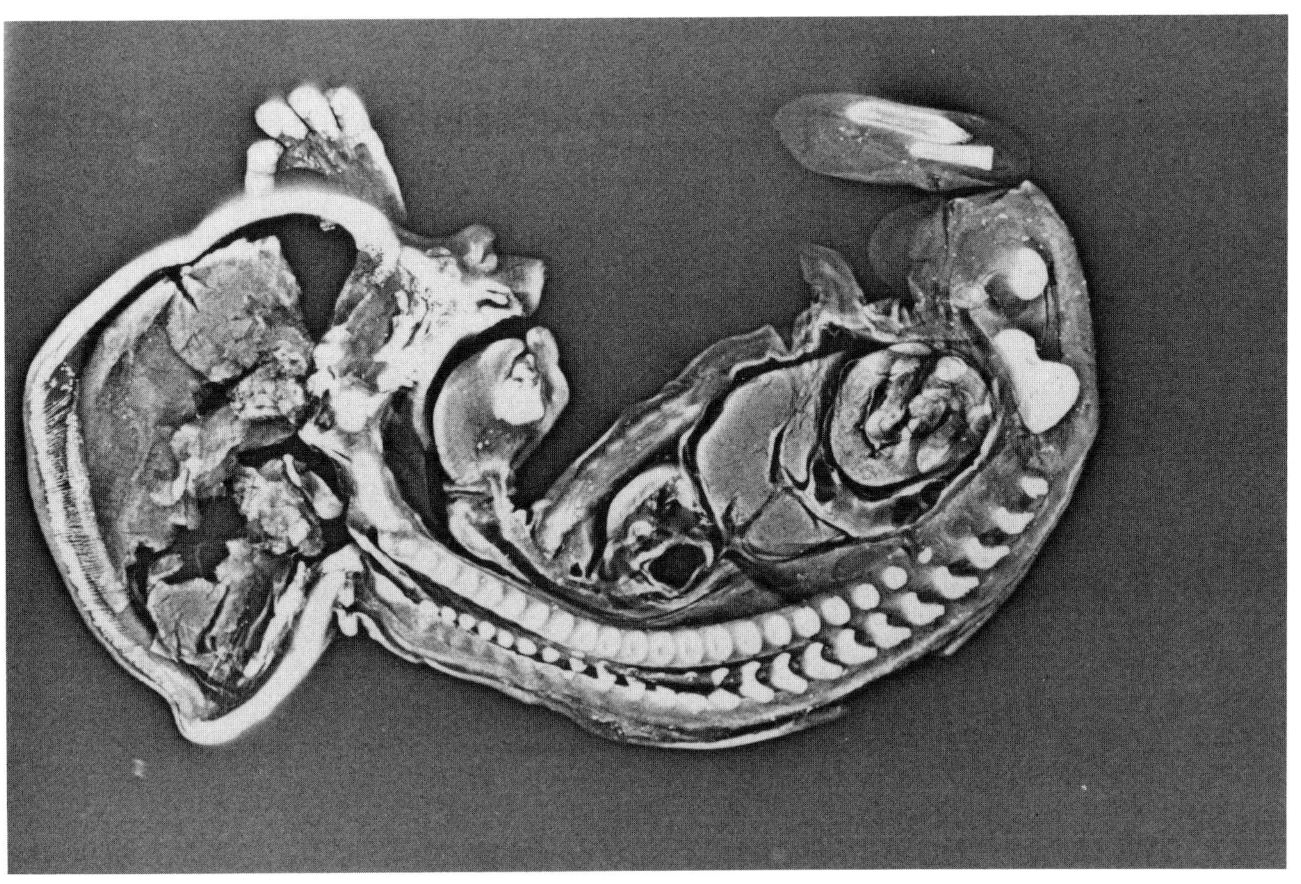

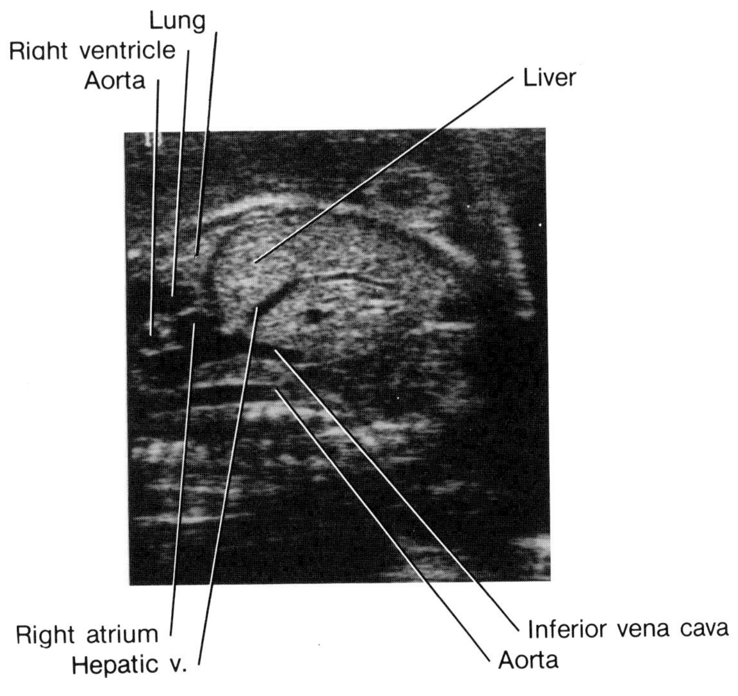

Lung
Right ventricle
Aorta
Liver
Right atrium
Hepatic v.
Inferior vena cava
Aorta

Pericardial cavity
Right ventricle
Ductus venosus
Transverse colon
Umbilical v.
Urinary bladder
Pubic bone
Ascending aorta
Manubrium
Clavicle
Tooth bud
Hyoid bone
Middle concha
Soft palate
Duodenum
Pancreas
Esophagus
Left atrium
Right bronchus
Aorta
Sella turcica
Nasopharynx
Thyroid cartilage
Cricoid cartilage
Left brachiocephalic v.
Pulmonary trunk

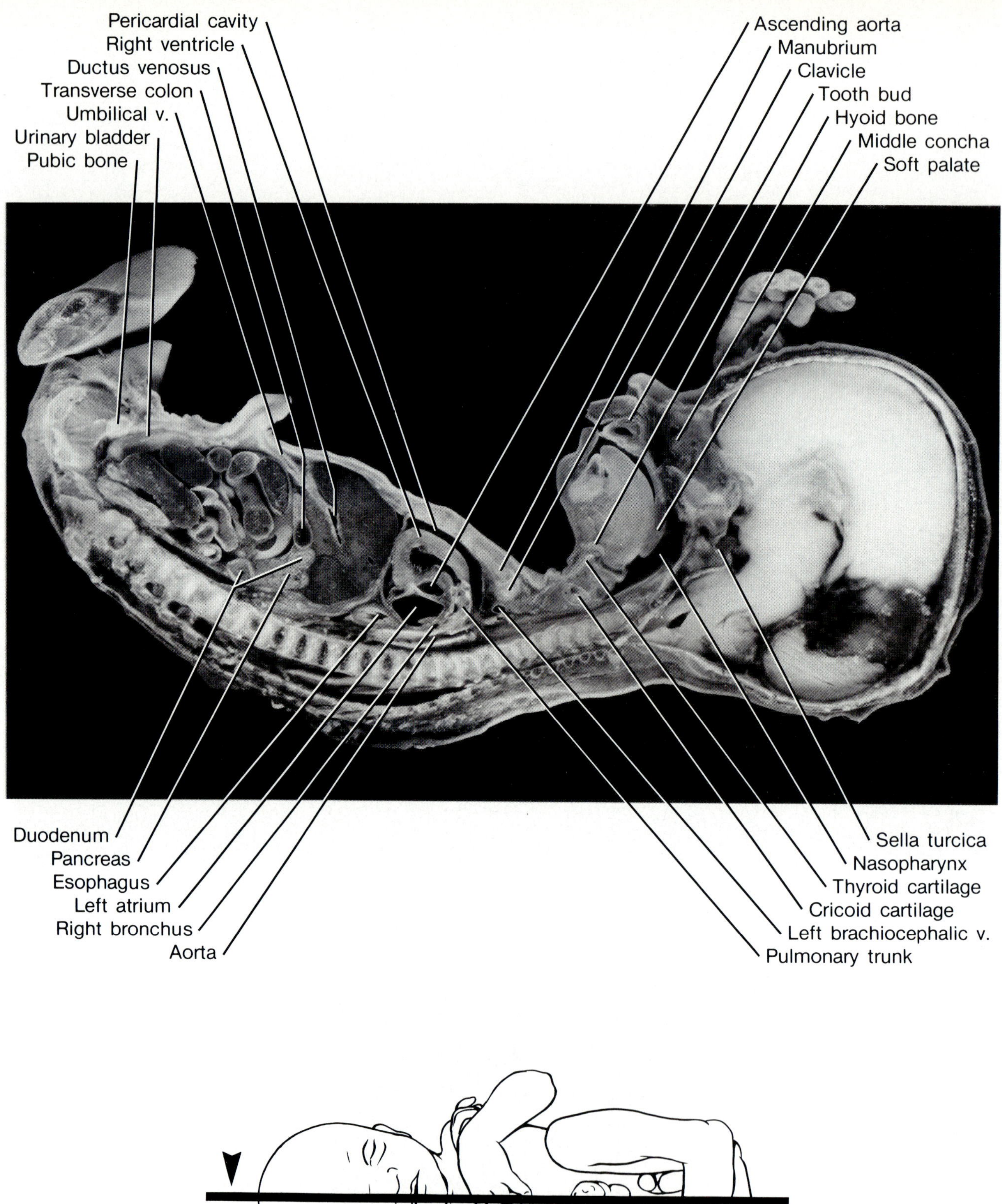

Figure 3.9

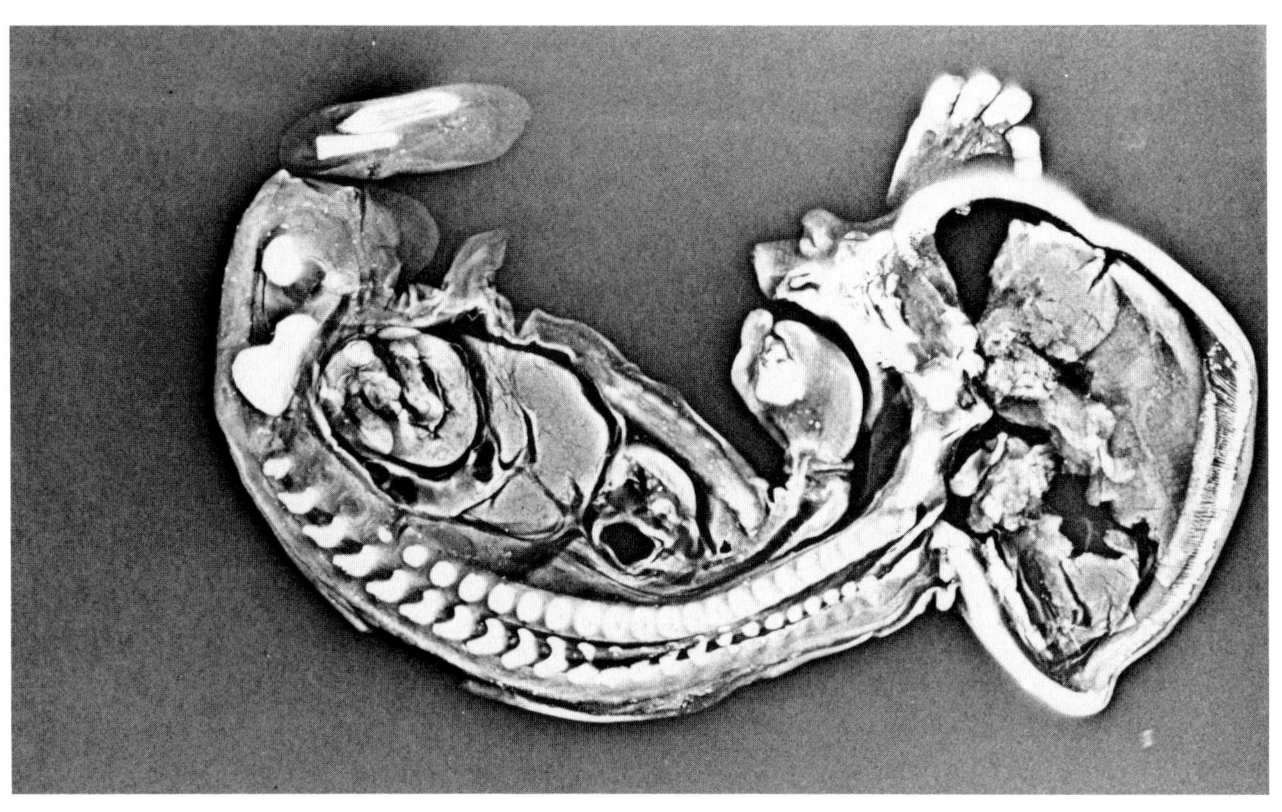

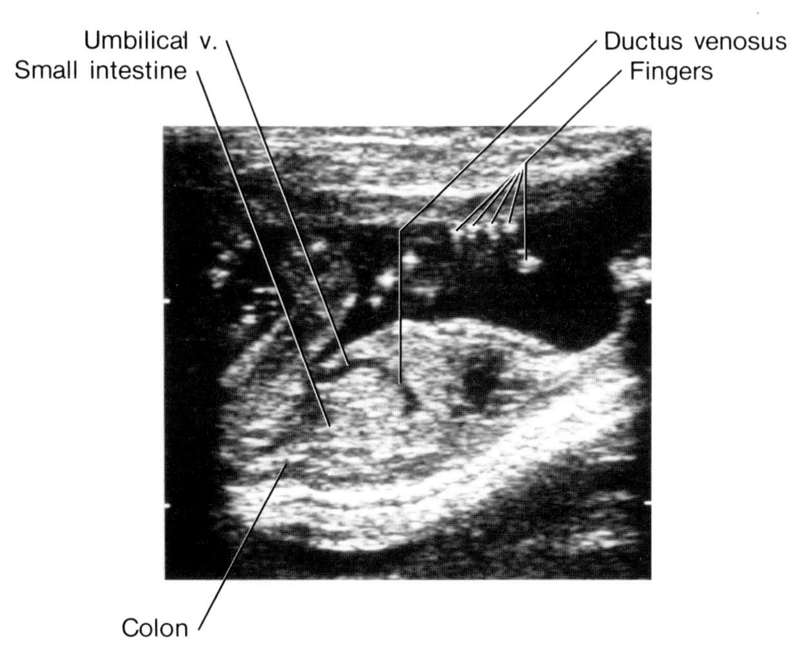
Umbilical v.
Small intestine
Ductus venosus
Fingers
Colon

Right ventricle
Thymus
Clavicle
Mandible
Tooth bud
Tongue
Nasal septum
Pituitary
Corpus callosum
Left ventricle
Diaphragm
Liver
Transverse colon
Jejunum
Penis
Urinary bladder
Scrotum
Rectum
Lateral ventricle
Dura mater
Tentorium cerebelli
Basioccipital bone
Nasopharynx
Soft palate
Hyoid bone
Thyroid gland
Left brachiocephalic v.
Pulmonary trunk
Intervertebral disc
Pancreas
Duodenum
Aorta
Vertebral canal
Esophagus
Mitral valve
Left atrium
Left bronchus
Left pulmonary v.

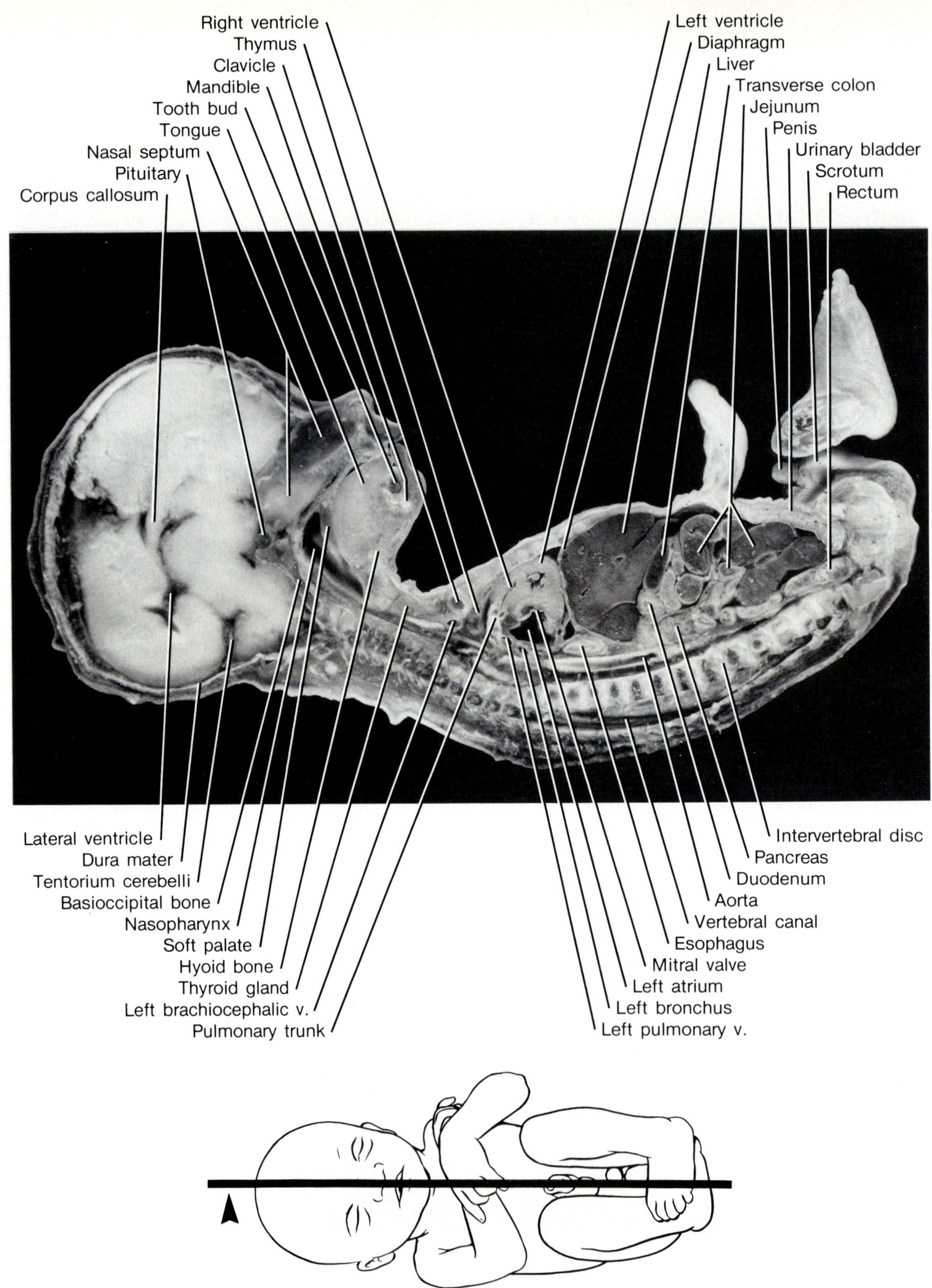

Figure 3.10

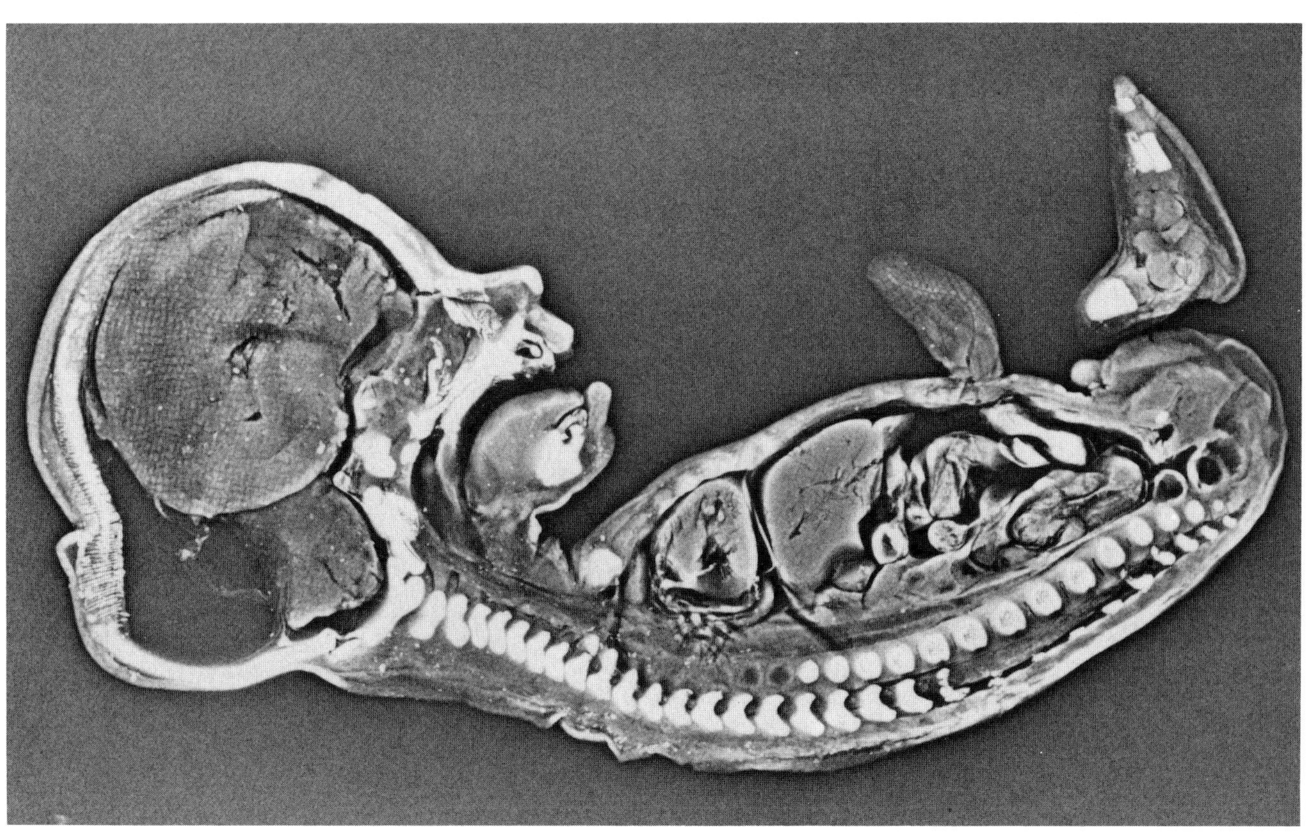

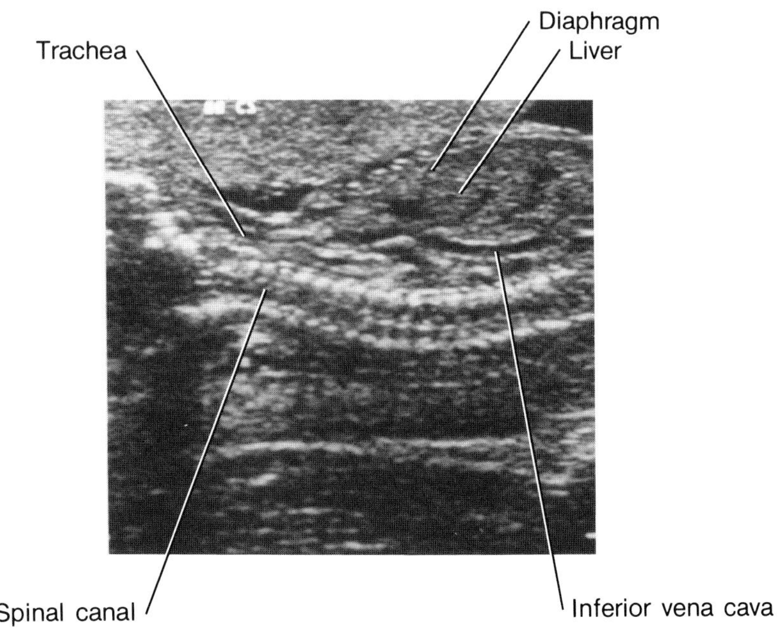
Trachea
Diaphragm
Liver
Spinal canal
Inferior vena cava

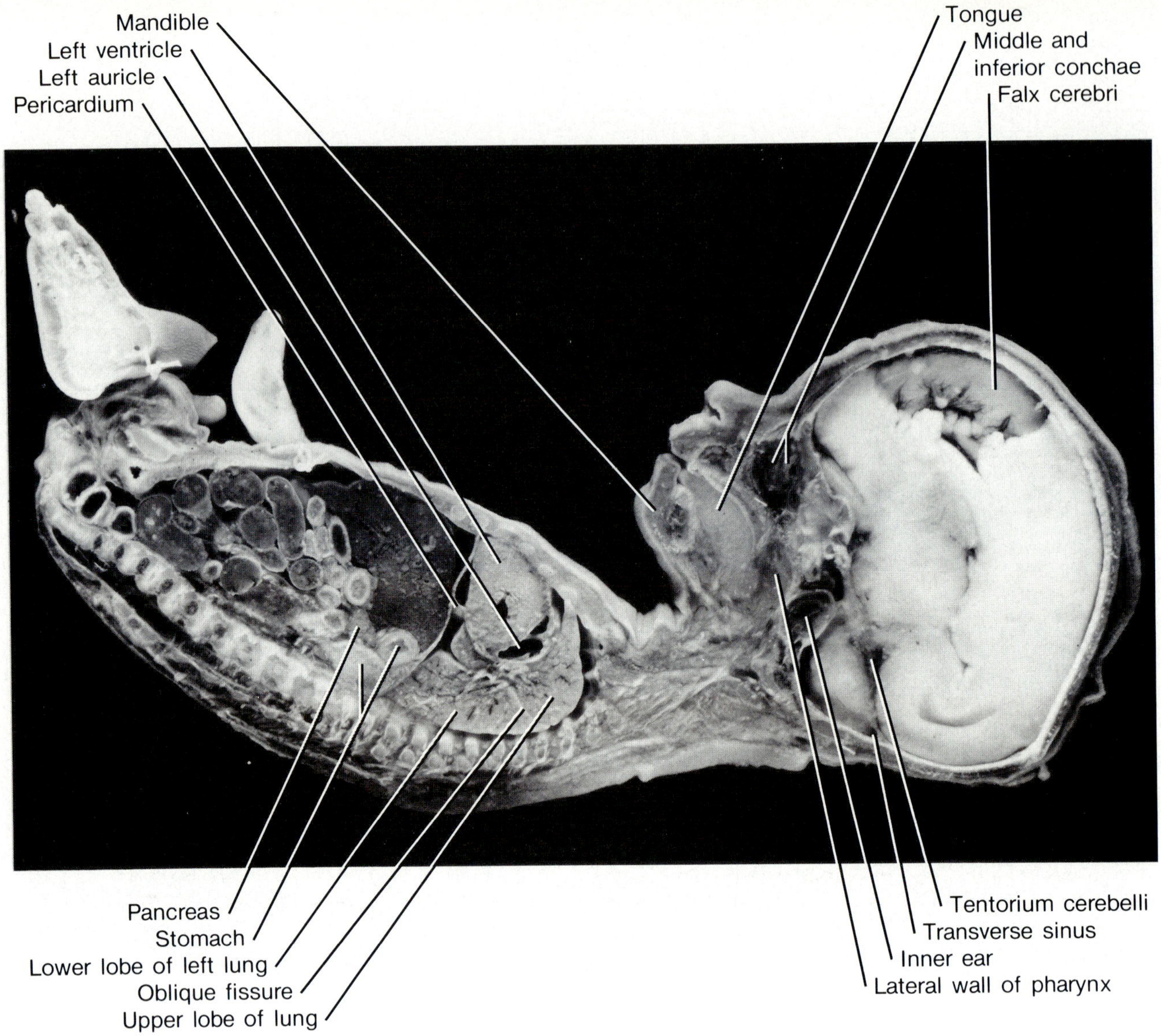

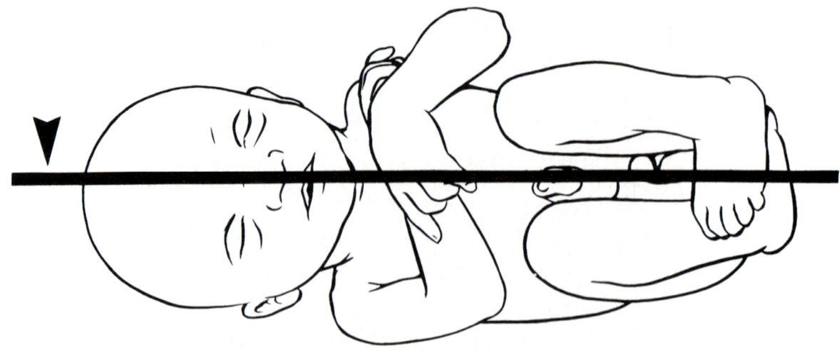

Mandible
Left ventricle
Left auricle
Pericardium

Tongue
Middle and inferior conchae
Falx cerebri

Pancreas
Stomach
Lower lobe of left lung
Oblique fissure
Upper lobe of lung

Tentorium cerebelli
Transverse sinus
Inner ear
Lateral wall of pharynx

Figure 3.11

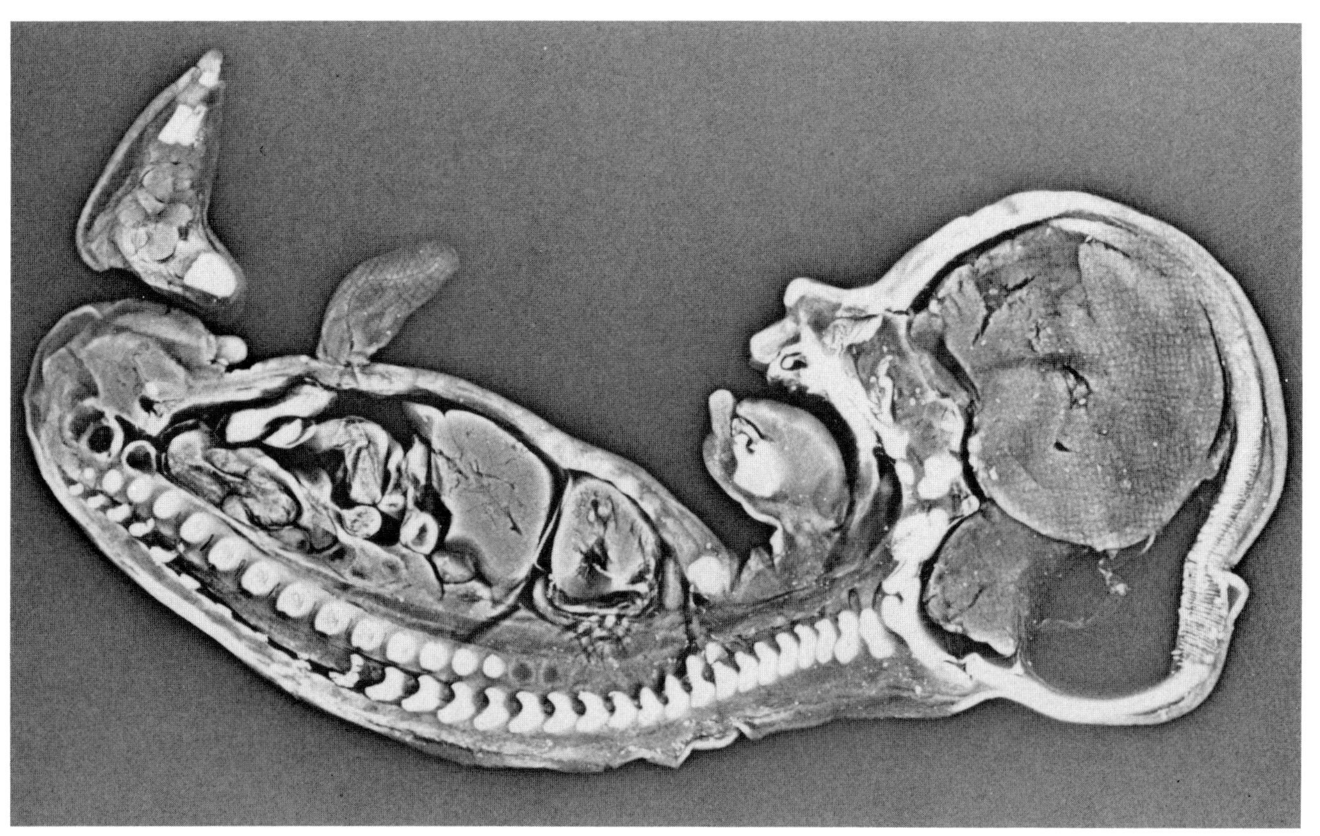

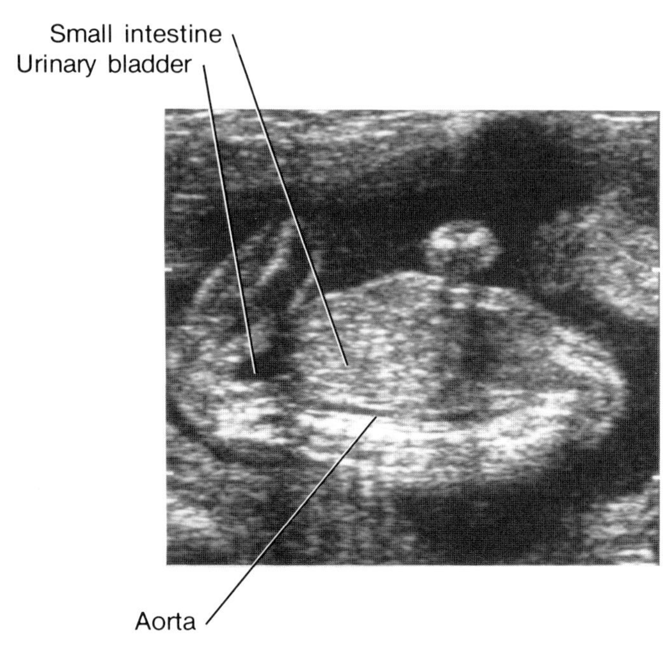
Small intestine
Urinary bladder
Aorta

Left ventricle
Maxilla
Hard palate
Tongue
Frontal bone
Medial rectus m.
Levator palpebrae m.
Dura mater
Pericardium
Diaphragm
Left lobe of liver
Duodenum
Jejunum
Urinary bladder
Symphysis pubis
Prostate
Lateral ventricle
Tentorium cerebelli
Cerebellum
Inner ear
Pharynx
Tooth bud
Upper lobe of left lung
Oblique fissure of left lung
Pleural cavity
Anal canal
Rectum
Ileum
Kidney
Suprarenal gland
Pancreas
Body of stomach
Lower lobe of left lung

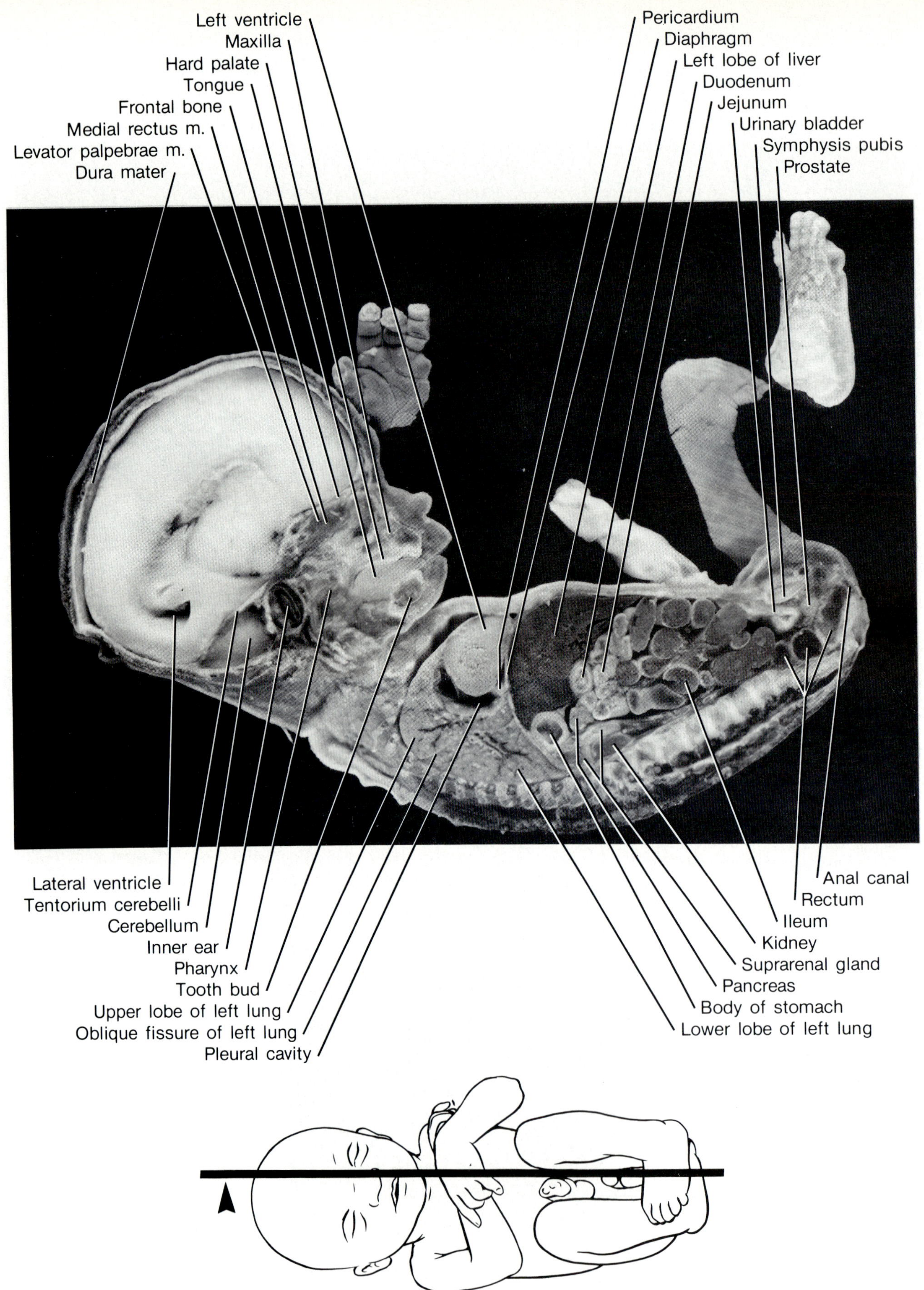

Figure 3.12

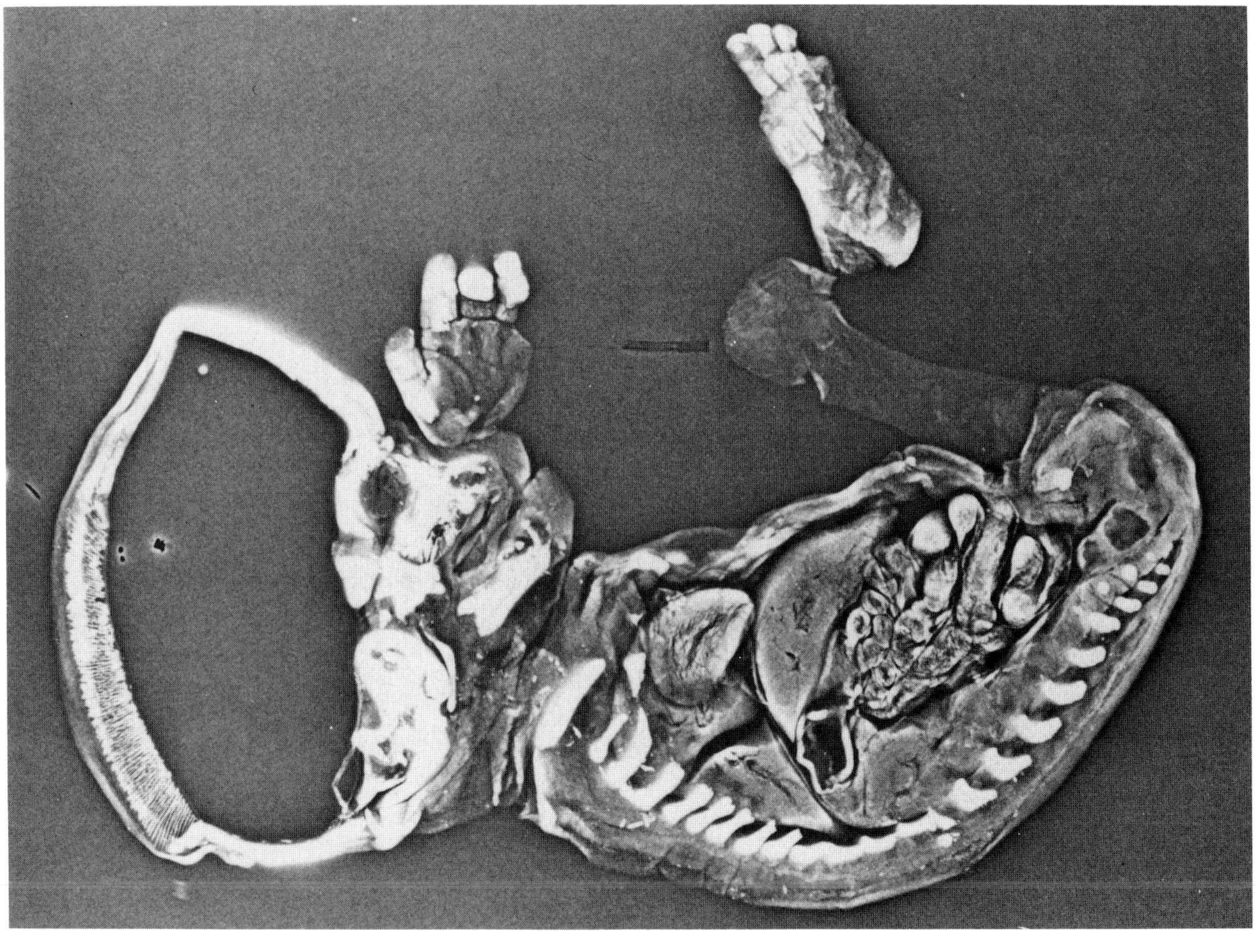

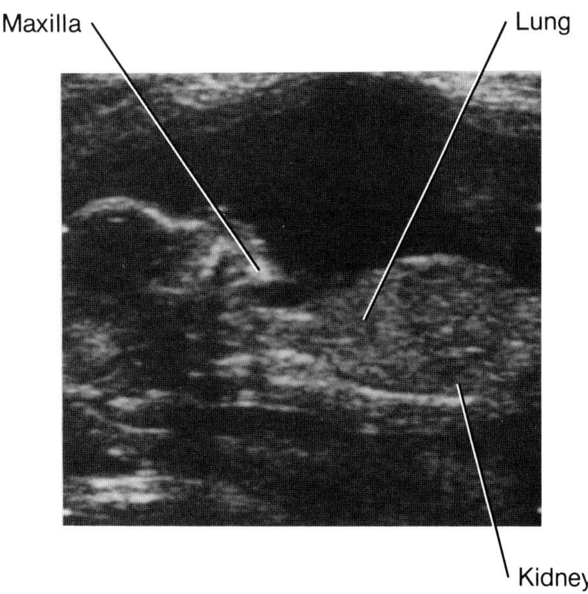

Maxilla
Lung
Kidney

Left ventricle
Duodenum
Pubic ramus
Ischiopubic ramus
Sclera
Middle cranial fossa
Temporal lobe
Sigmoid sinus
Obturator n.
Psoas m.
Pyramid of left kidney
Pancreas
Suprarenal gland
Spleen
Lateral pterygoid m.
Upper lobe of lung
Pylorus
Oblique fissure
Lower lobe of lung
Body of stomach

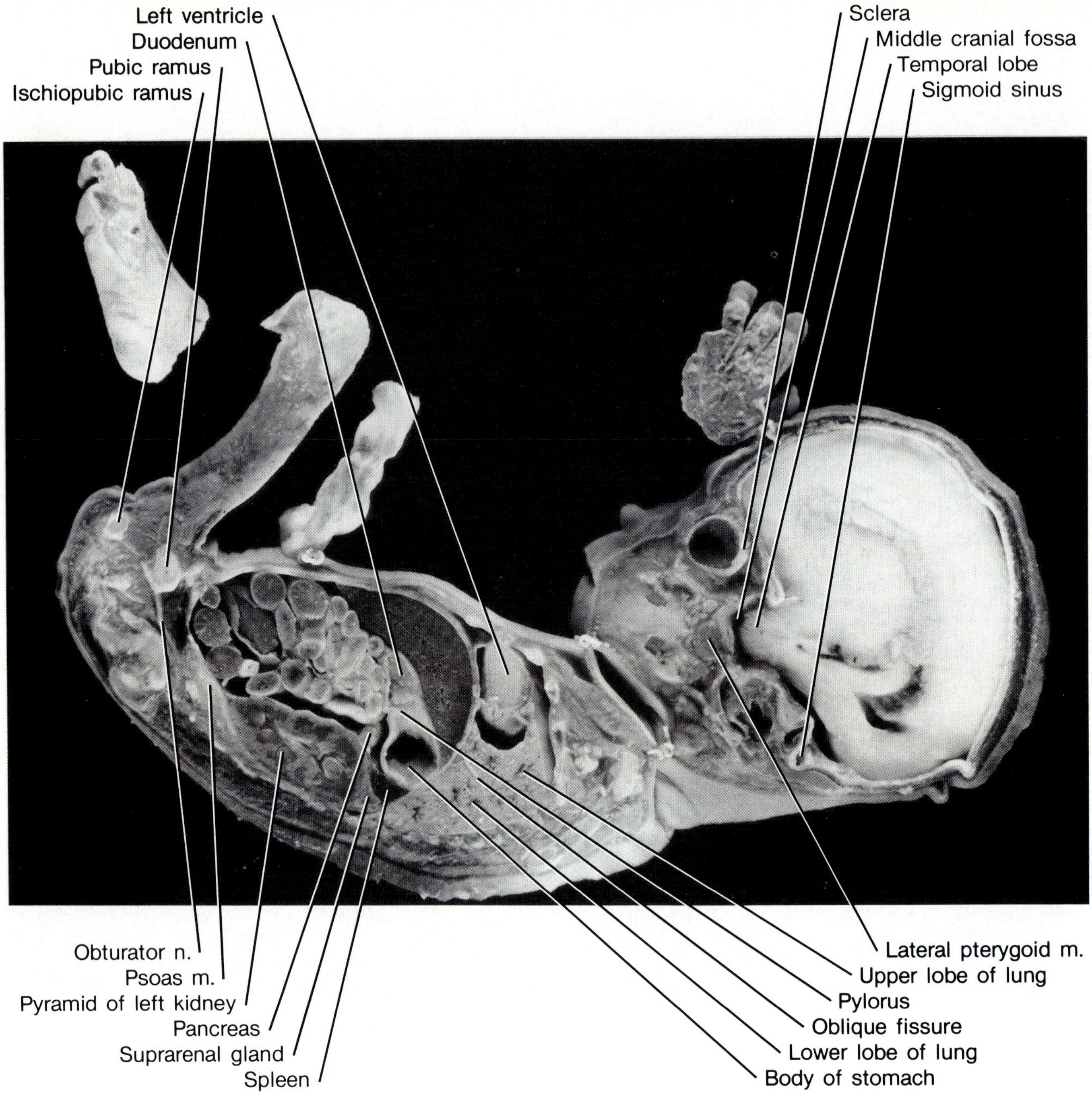

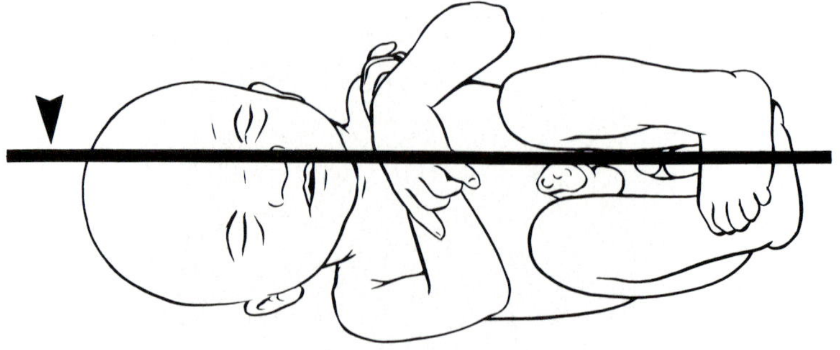

Figure 3.13

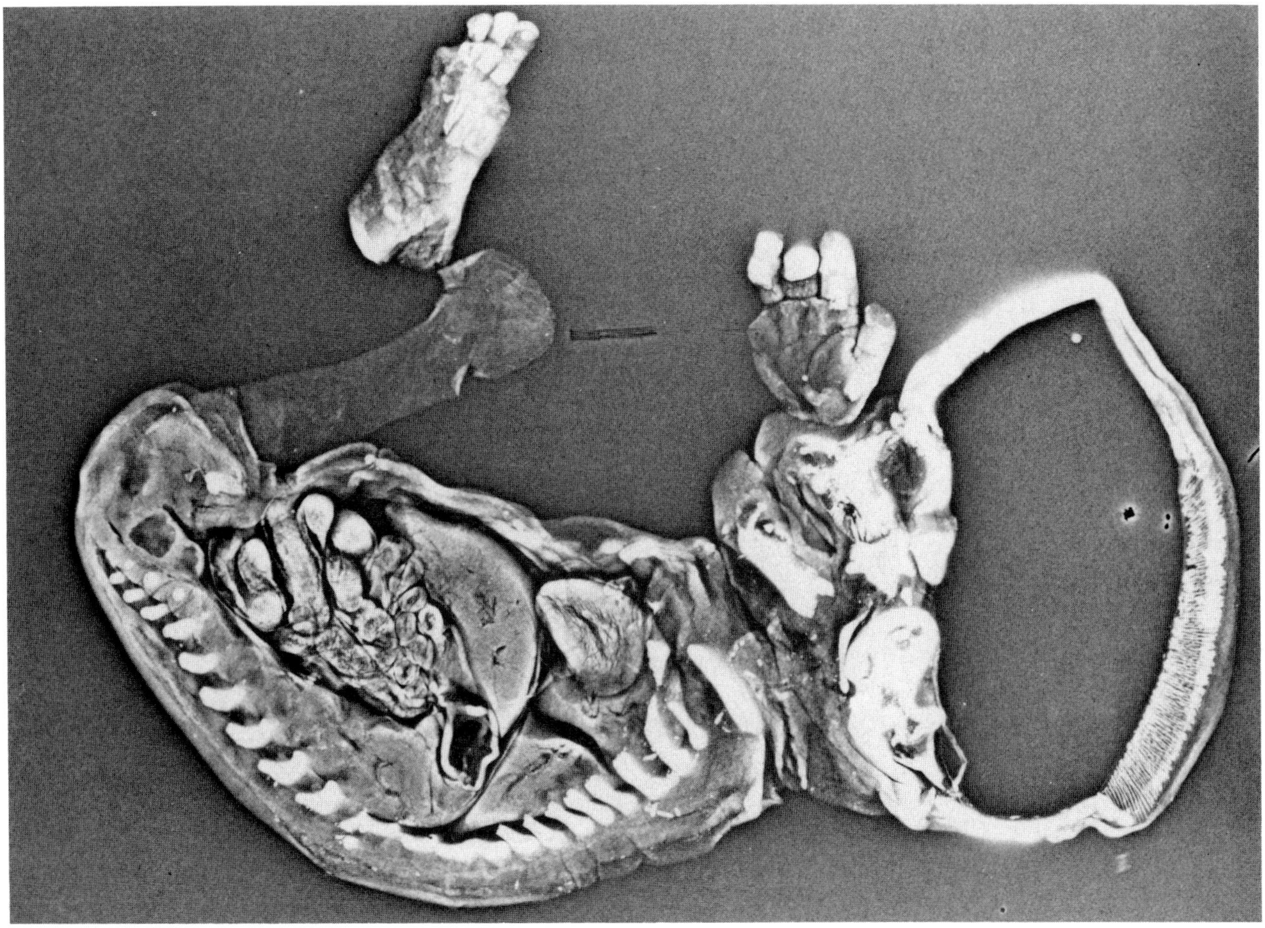

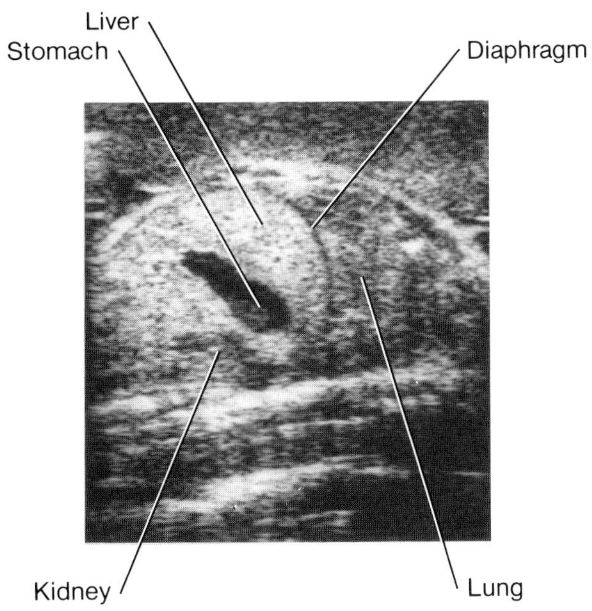

Liver
Stomach
Diaphragm
Kidney
Lung

Liver
Diaphragm
Pectoralis major m.
Brachial plexus
Acromion
Zygoma
Lens
Lateral pterygoid m.
Jejunum
Ileum
Iliacus m.
Testis
Quadriceps femoris tendon
Medial condyle of femur
Medial condyle of tibia
Hamstring m.
Transverse venous sinus
Middle ear
Clavicle
Subscapularis m.
Scapula
Upper lobe of left lung
Oblique fissure
Stomach
Gluteus maximus m.
Head of femur
Ilium
Renal cortex
Major calyx
Costodiaphragmatic recess
Suprarenal gland
Spleen

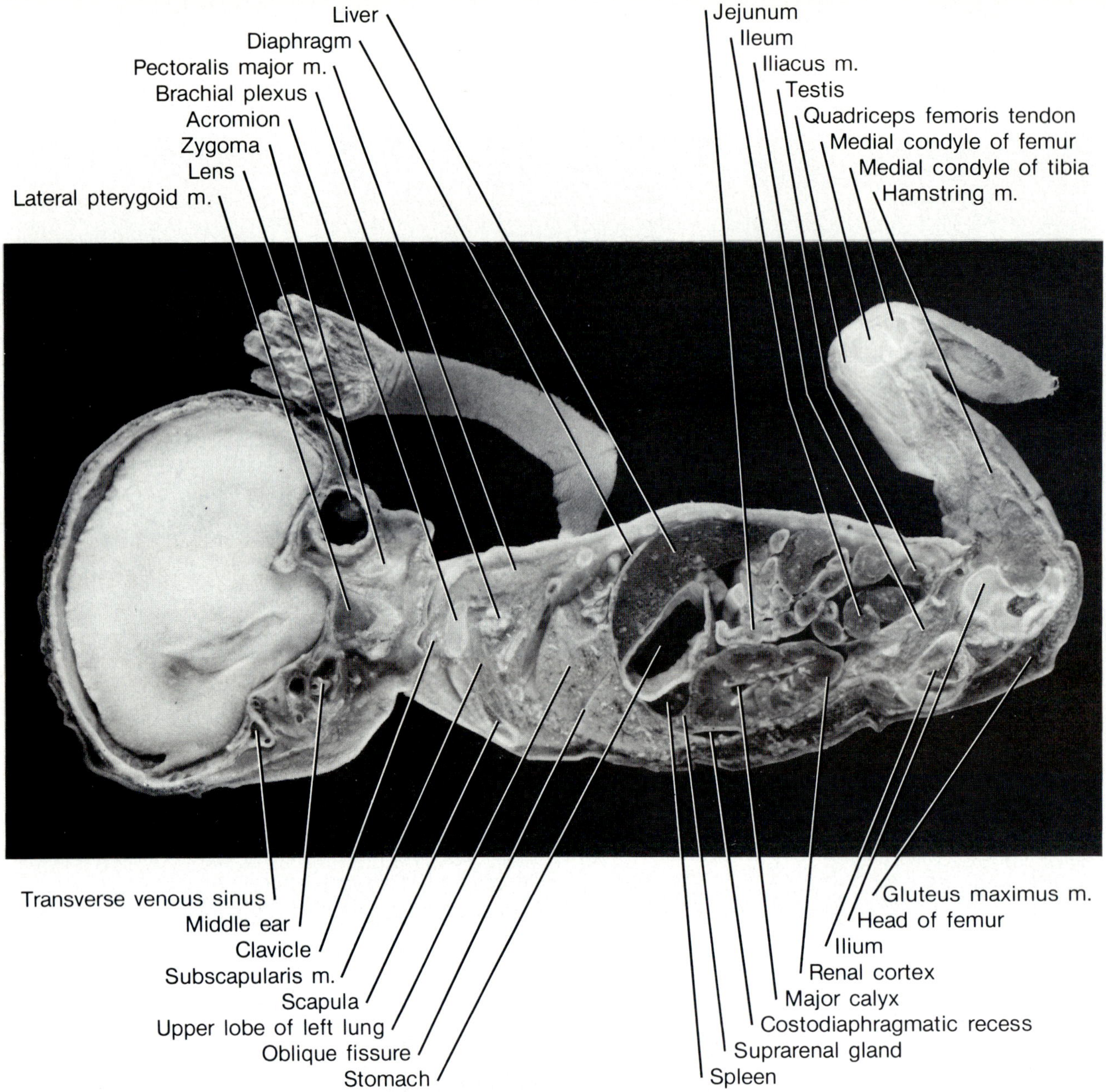

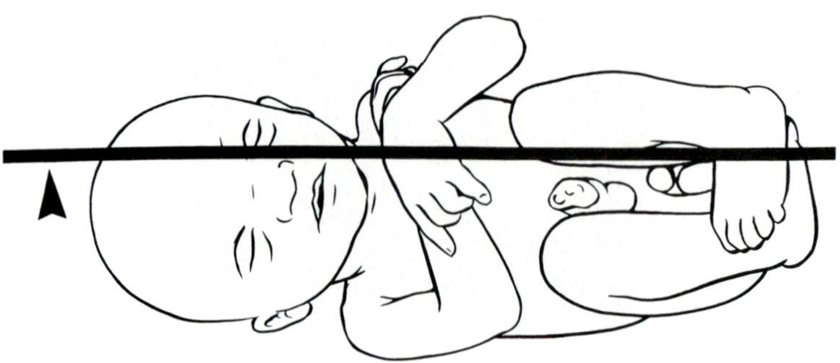

Figure 3.14

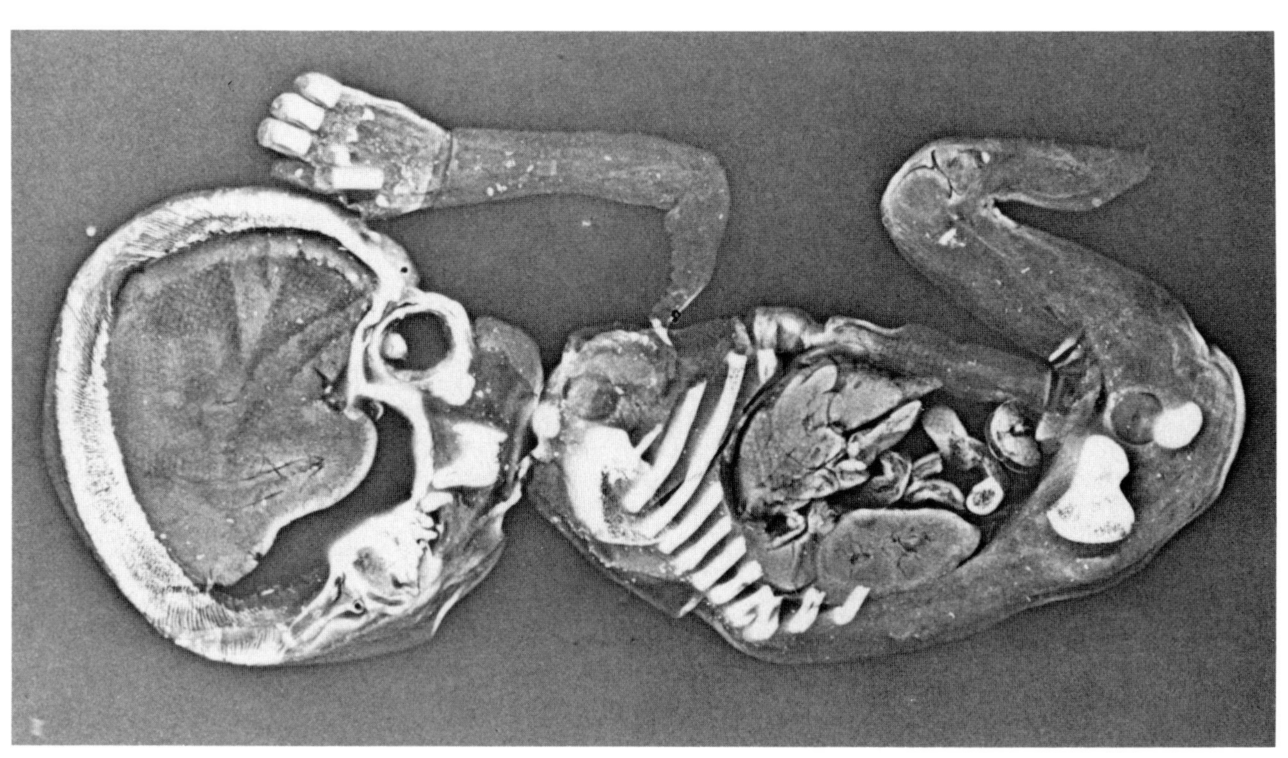

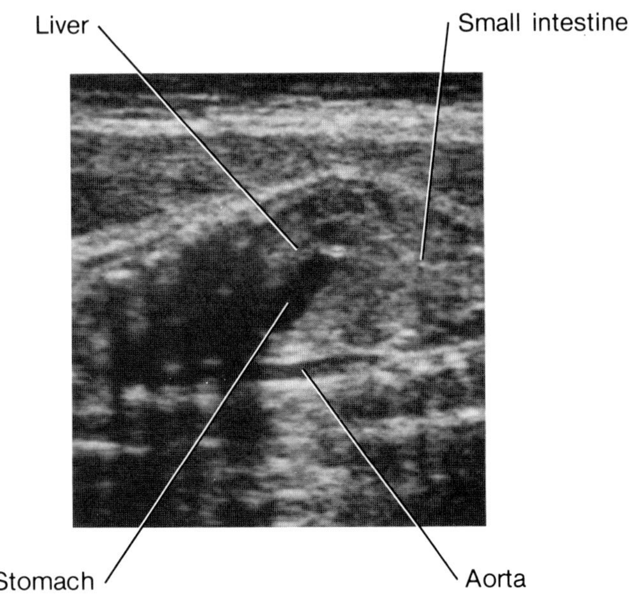

Liver
Small intestine
Stomach
Aorta

Head of femur
Temporalis m.
Sclera
Gluteus maximus m.
Gluteus medius m.
Ilium
Sigmoid colon
Middle ear
Condyle of mandible
Head of humerus
Transverse colon

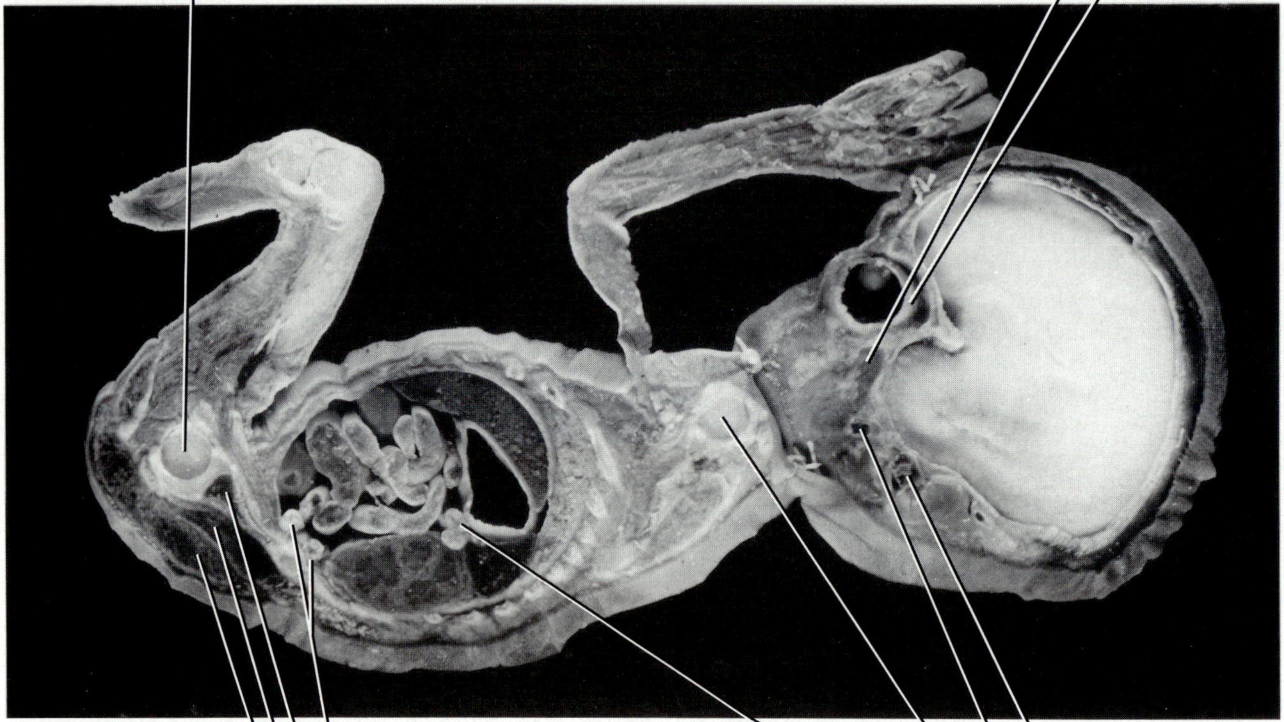

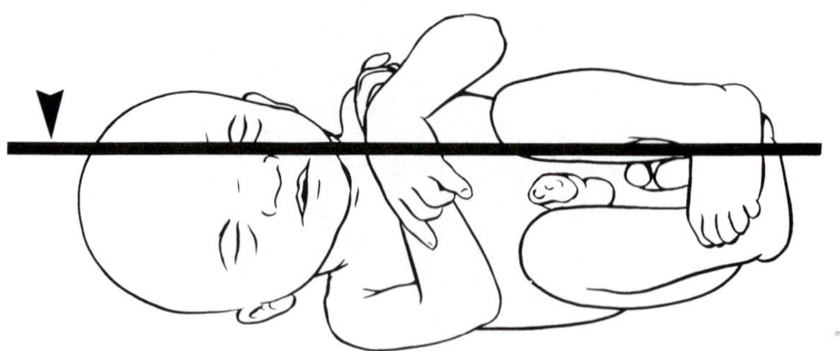

Figure 3.15

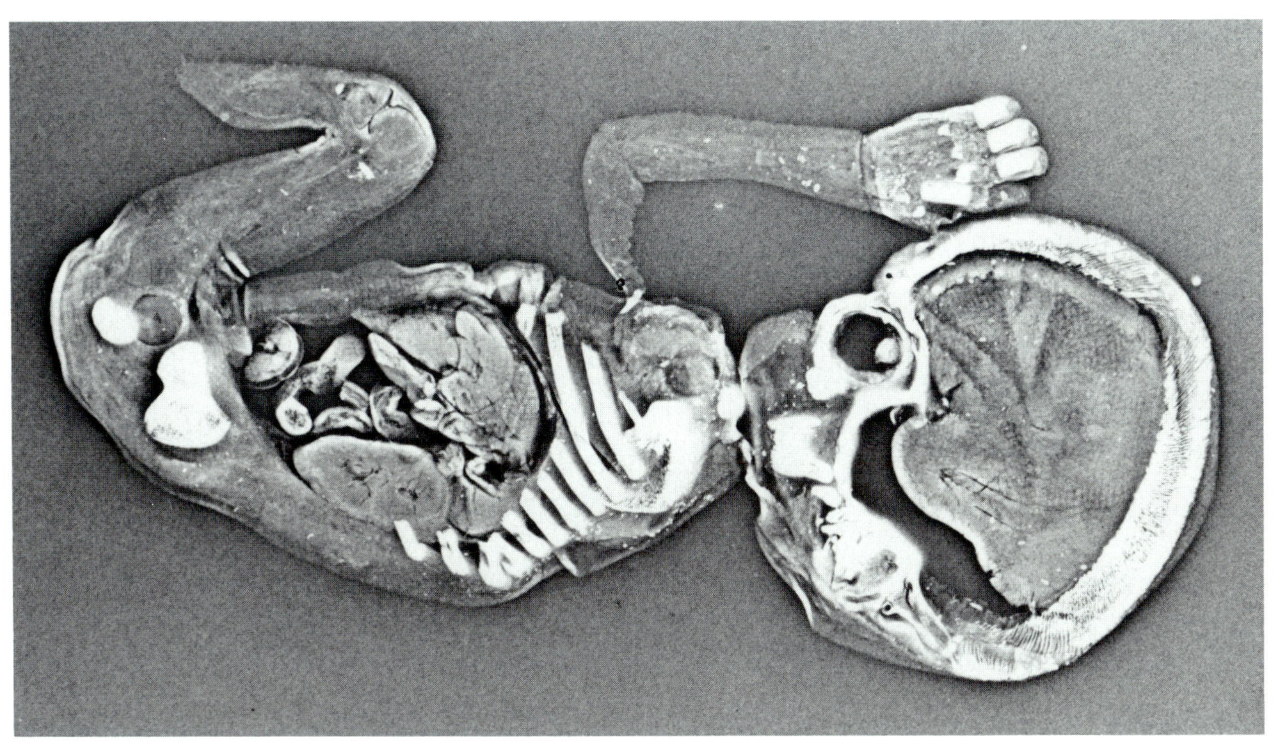

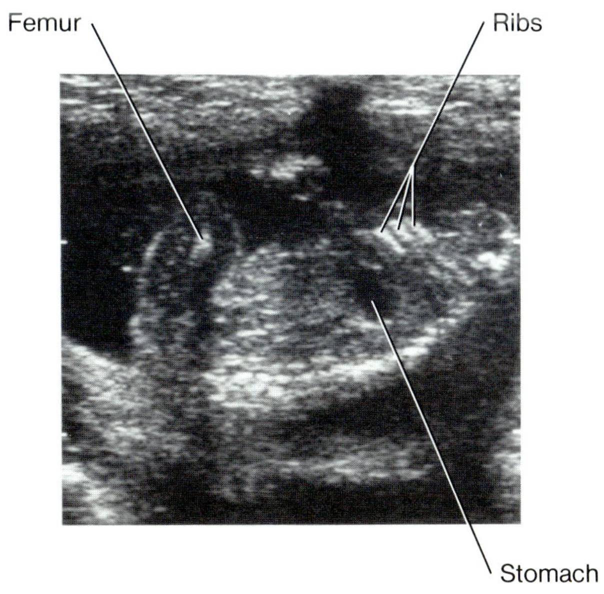
Femur
Ribs
Stomach

Quadriceps femoris tendon
Small intestine
Liver
Stomach
Diaphragm
Medial epicondyle
Femur
Tibia
Gastrocnemius m.
Hamstring m.
Talus
Navicular
Cuneiform
External auditory meatus
Head of humerus
Scapula
Spleen
Splenic flexure
Head of femur
in acetabulum
Gluteus medius m.
Iliacus m.
Ilium
Descending colon

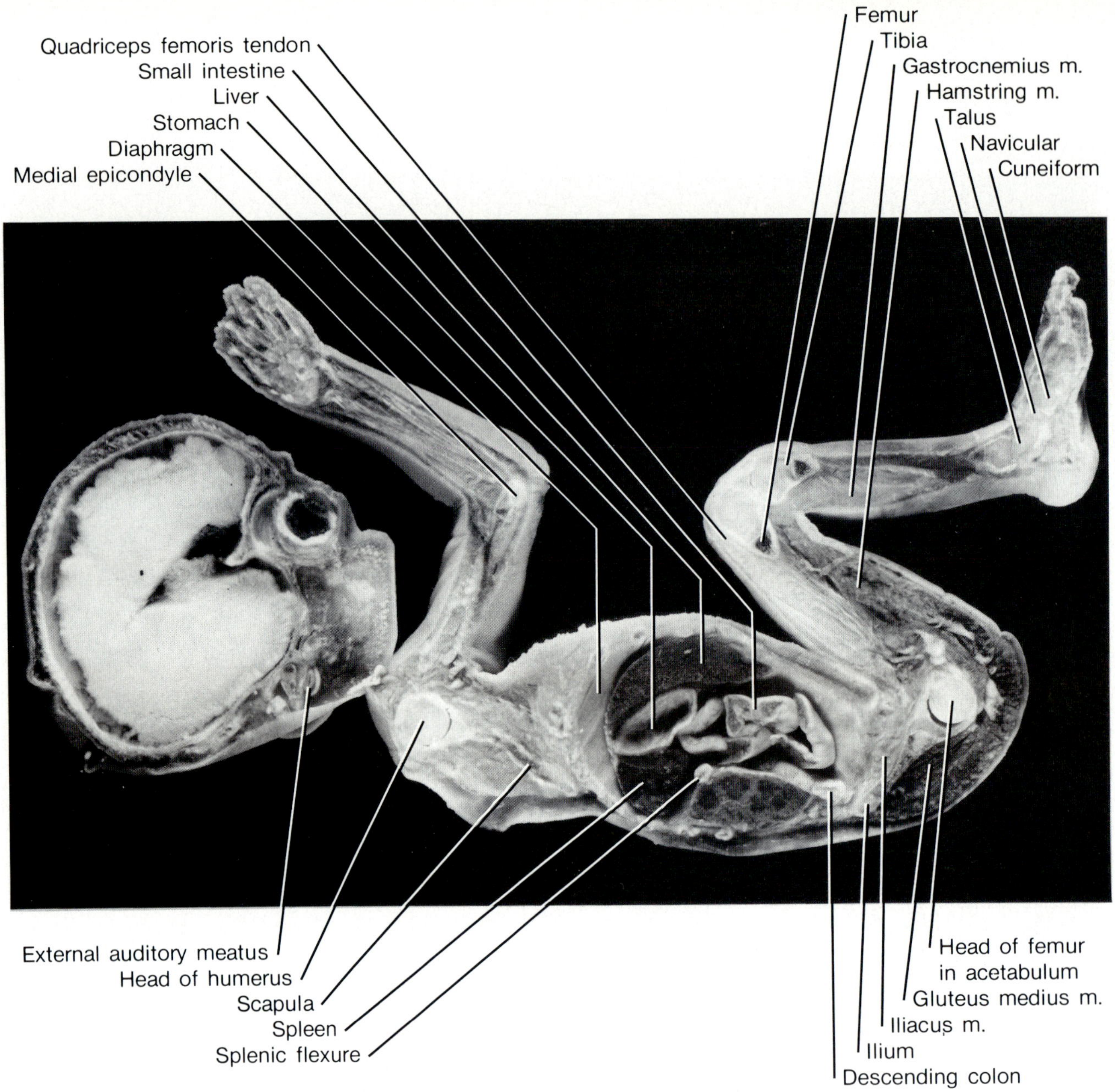

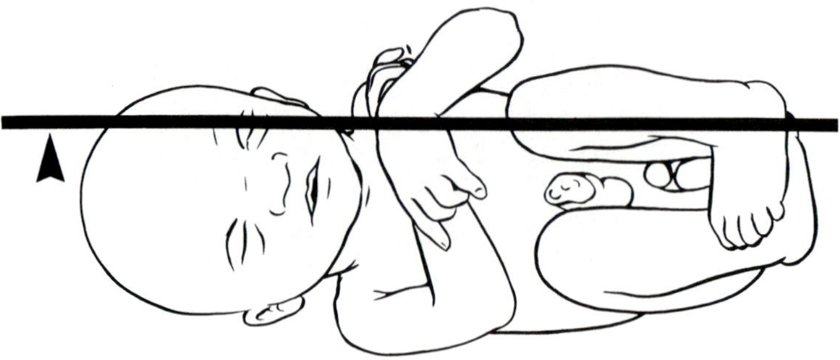

Figure 3.16

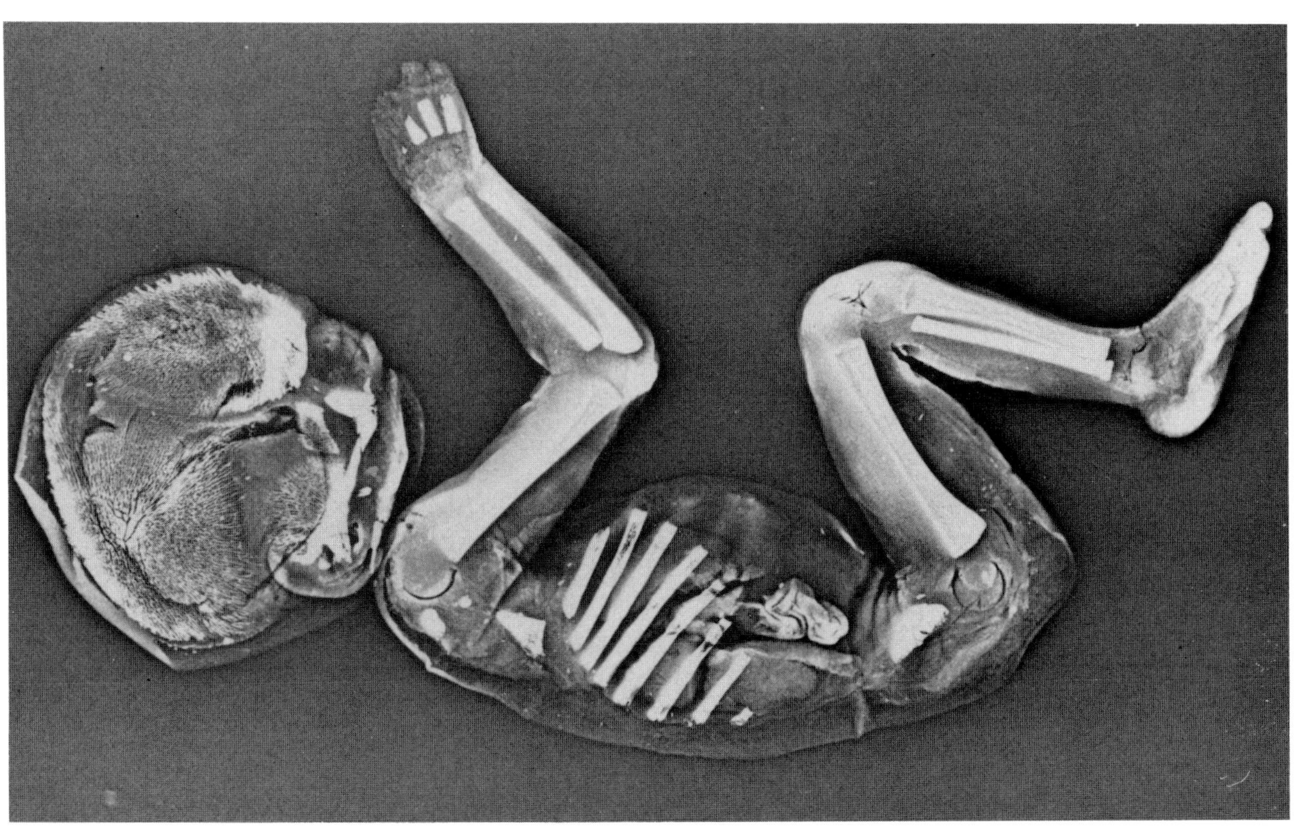

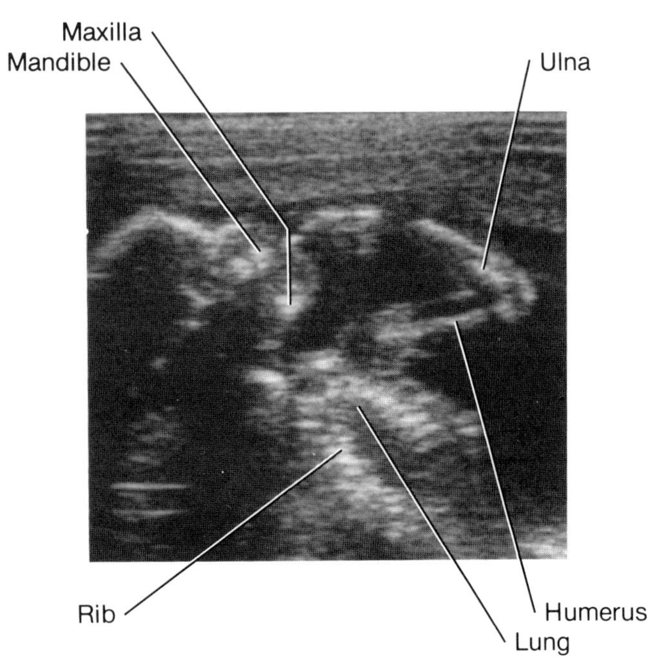

Maxilla
Mandible
Ulna
Rib
Humerus
Lung

4

SAGITTAL SECTIONS

36-week fetus

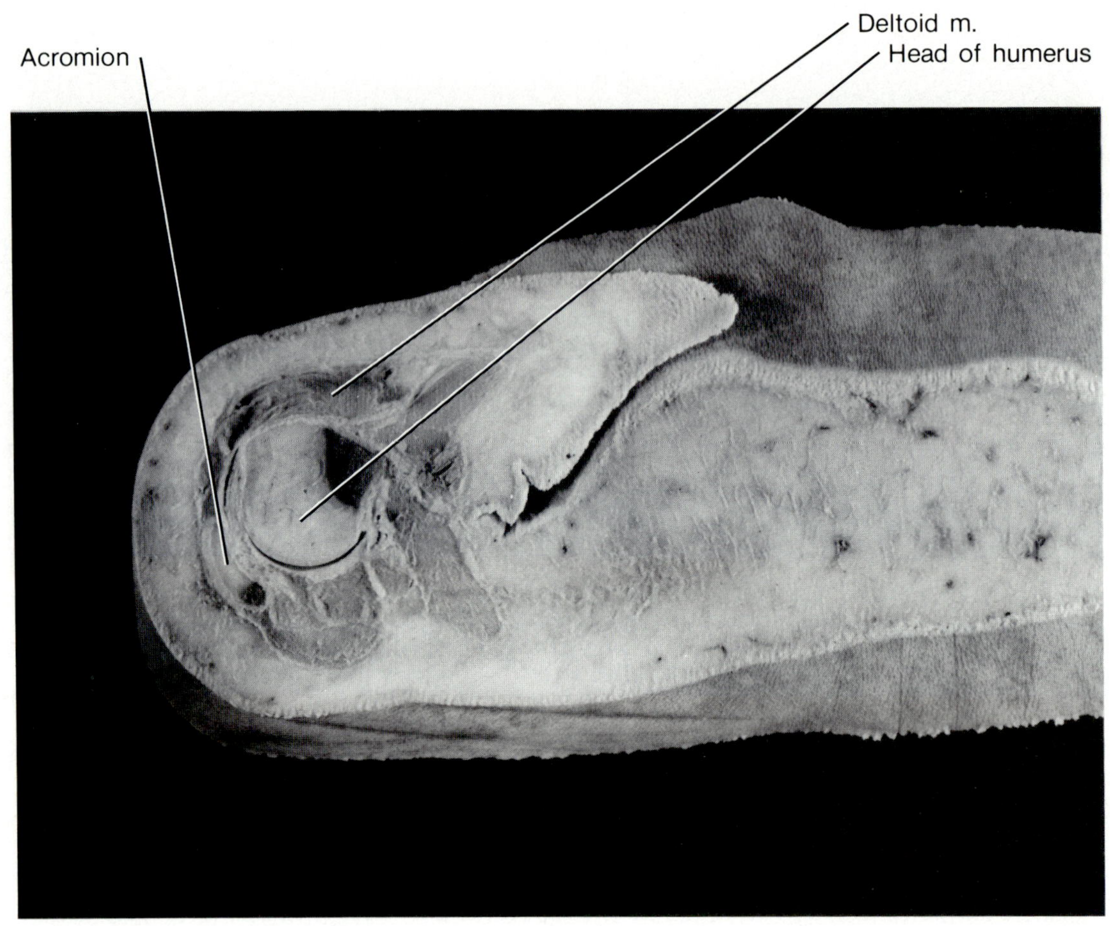

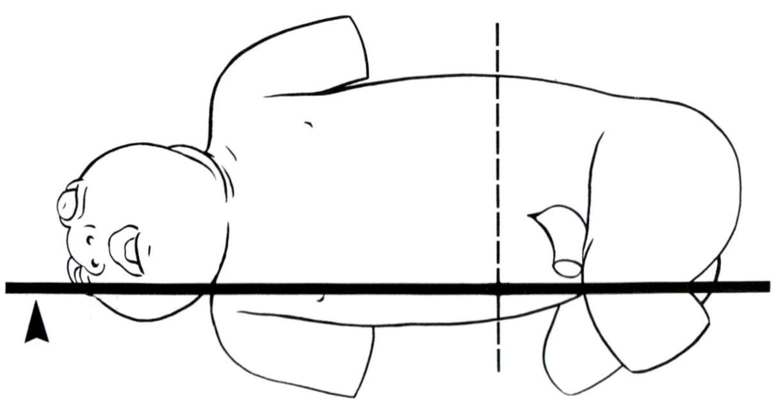

Figure 4.1

    FETAL SECTIONAL ANATOMY AND ULTRASONOGRAPHY

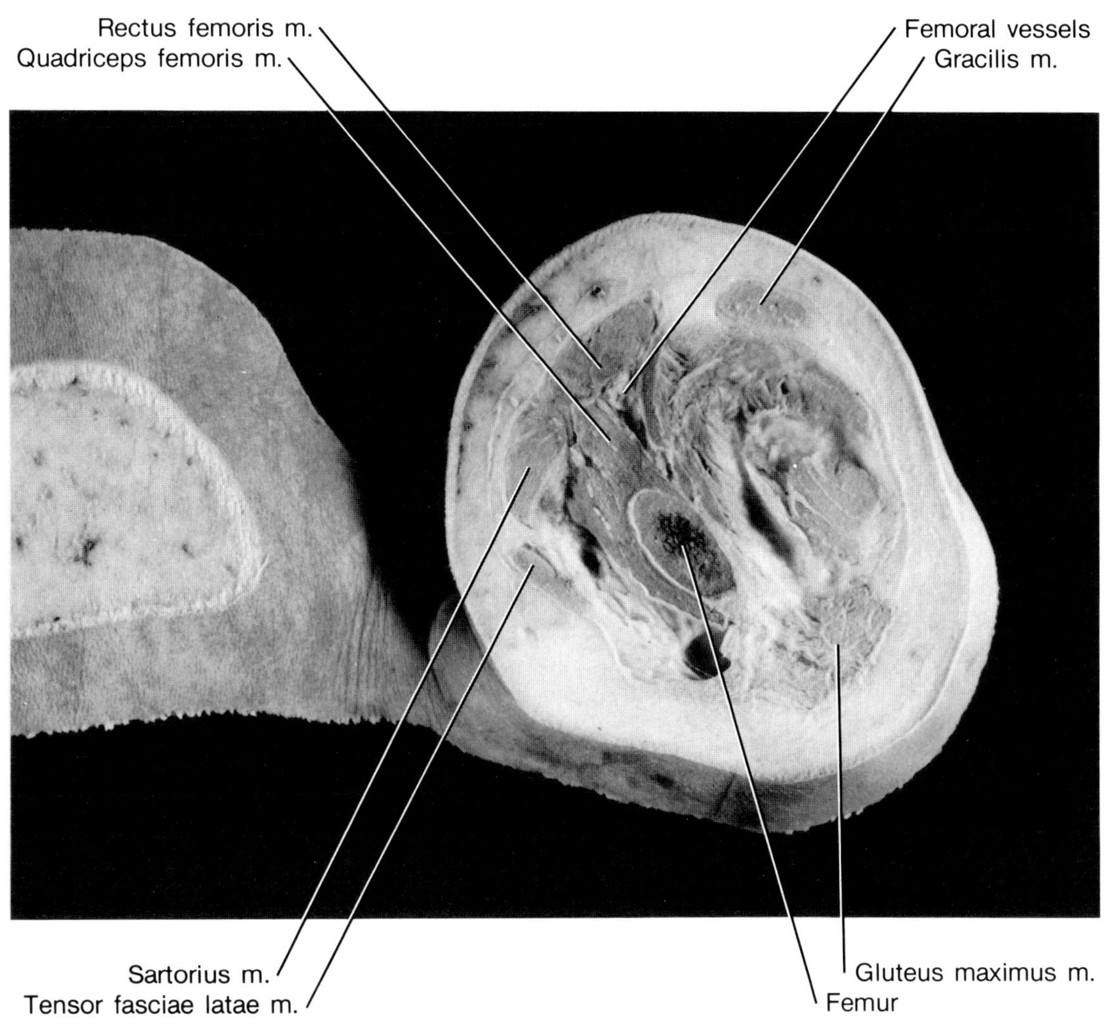

Rectus femoris m.
Quadriceps femoris m.
Femoral vessels
Gracilis m.
Sartorius m.
Tensor fasciae latae m.
Gluteus maximus m.
Femur

External oblique m.
Internal oblique m.
Transversus abdominis m.

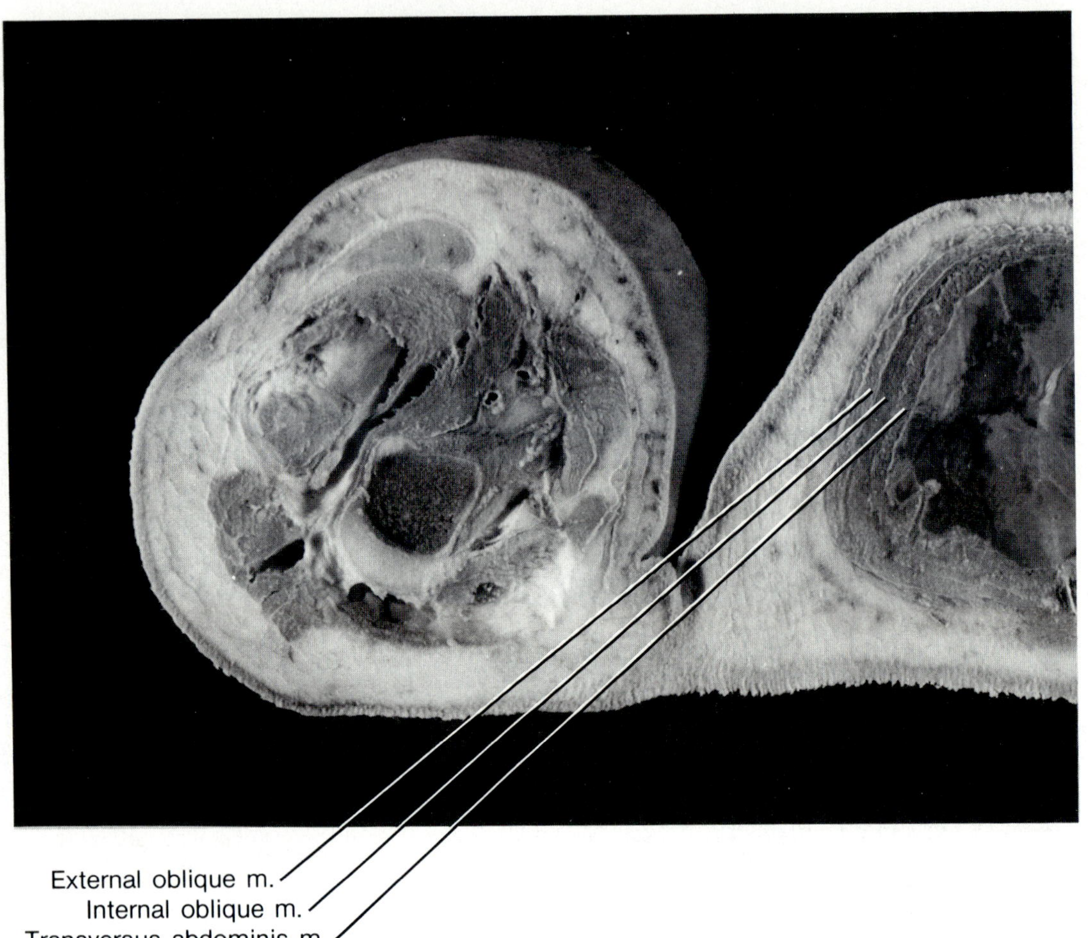

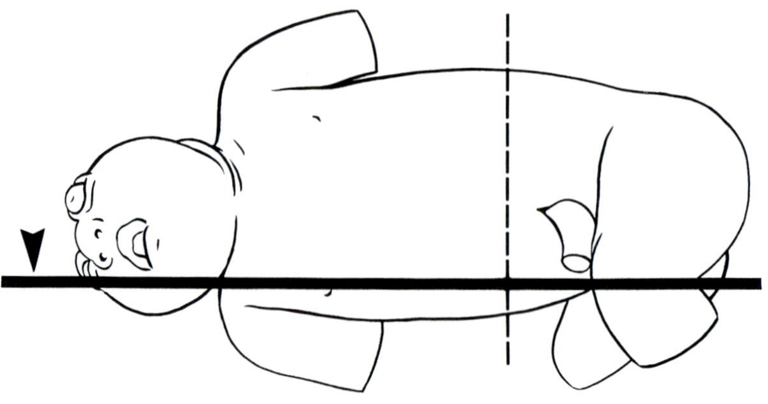

Figure 4.2

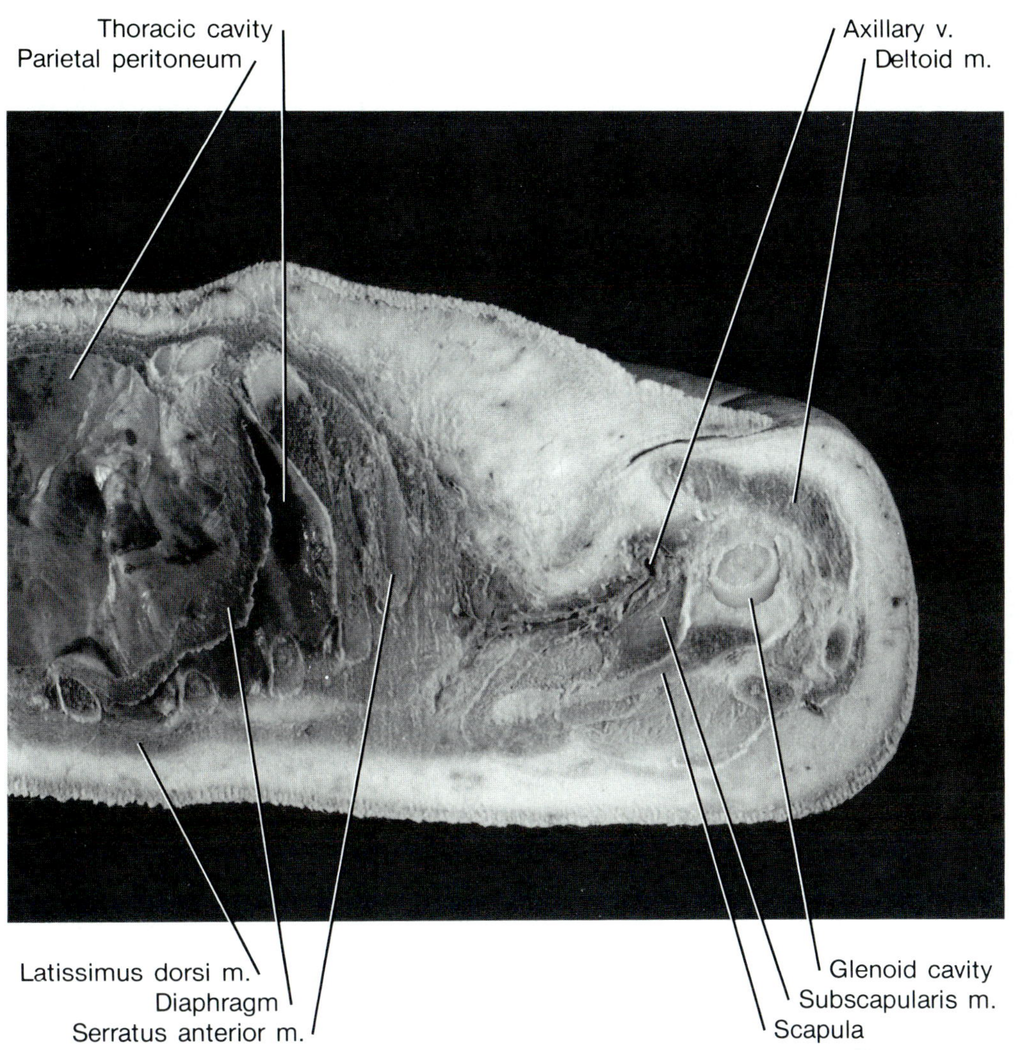

Thoracic cavity
Parietal peritoneum
Axillary v.
Deltoid m.
Latissimus dorsi m.
Diaphragm
Serratus anterior m.
Glenoid cavity
Subscapularis m.
Scapula

Cords of brachial plexus
Pectoralis major m.
Supraspinatus m.
Clavicle
Axillary a.
Subscapularis m.
Intercostal m.
Ribs
Spine of scapula
Infraspinatus m.
Scapula
Thoracic cavity
Serratus anterior m.

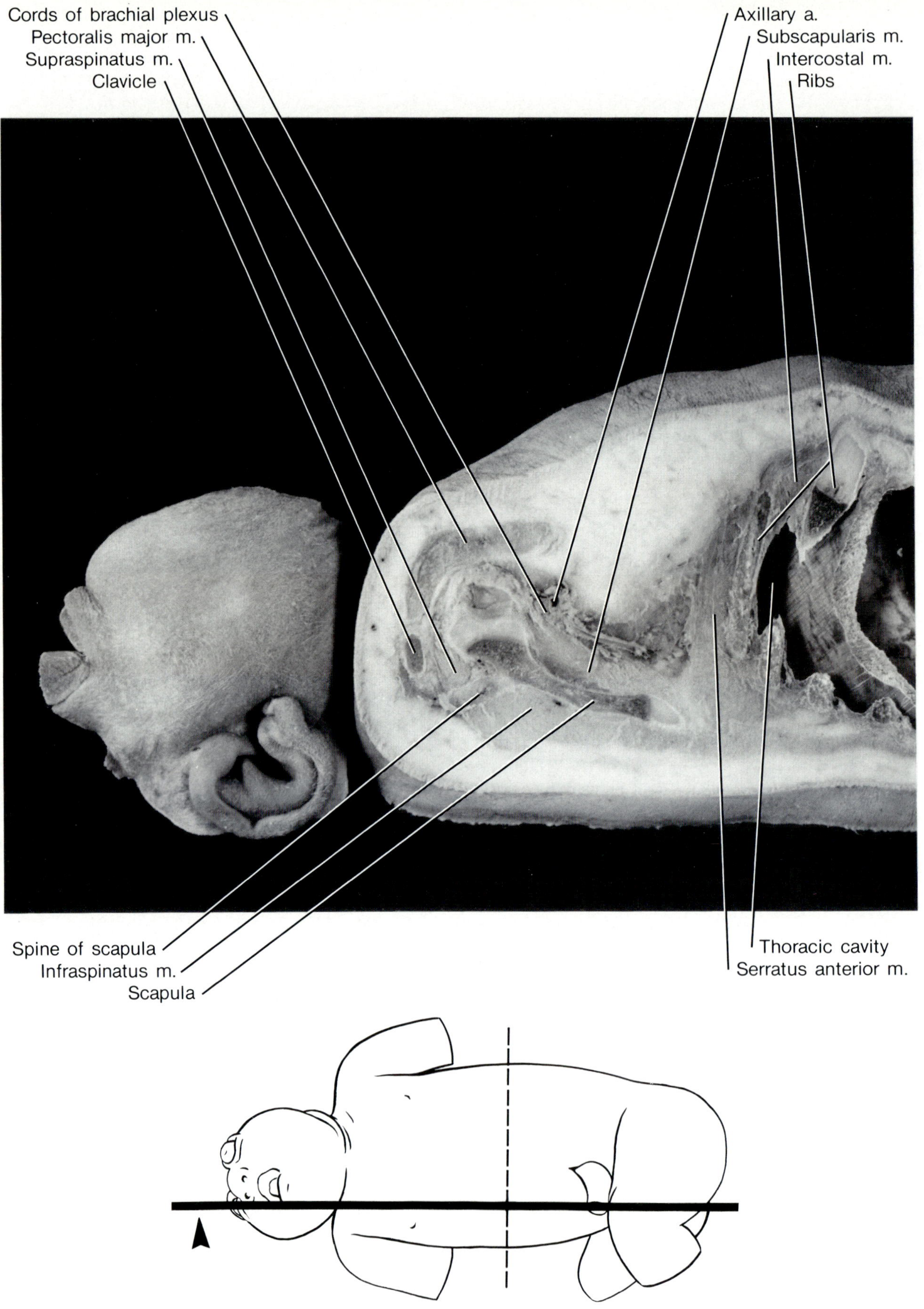

Figure 4.3

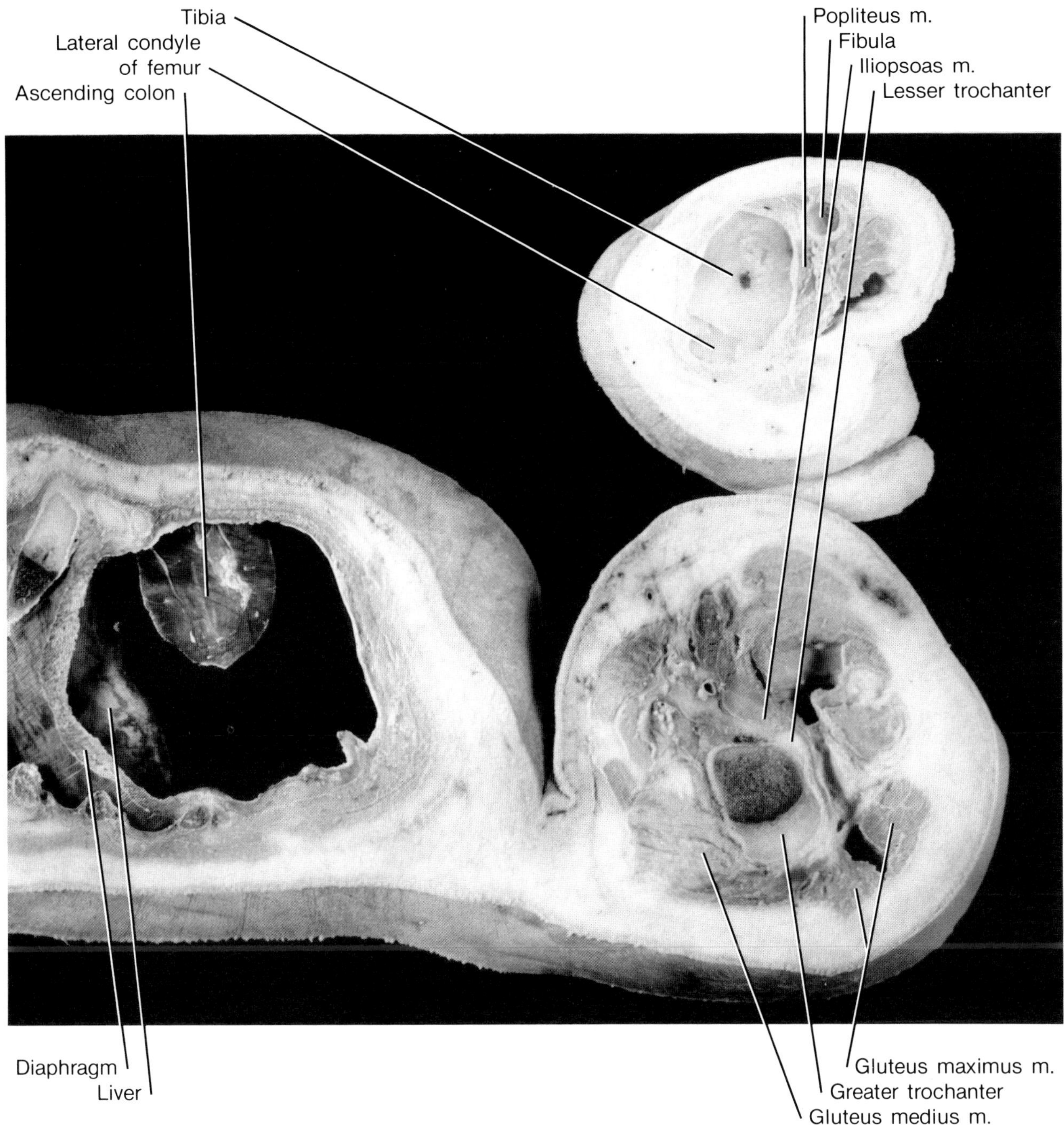

Tibia
Lateral condyle
of femur
Ascending colon
Popliteus m.
Fibula
Iliopsoas m.
Lesser trochanter
Diaphragm
Liver
Gluteus maximus m.
Greater trochanter
Gluteus medius m.

Patella
Tibia
Femur
Parietal peritoneum
Ascending colon
Femur
Gluteus maximus m.
Ilium
Gluteus minimus m.
Gluteus medius m.

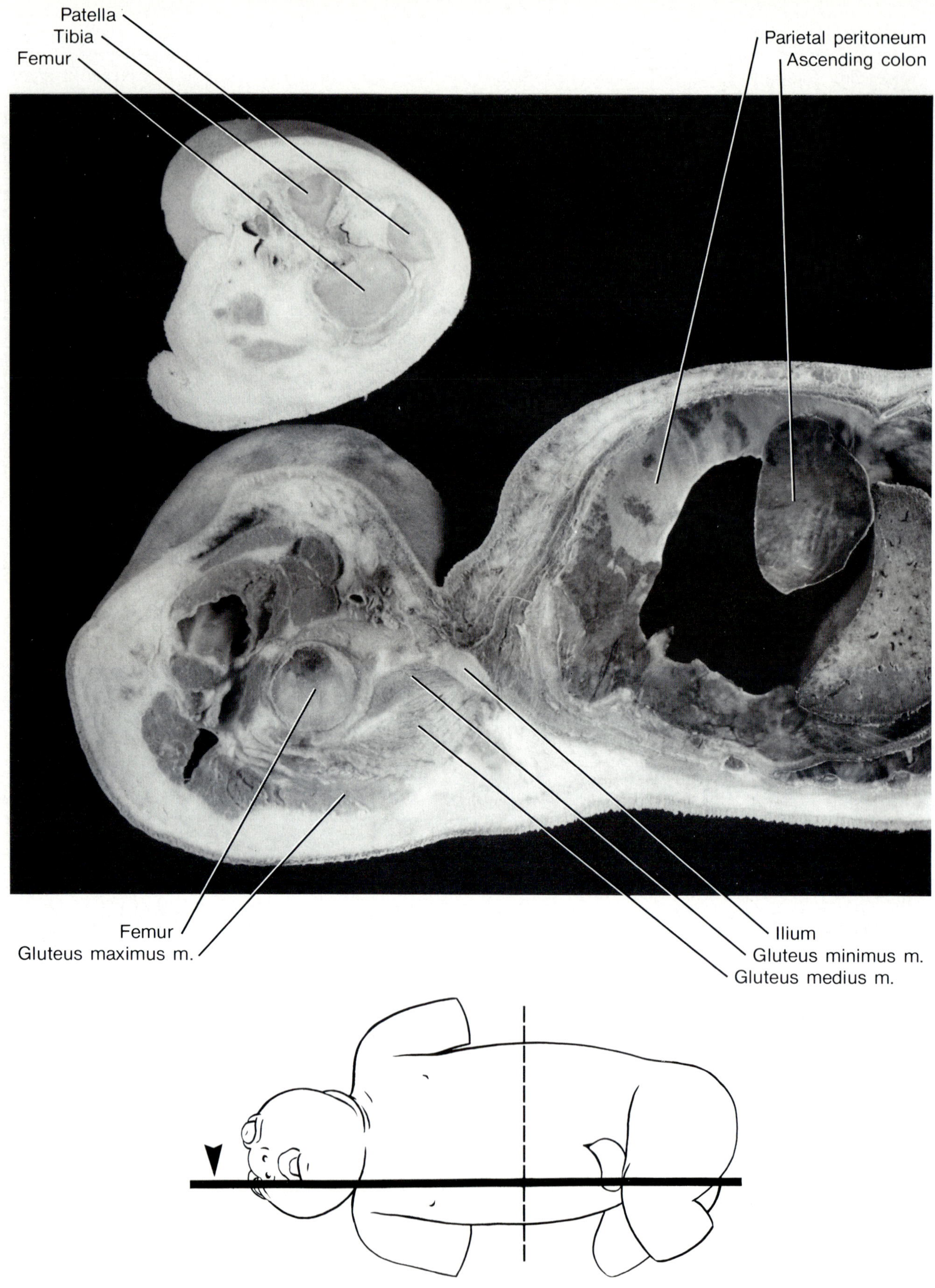

Figure 4.4

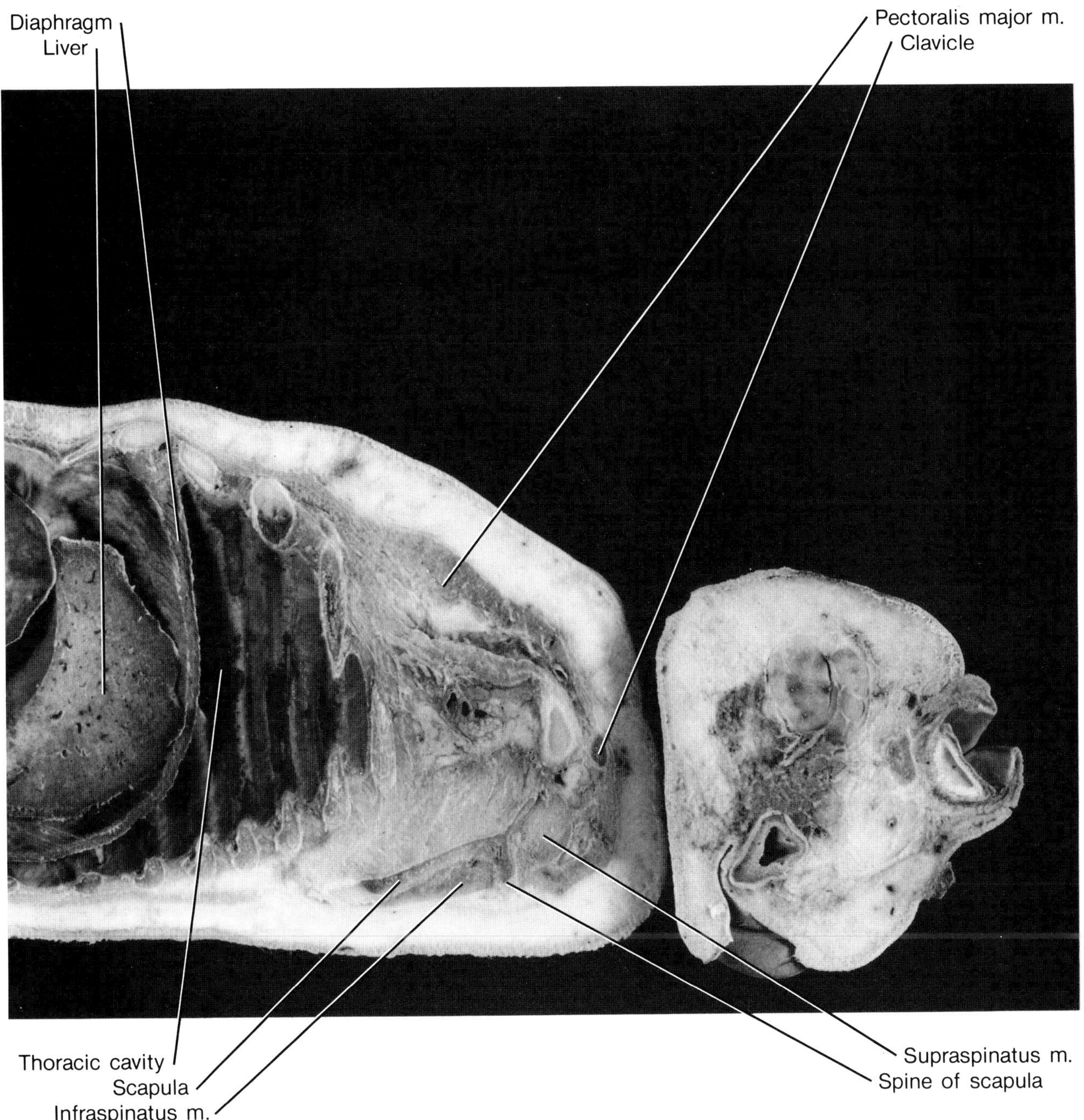

Diaphragm
Liver
Pectoralis major m.
Clavicle
Thoracic cavity
Scapula
Infraspinatus m.
Supraspinatus m.
Spine of scapula

Pectoralis major m.
Right subclavian v.
Clavicle
Diaphragm
Liver
Scapula
Oblique fissure of lung

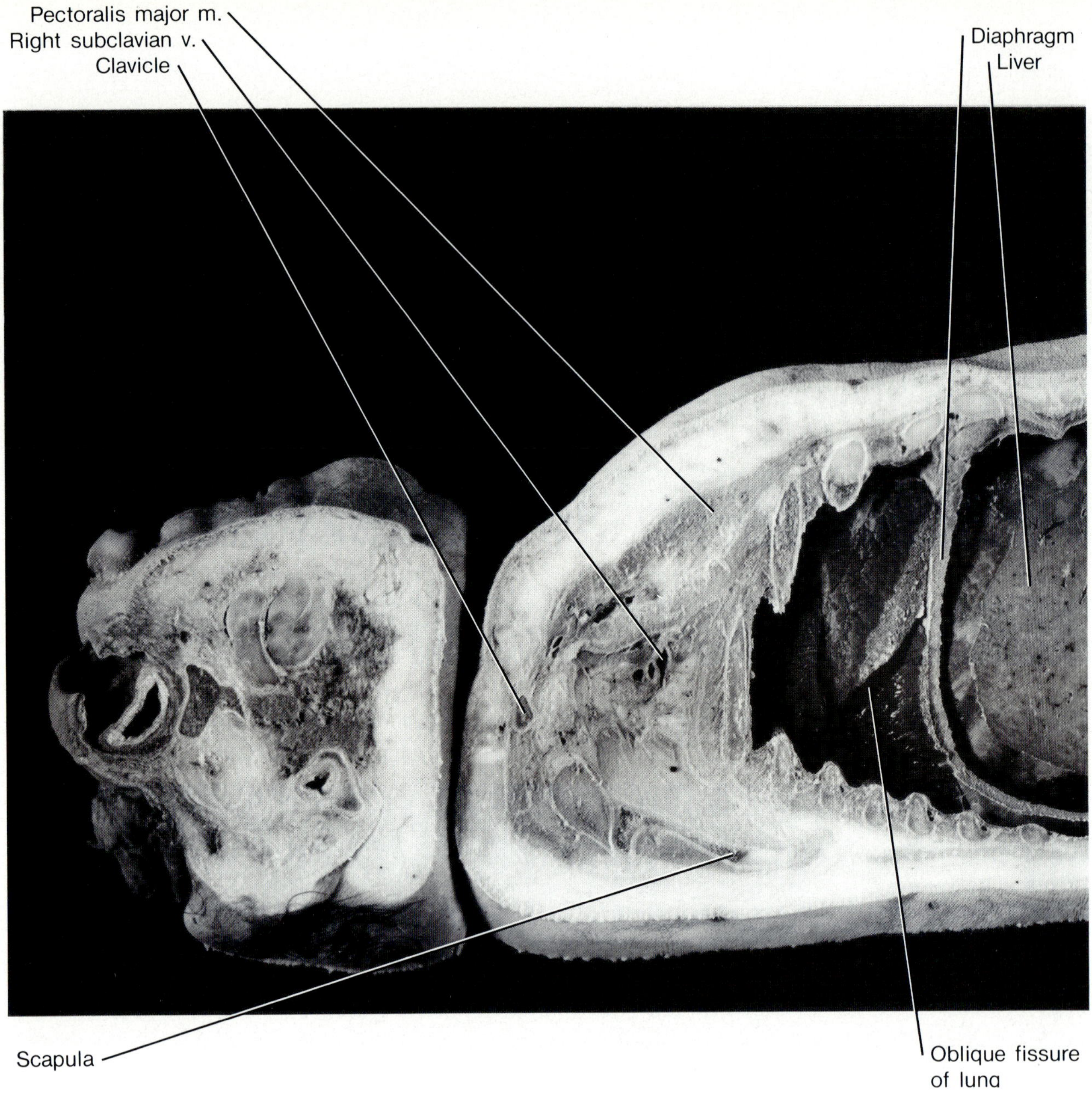

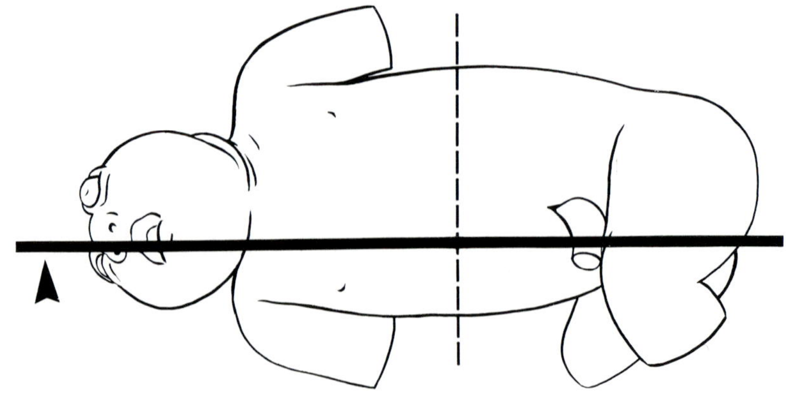

Figure 4.5

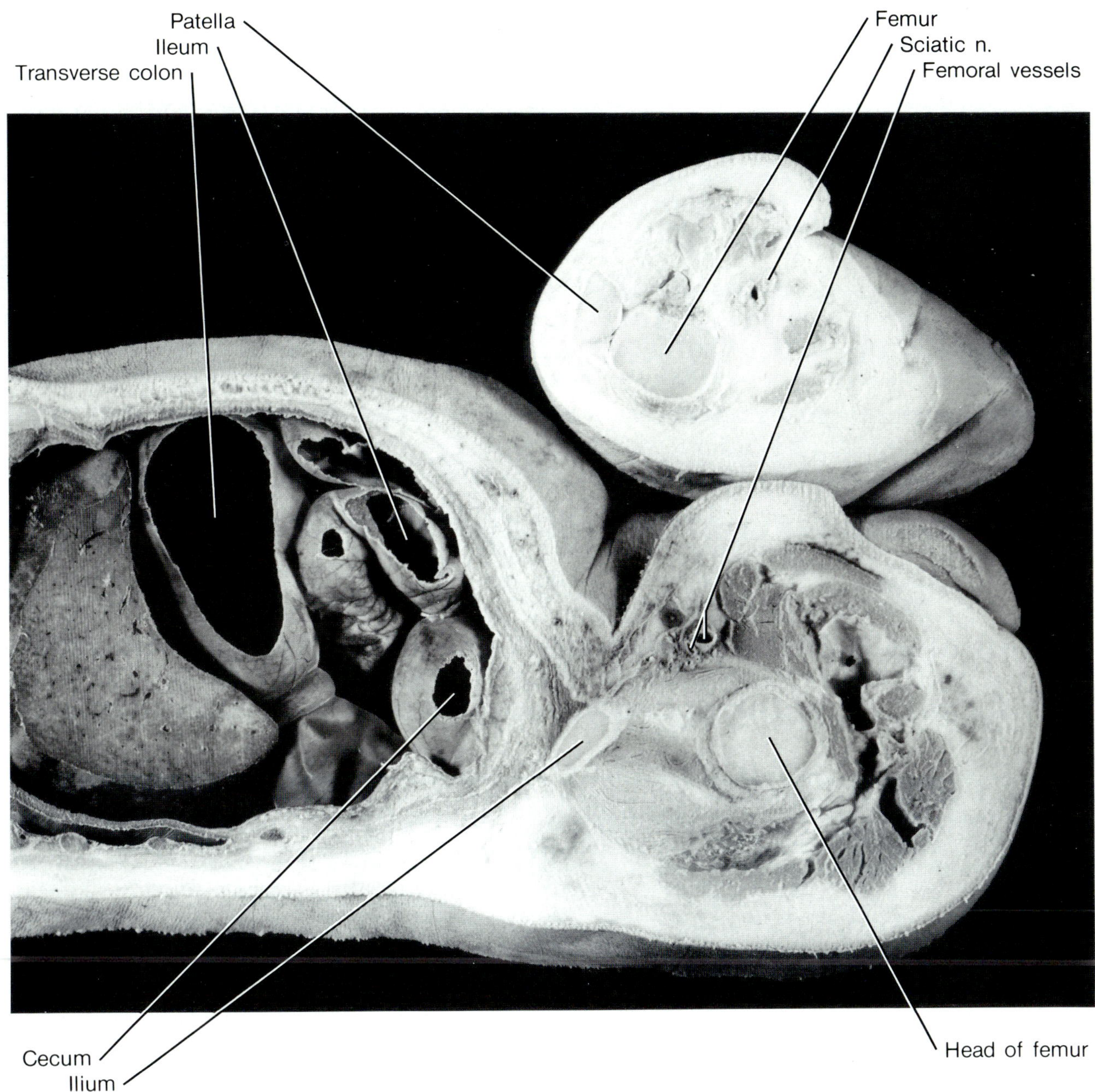

Patella
Ileum
Transverse colon
Femur
Sciatic n.
Femoral vessels
Cecum
Ilium
Head of femur

Femoral vessels
Fovea of head of femur
Transverse colon
Gall bladder
Acetabulum
Iliacus abdominis m.
Ilium
Cecum
Liver
Hepatic flexure
of colon
Ascending colon

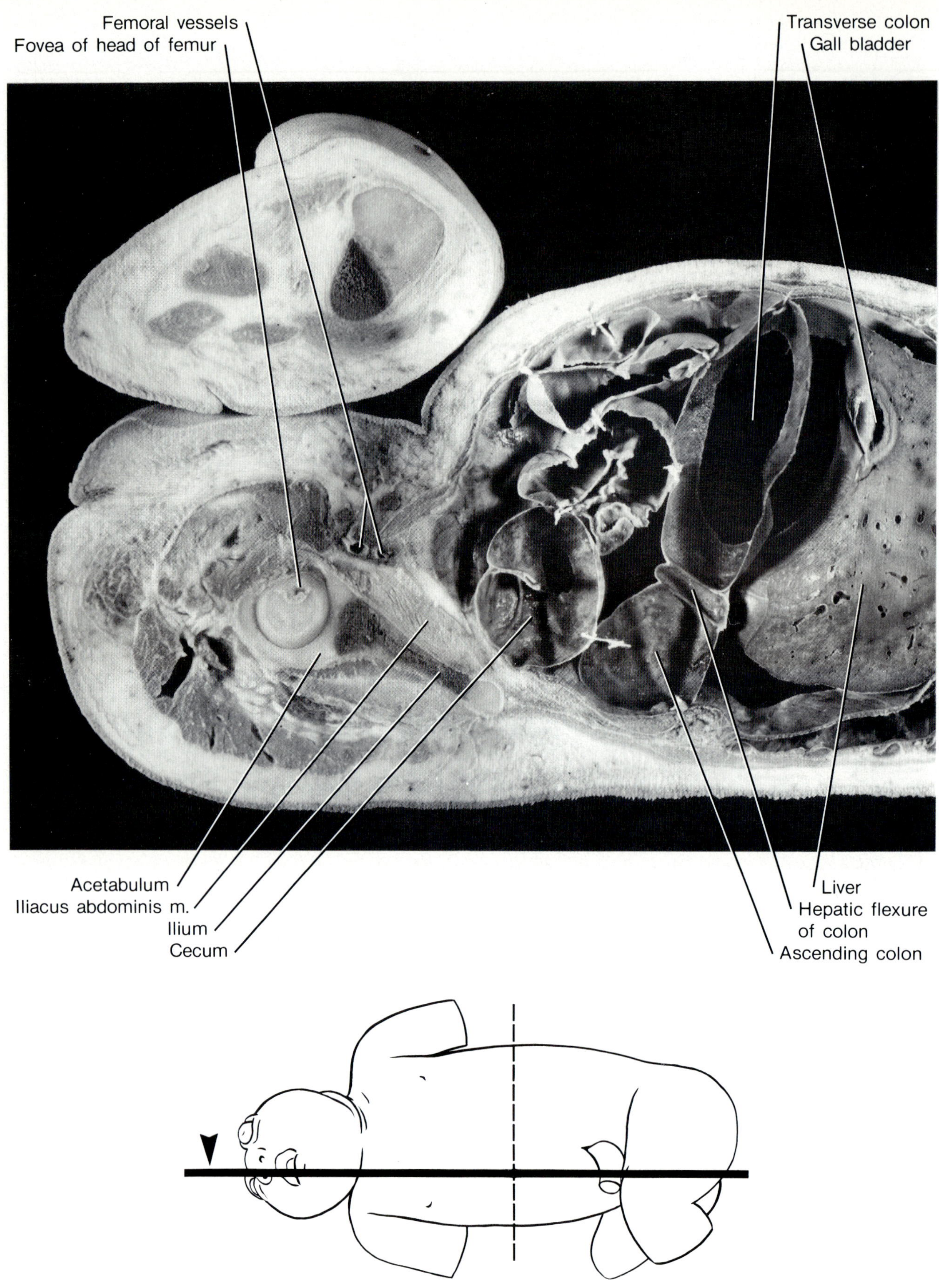

Figure 4.6

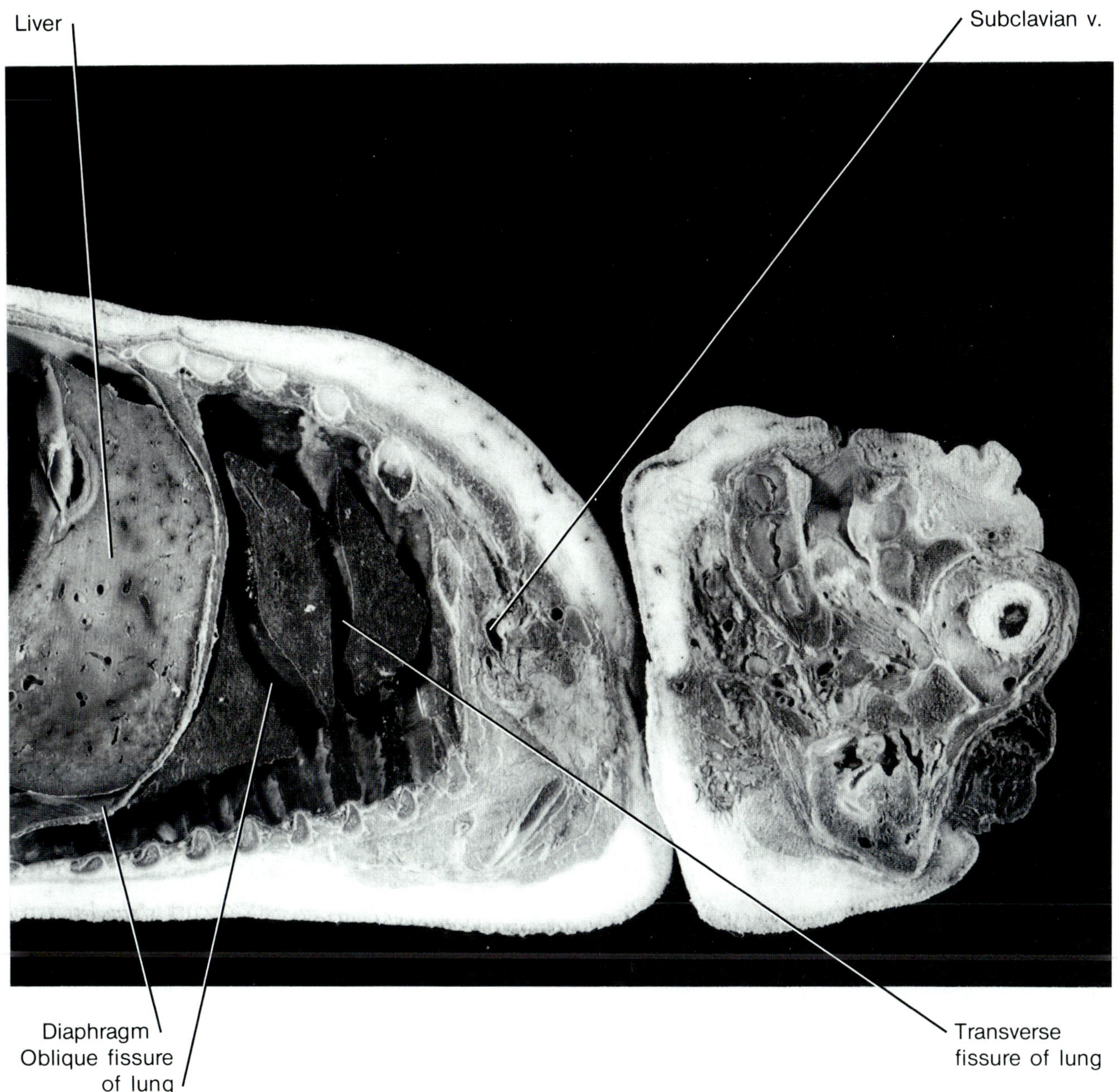

Liver
Subclavian v.
Diaphragm
Oblique fissure
of lung
Transverse
fissure of lung

Right subclavian v.
Clavicle
Middle lobe of lung
Diaphragm
Scapula
Upper lobe
of right lung
Lower lobe
of lung

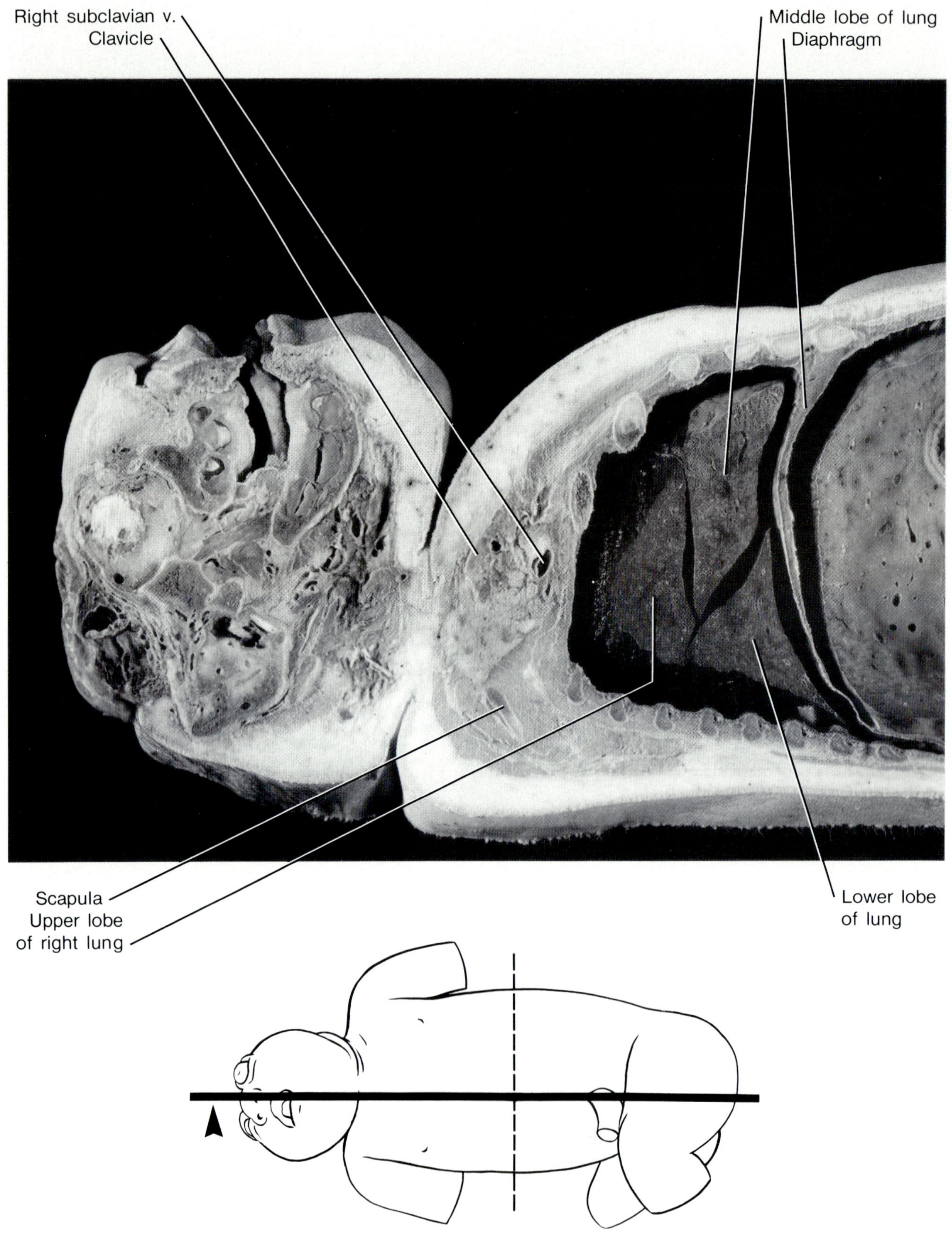

Figure 4.7

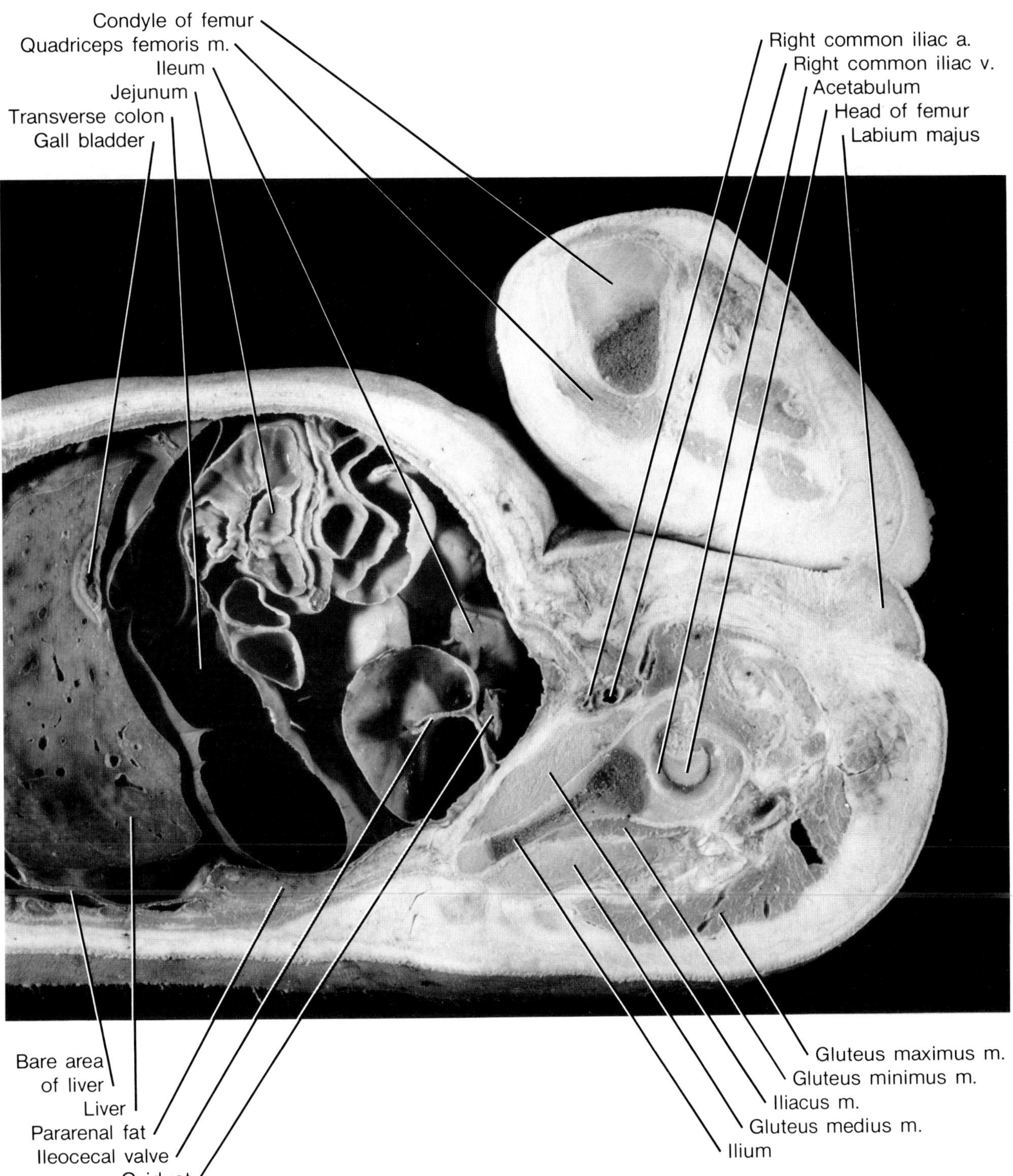

Condyle of femur
Quadriceps femoris m.
Ileum
Jejunum
Transverse colon
Gall bladder
Right common iliac a.
Right common iliac v.
Acetabulum
Head of femur
Labium majus
Bare area
of liver
Liver
Pararenal fat
Ileocecal valve
Oviduct
Gluteus maximus m.
Gluteus minimus m.
Iliacus m.
Gluteus medius m.
Ilium

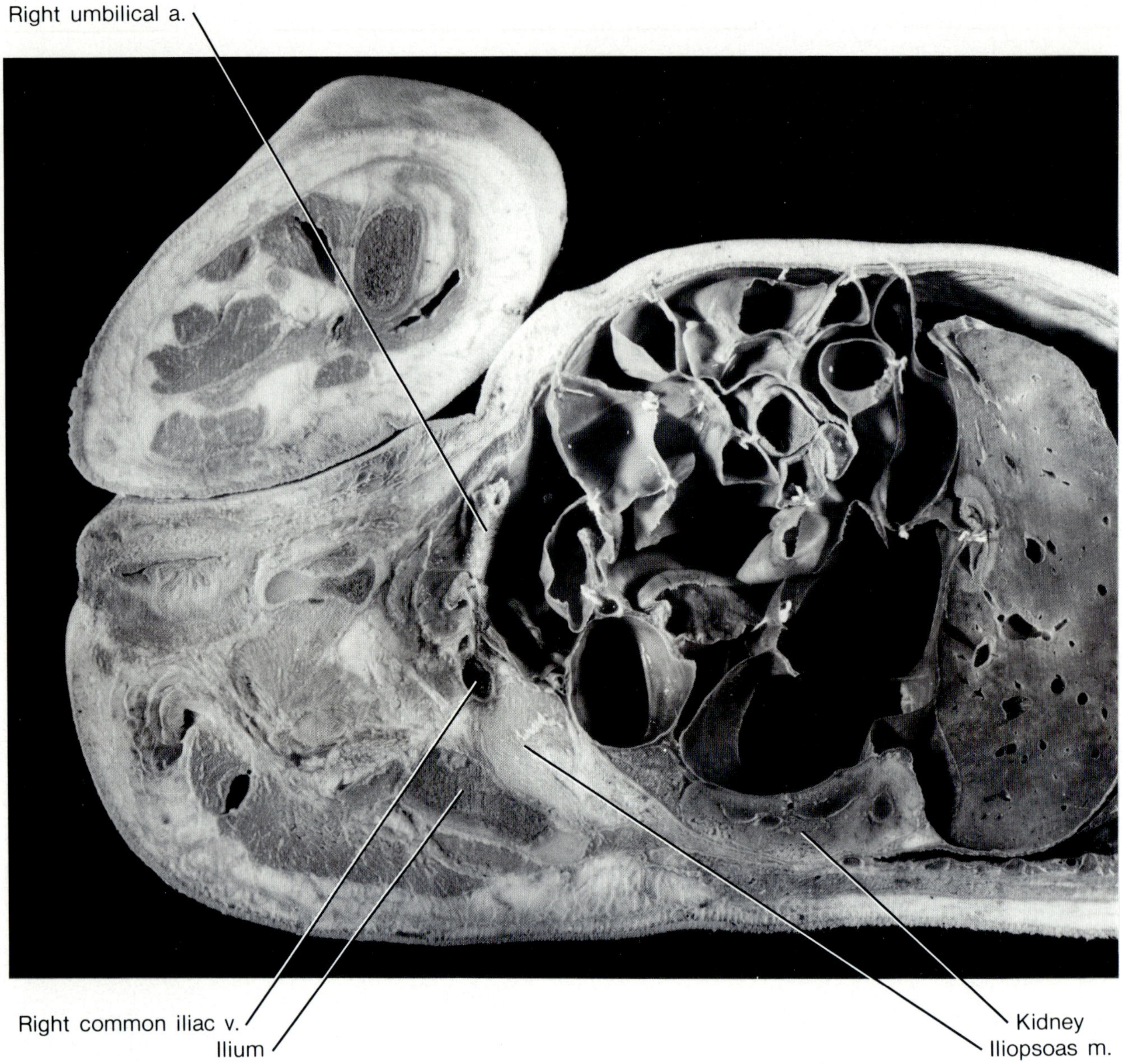

Right umbilical a.

Right common iliac v.
Ilium

Kidney
Iliopsoas m.

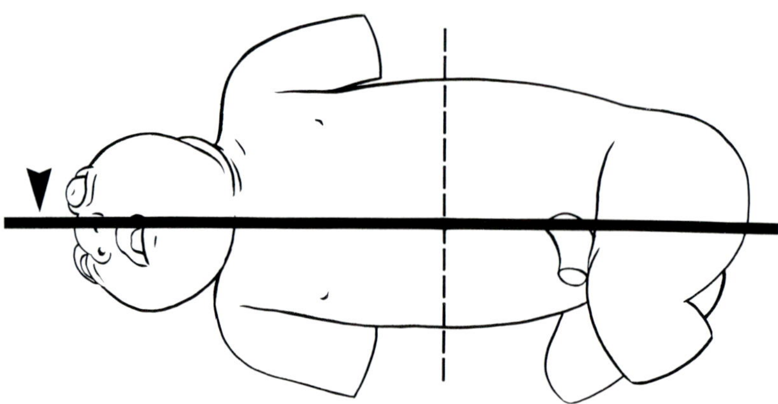

Figure 4.8

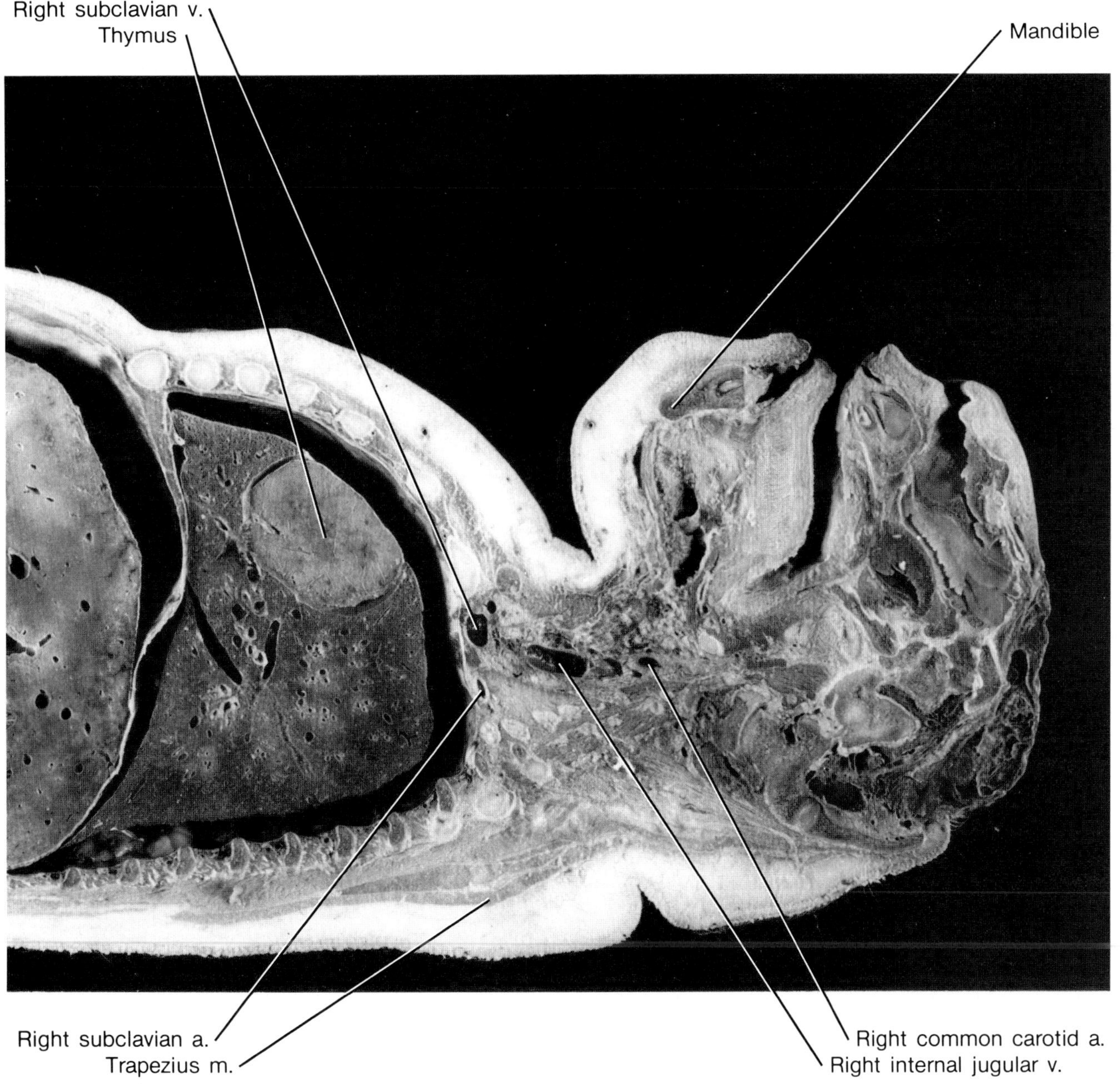

Right subclavian v.
Thymus
Mandible
Right subclavian a.
Trapezius m.
Right common carotid a.
Right internal jugular v.

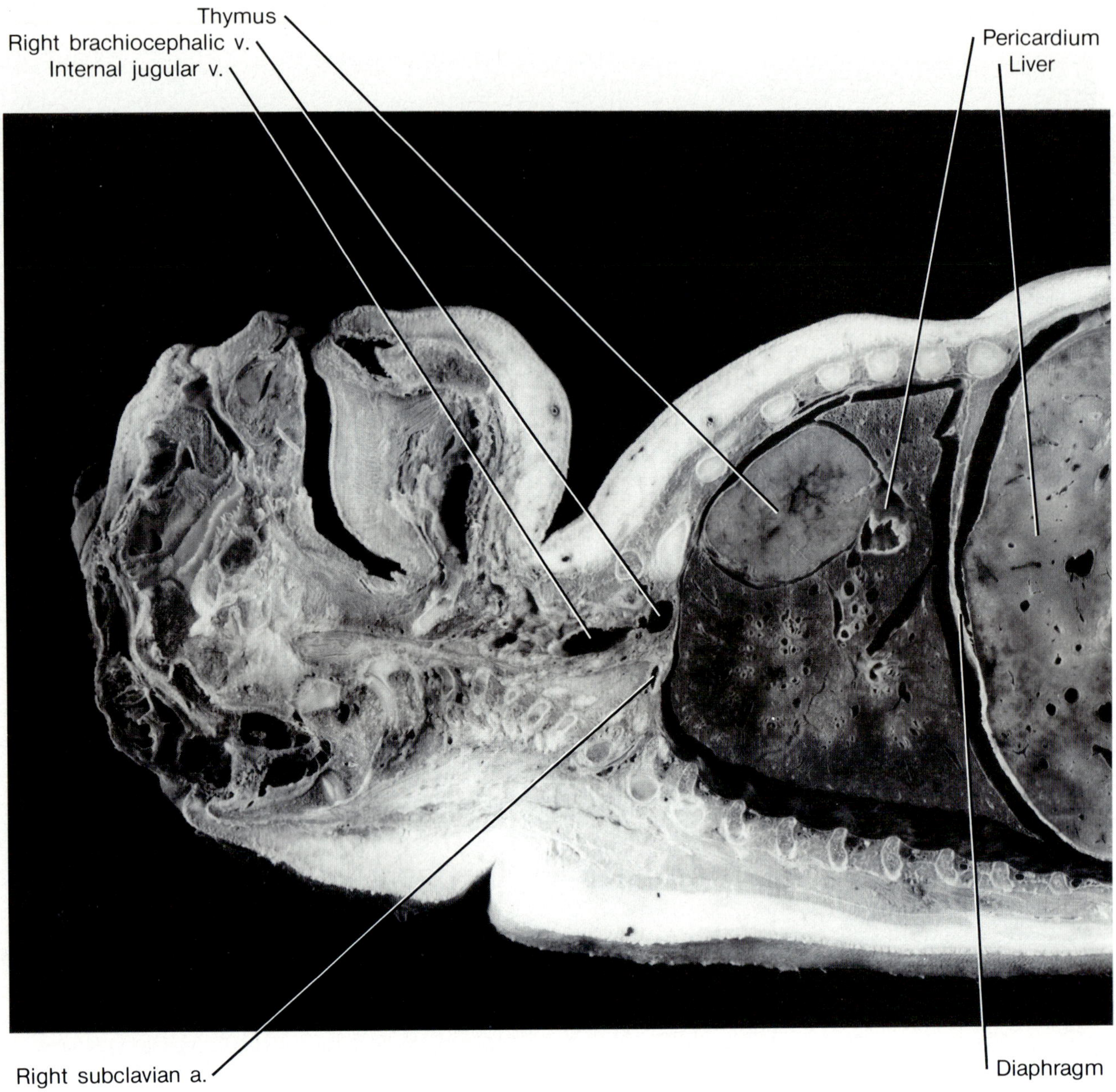

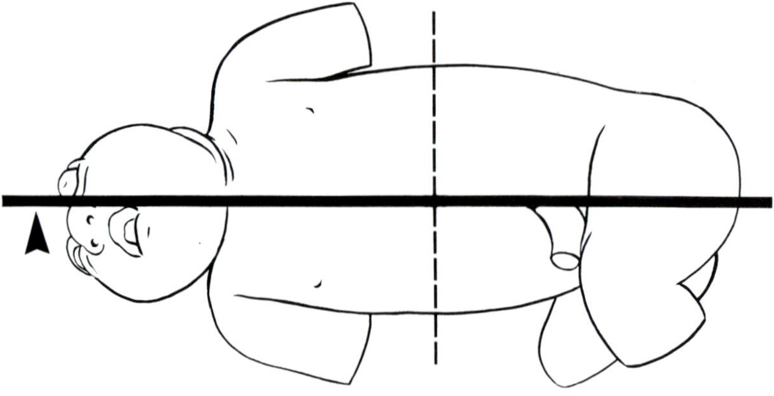

Figure 4.9

    FETAL SECTIONAL ANATOMY AND ULTRASONOGRAPHY

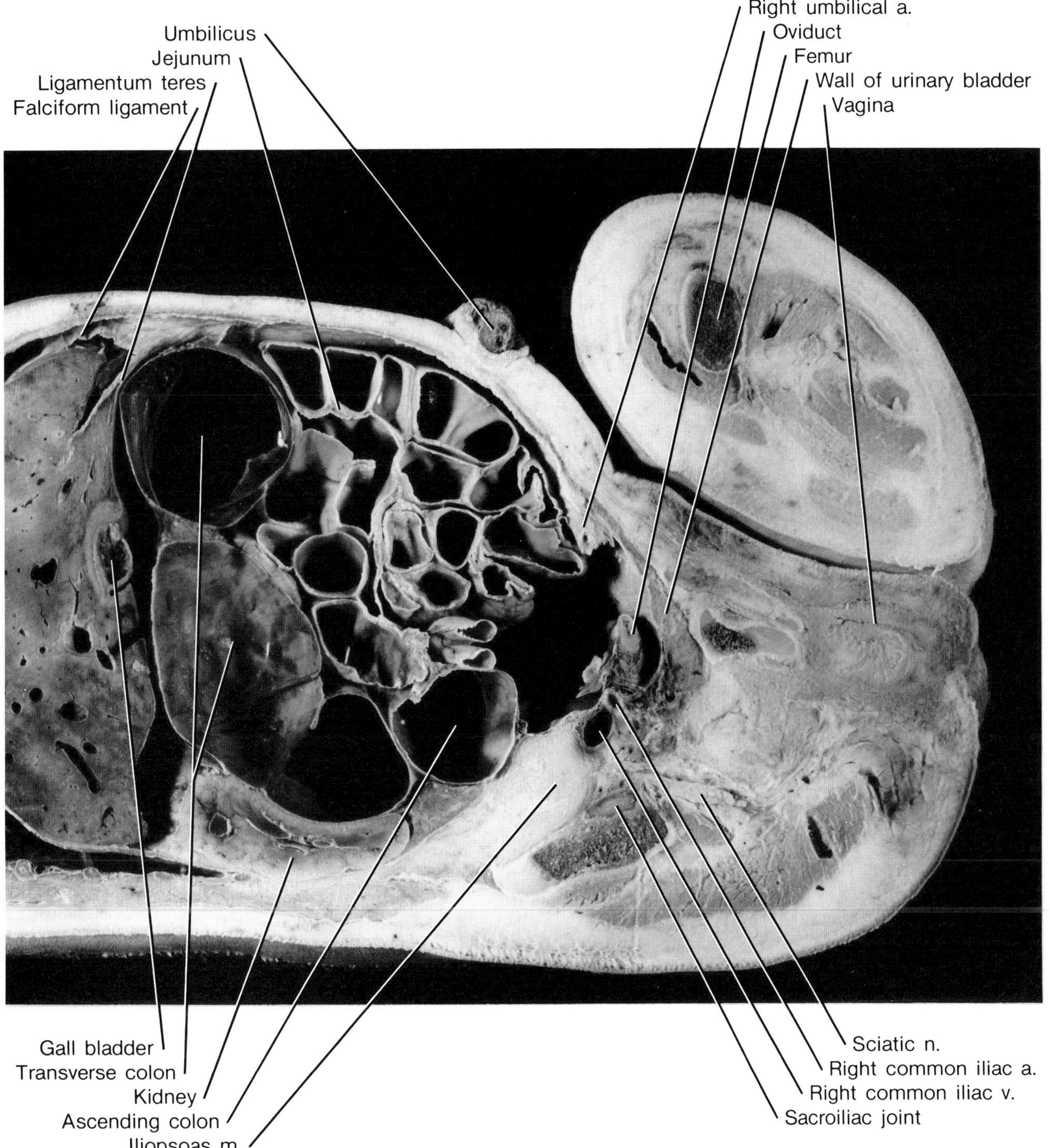

Umbilicus
Jejunum
Ligamentum teres
Falciform ligament
Right umbilical a.
Oviduct
Femur
Wall of urinary bladder
Vagina
Gall bladder
Transverse colon
Kidney
Ascending colon
Iliopsoas m.
Sciatic n.
Right common iliac a.
Right common iliac v.
Sacroiliac joint

Bladder
Pubis
Anterior and
posterior fornices
Vagina
Renal v.
Transverse colon
Superior portion
of duodenum
Ligamentum teres
Anal canal
Rectum
Sigmoid colon
Common iliac vessels
Ureter
Portal v.
Right suprarenal gland
Kidney
Ascending colon
Ileum

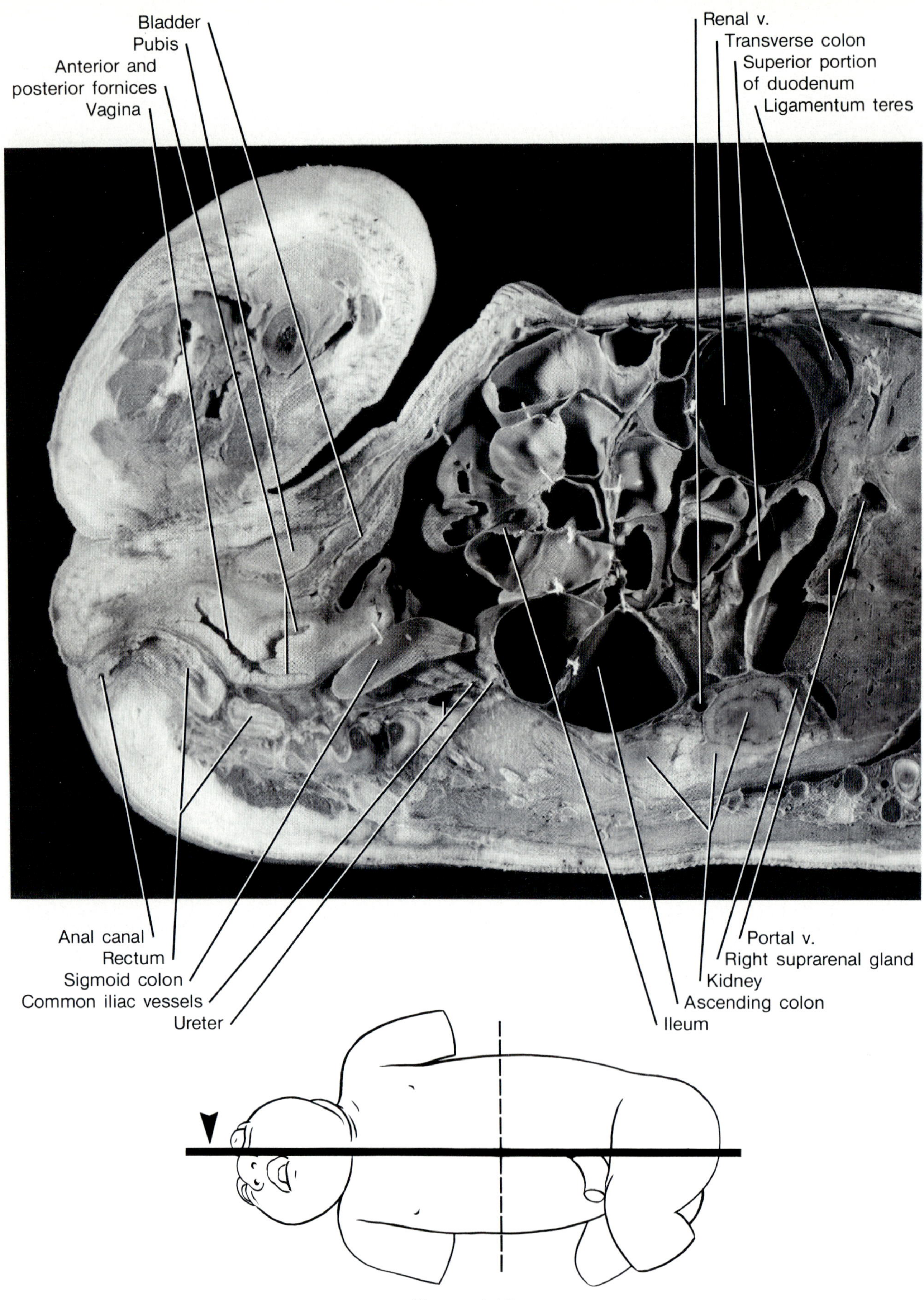

Figure 4.10

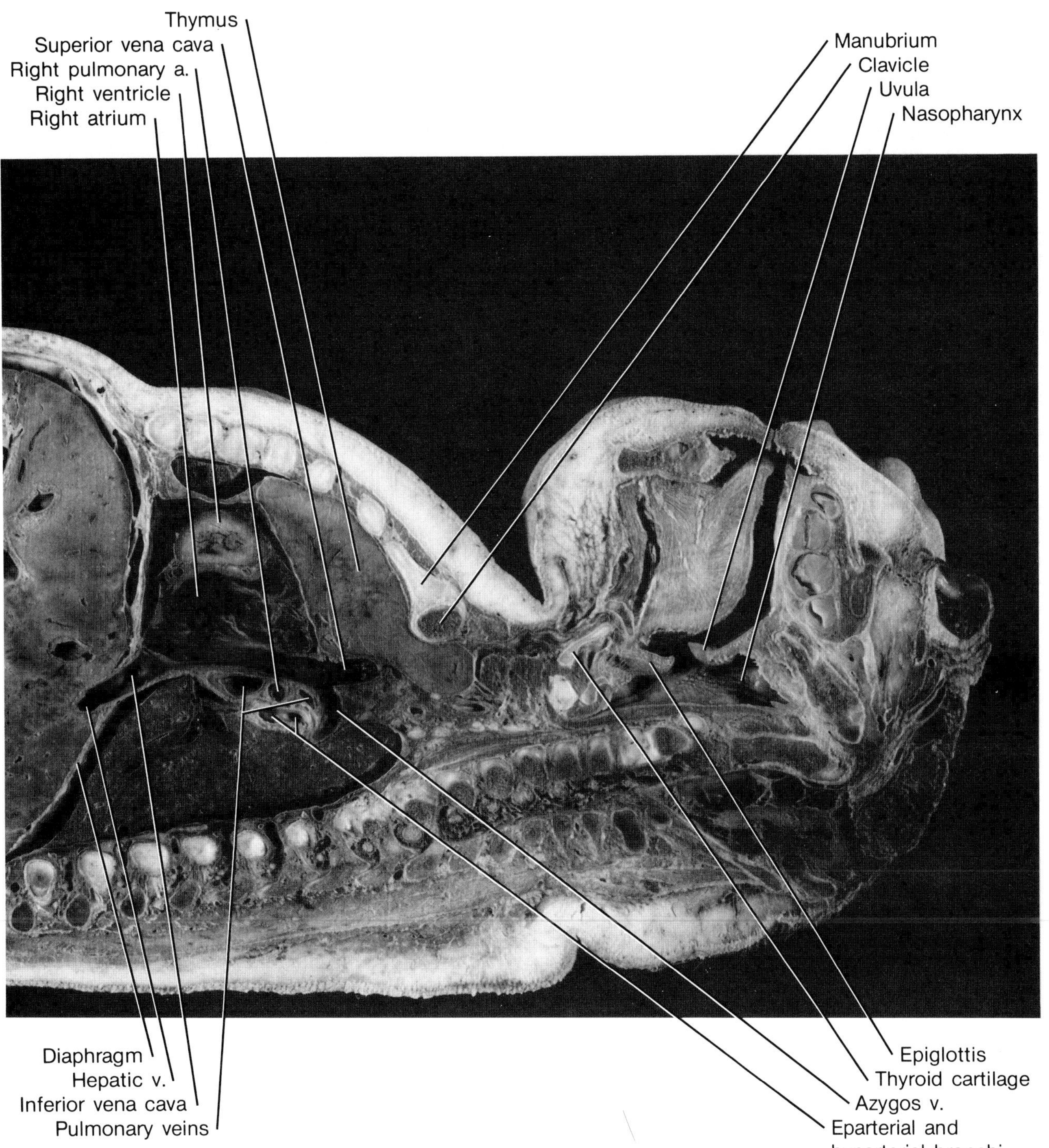

Thymus
Superior vena cava
Right pulmonary a.
Right ventricle
Right atrium
Manubrium
Clavicle
Uvula
Nasopharynx
Diaphragm
Hepatic v.
Inferior vena cava
Pulmonary veins
Epiglottis
Thyroid cartilage
Azygos v.
Eparterial and
hyparterial bronchi

Thymus
Manubrium
Pulmonary arteries
Clavicle
Tongue
Right auricle
Pulmonary veins
Right ventricle
Hepatic v.
Epiglottis
Thyroid cartilage
Cricoid cartilage
Brachiocephalic a.
Superior vena cava
Inferior vena cava
Lung
Right atrium
Right main bronchus
Arch of azygos v.

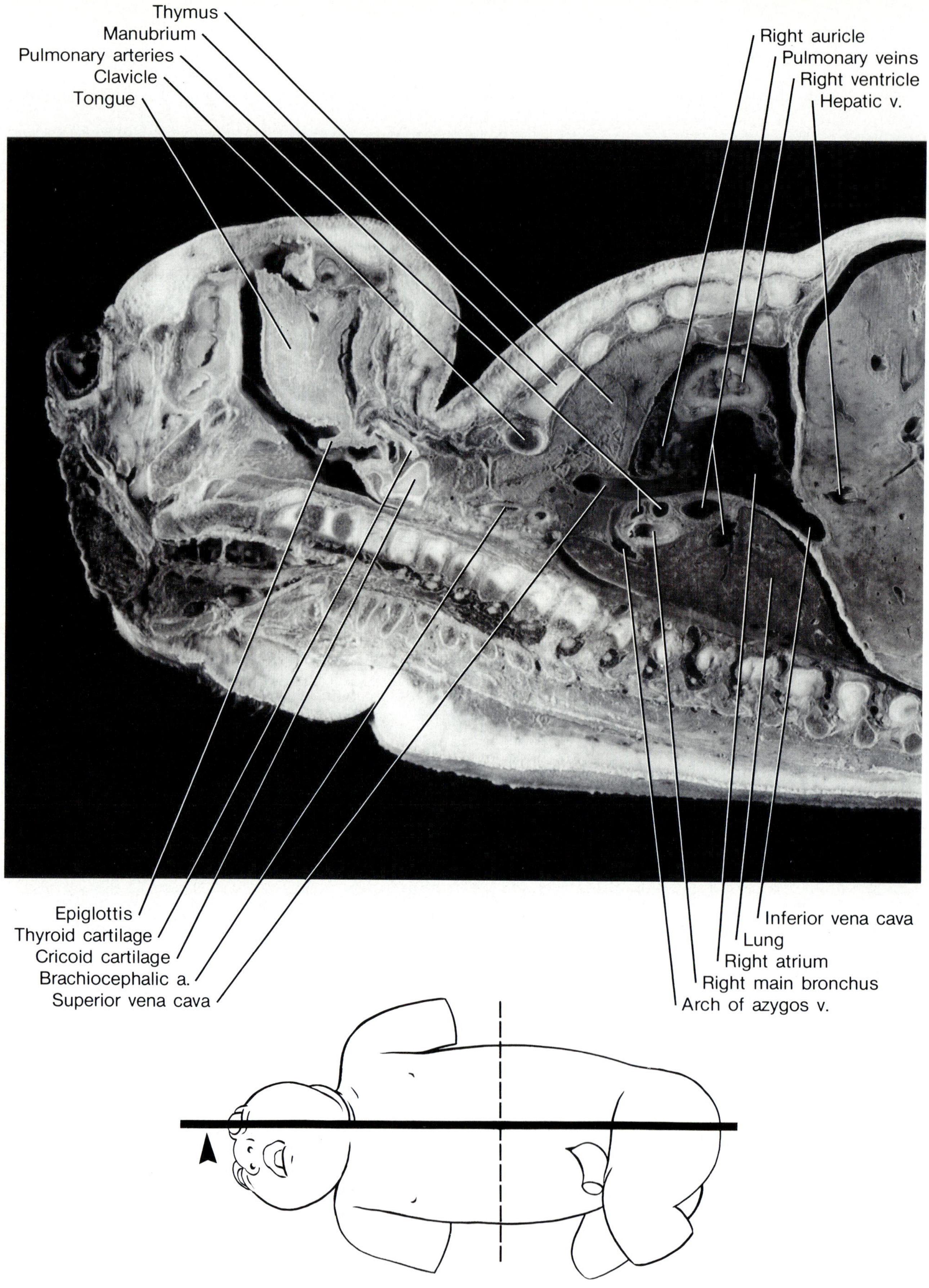

Figure 4.11

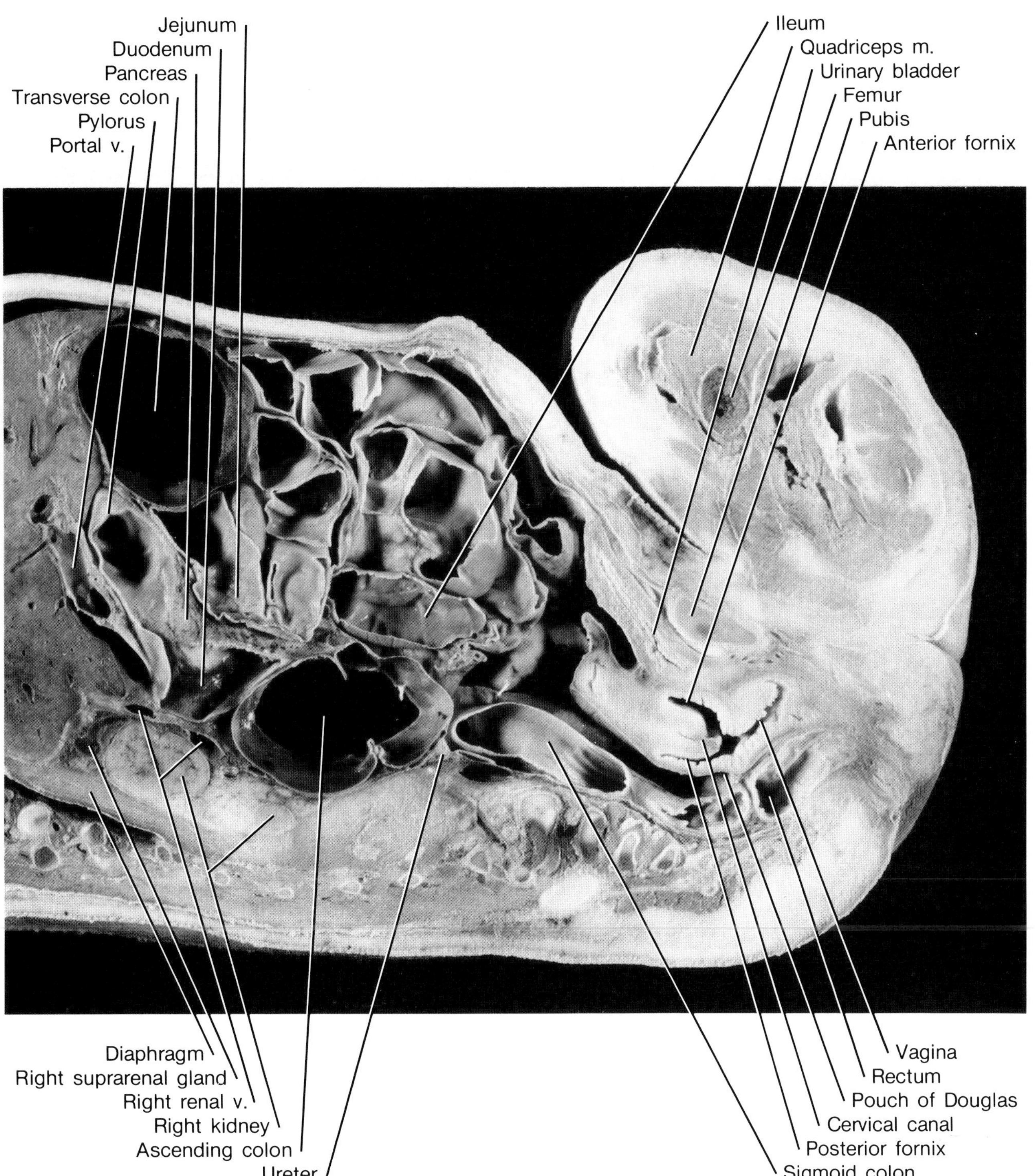

Jejunum
Duodenum
Pancreas
Transverse colon
Pylorus
Portal v.
Ileum
Quadriceps m.
Urinary bladder
Femur
Pubis
Anterior fornix
Diaphragm
Right suprarenal gland
Right renal v.
Right kidney
Ascending colon
Ureter
Vagina
Rectum
Pouch of Douglas
Cervical canal
Posterior fornix
Sigmoid colon

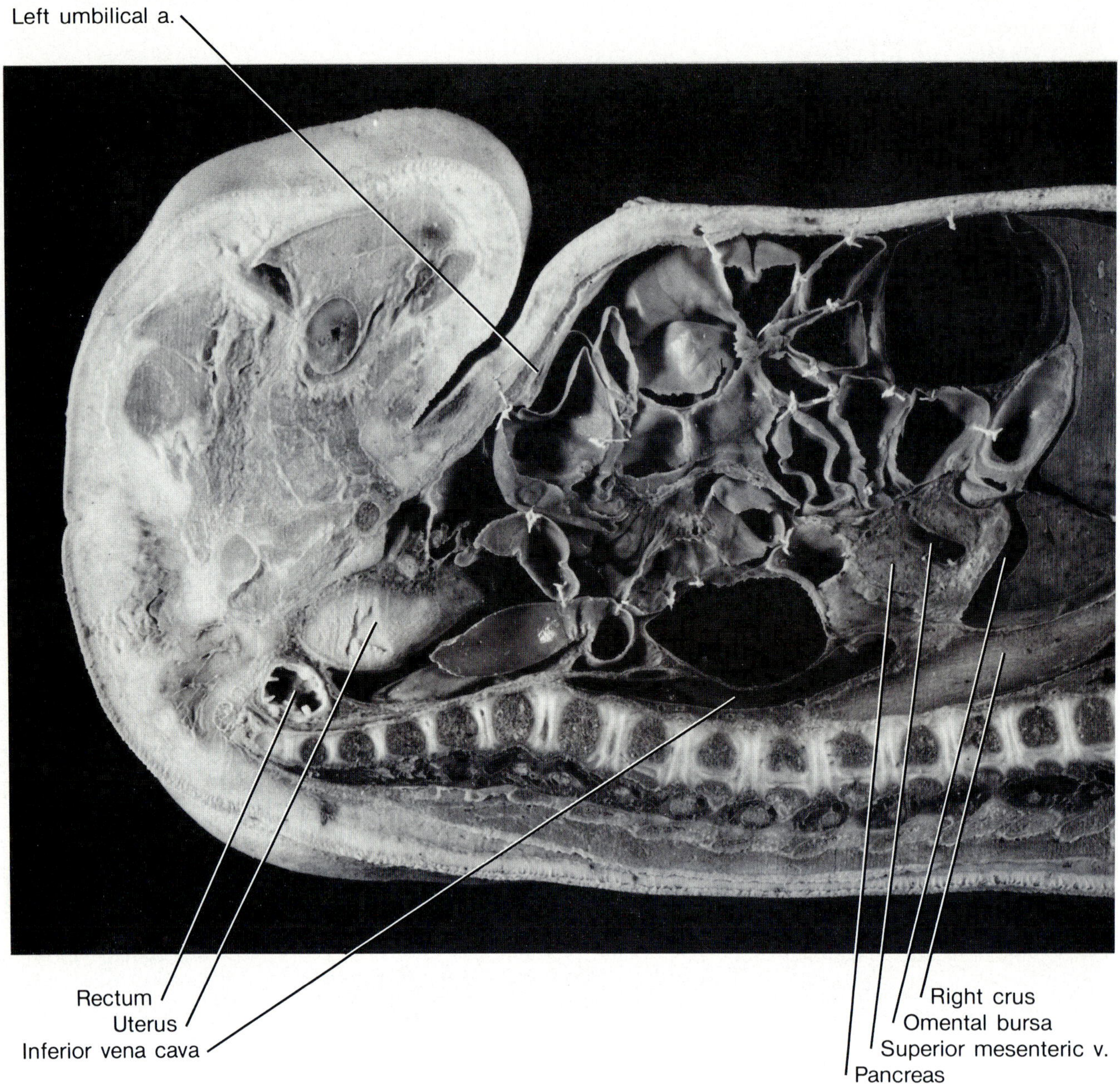

Left umbilical a.
Rectum
Uterus
Inferior vena cava
Right crus
Omental bursa
Superior mesenteric v.
Pancreas

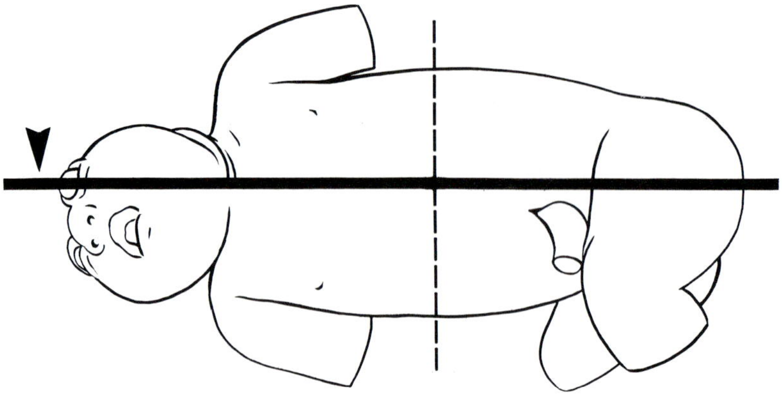

Figure 4.12

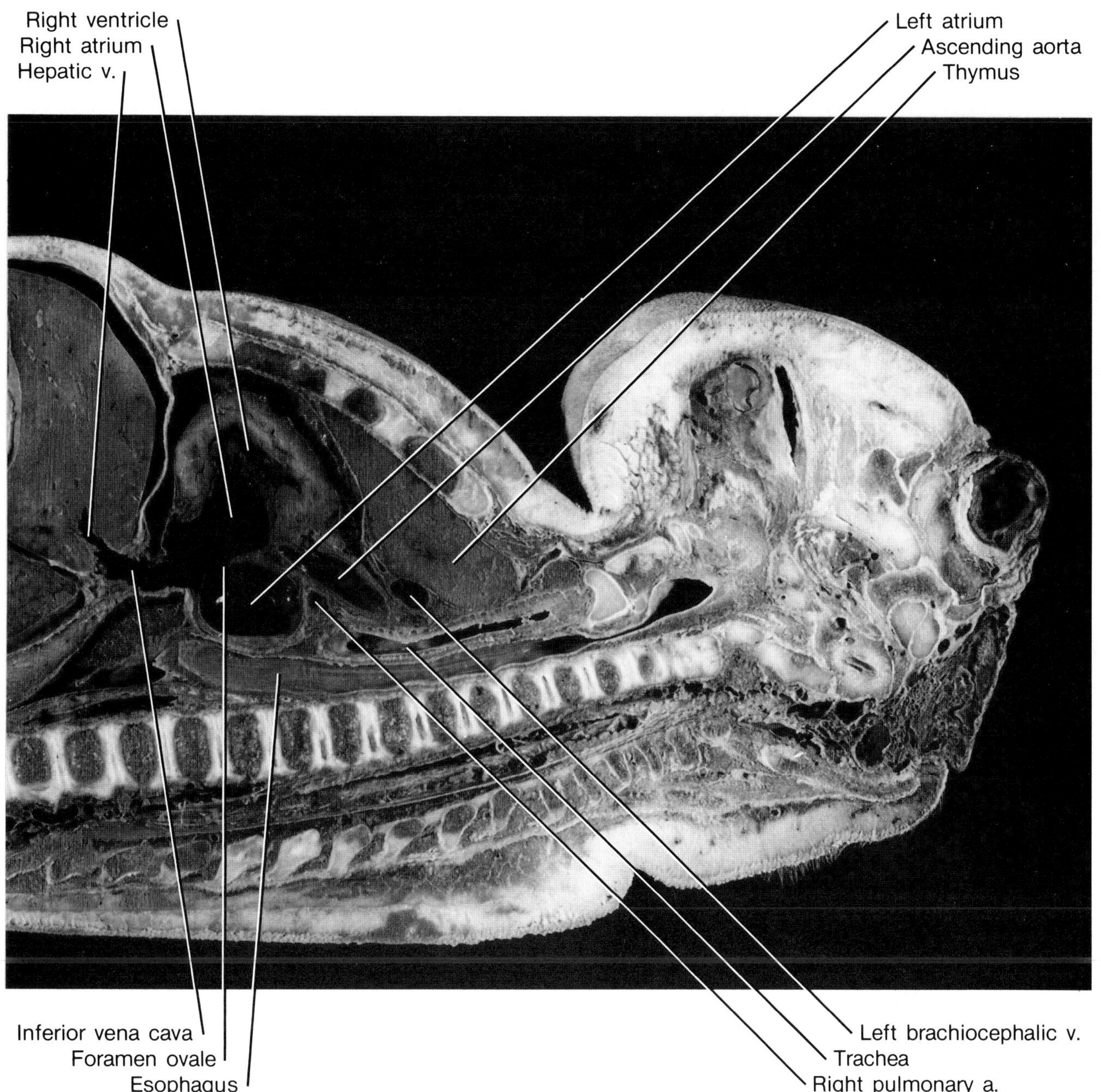

Right ventricle
Right atrium
Hepatic v.
Left atrium
Ascending aorta
Thymus
Inferior vena cava
Foramen ovale
Esophagus
Left brachiocephalic v.
Trachea
Right pulmonary a.

Ascending aorta
Trachea
Esophagus
Right ventricle
Right atrium
Opening of
coronary sinus
Left brachiocephalic v.
Right pulmonary a.
Left main bronchus
Lesser omentum
Spinal cord
Left atrium

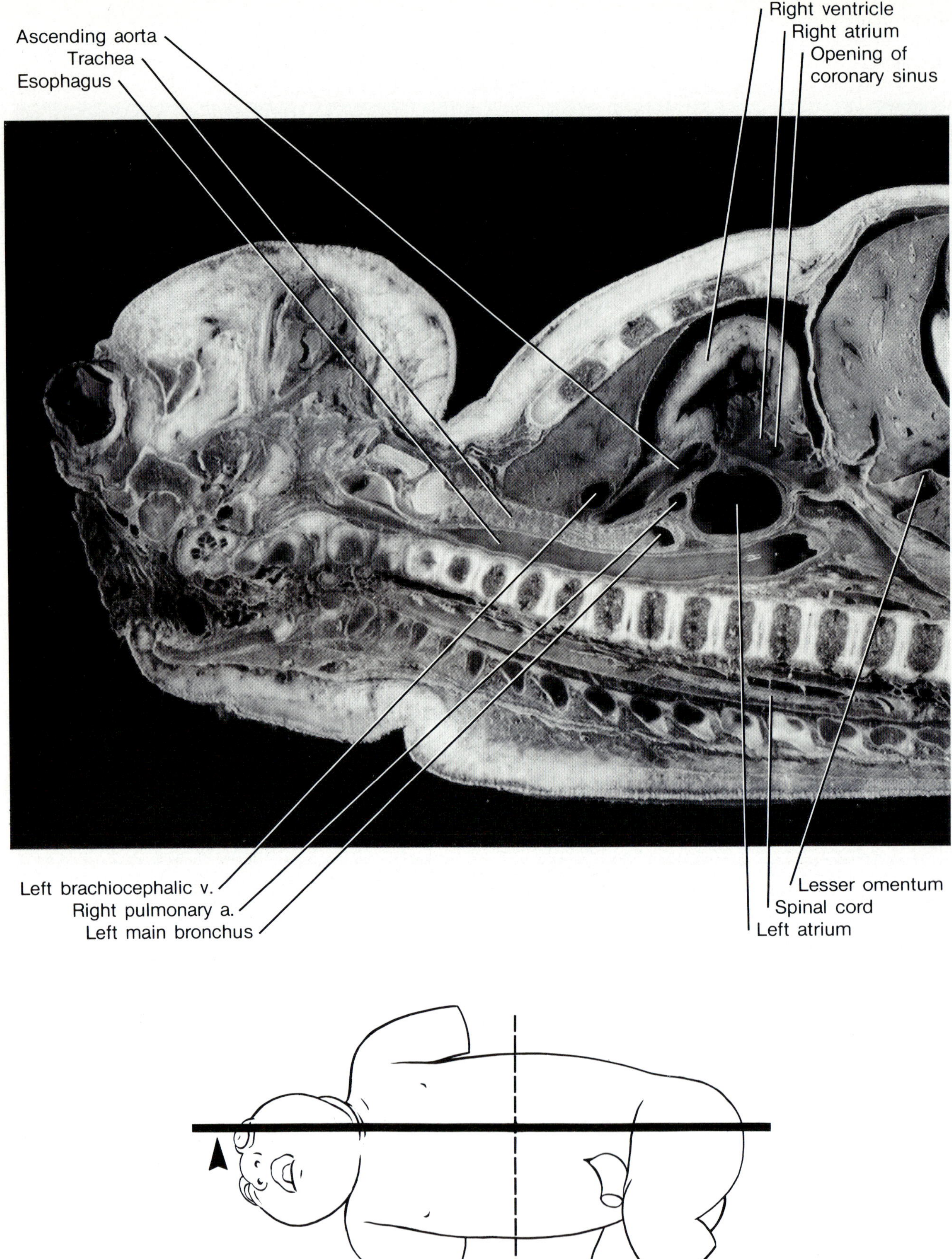

Figure 4.13

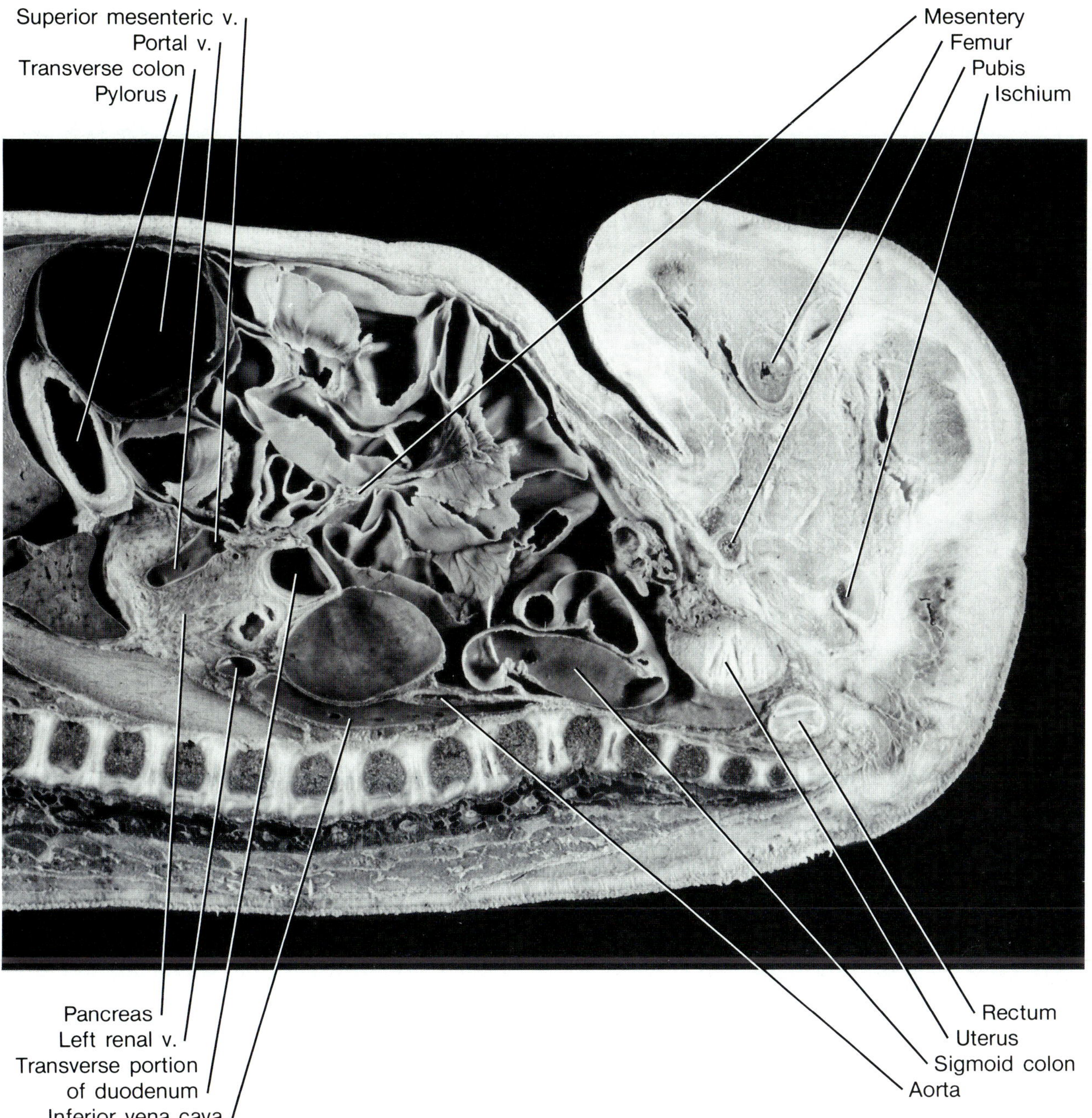

Superior mesenteric v.
Portal v.
Transverse colon
Pylorus
Mesentery
Femur
Pubis
Ischium
Pancreas
Left renal v.
Transverse portion
of duodenum
Inferior vena cava
Rectum
Uterus
Sigmoid colon
Aorta

Common iliac a.
Common iliac v.
Sigmoid colon
Pancreas
Left crus
of diaphragm

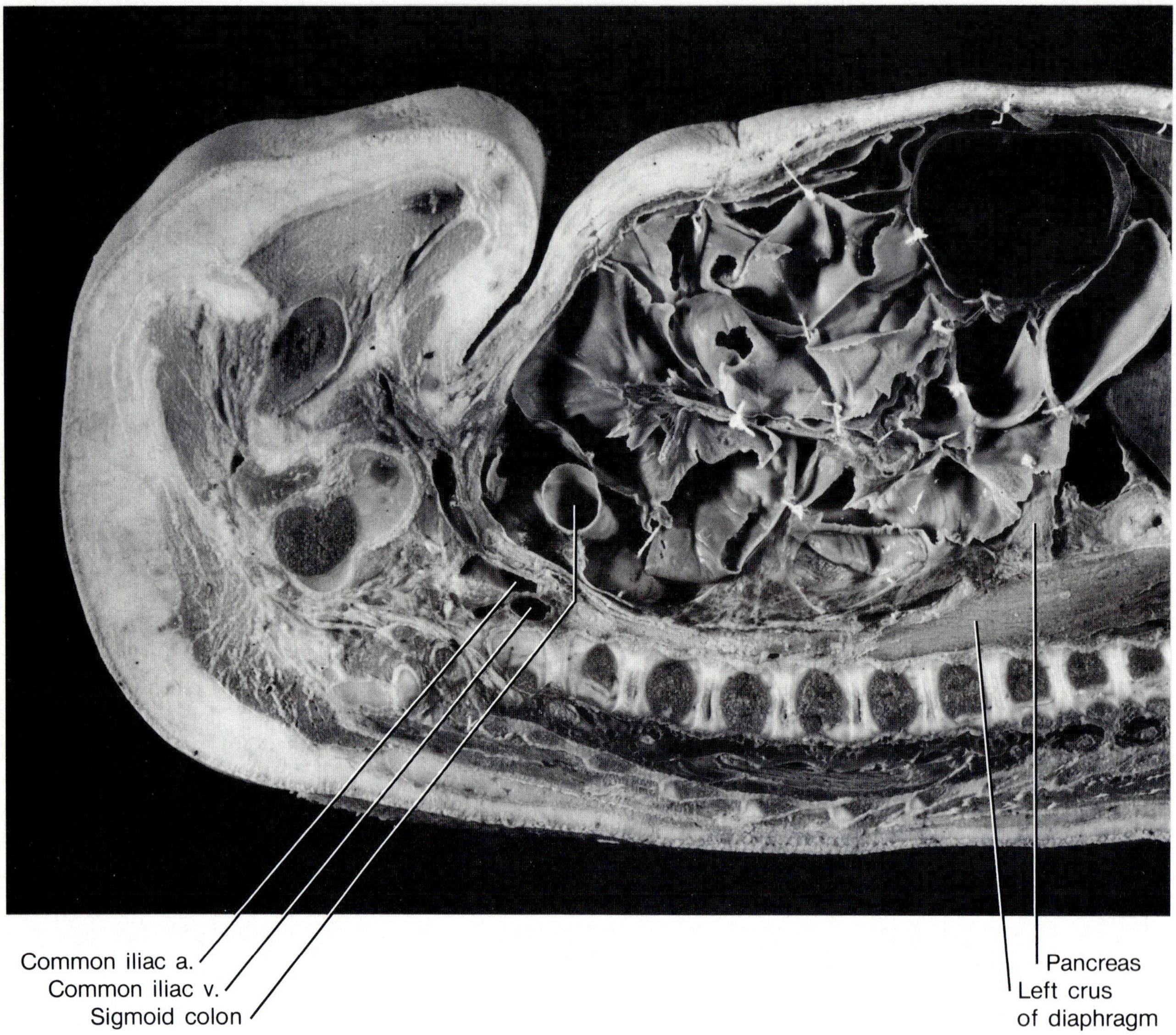

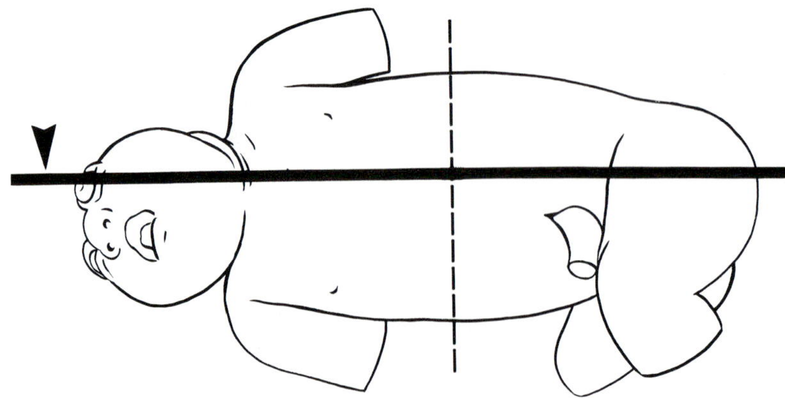

Figure 4.14

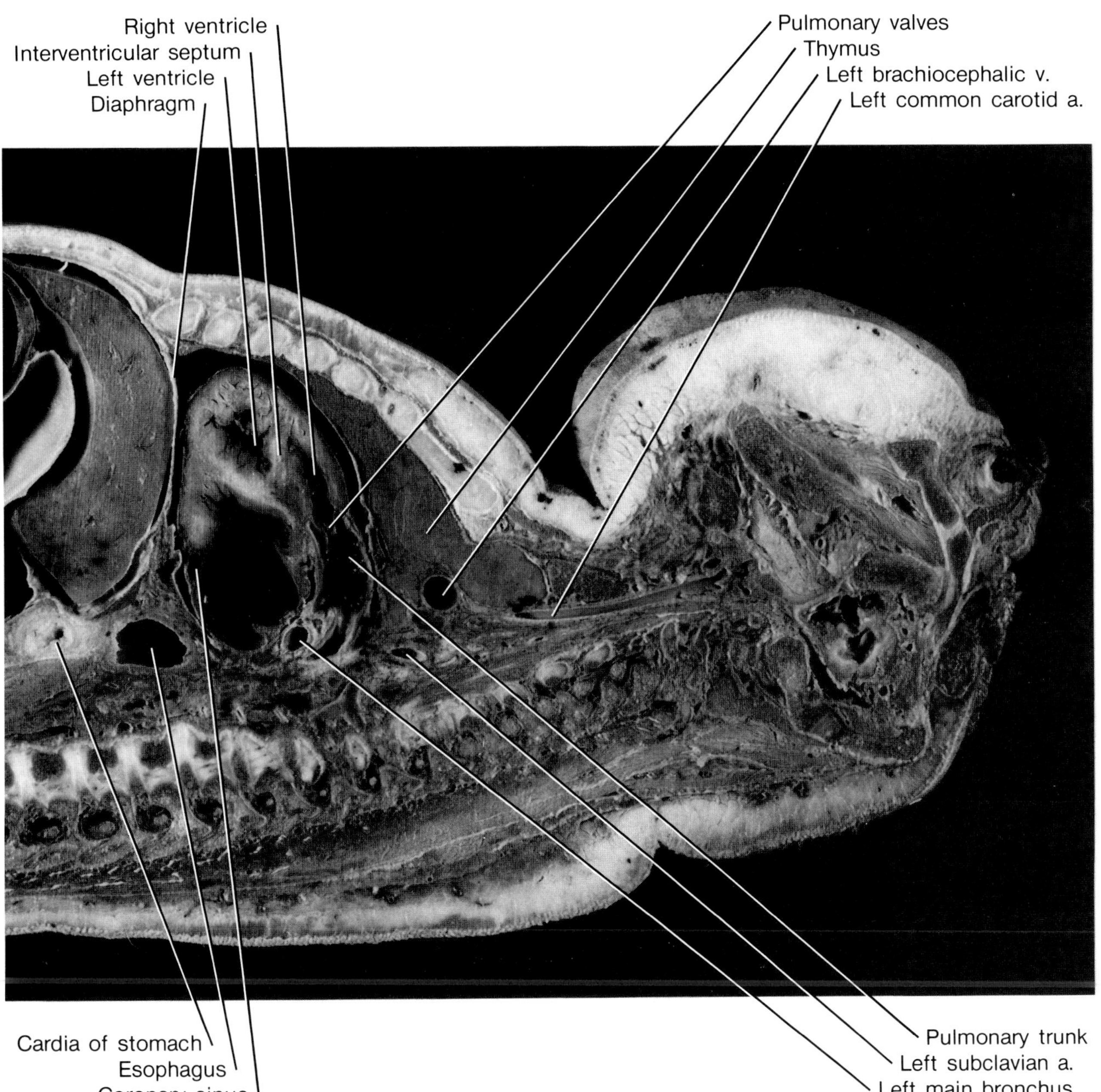

Right ventricle
Interventricular septum
Left ventricle
Diaphragm
Pulmonary valves
Thymus
Left brachiocephalic v.
Left common carotid a.
Cardia of stomach
Esophagus
Coronary sinus
Pulmonary trunk
Left subclavian a.
Left main bronchus

Right ventricle
Thymus
Manubrium
Pulmonary trunk
Left ventricle
Diaphragm
Lung
Liver
Left brachiocephalic v.
Left subclavian a.
Pleural cavity
Accessory hemiazygos v.
Left main bronchus
Cardia of stomach
Esophagus
Coronary sinus
Pulmonary v.
Left atrium

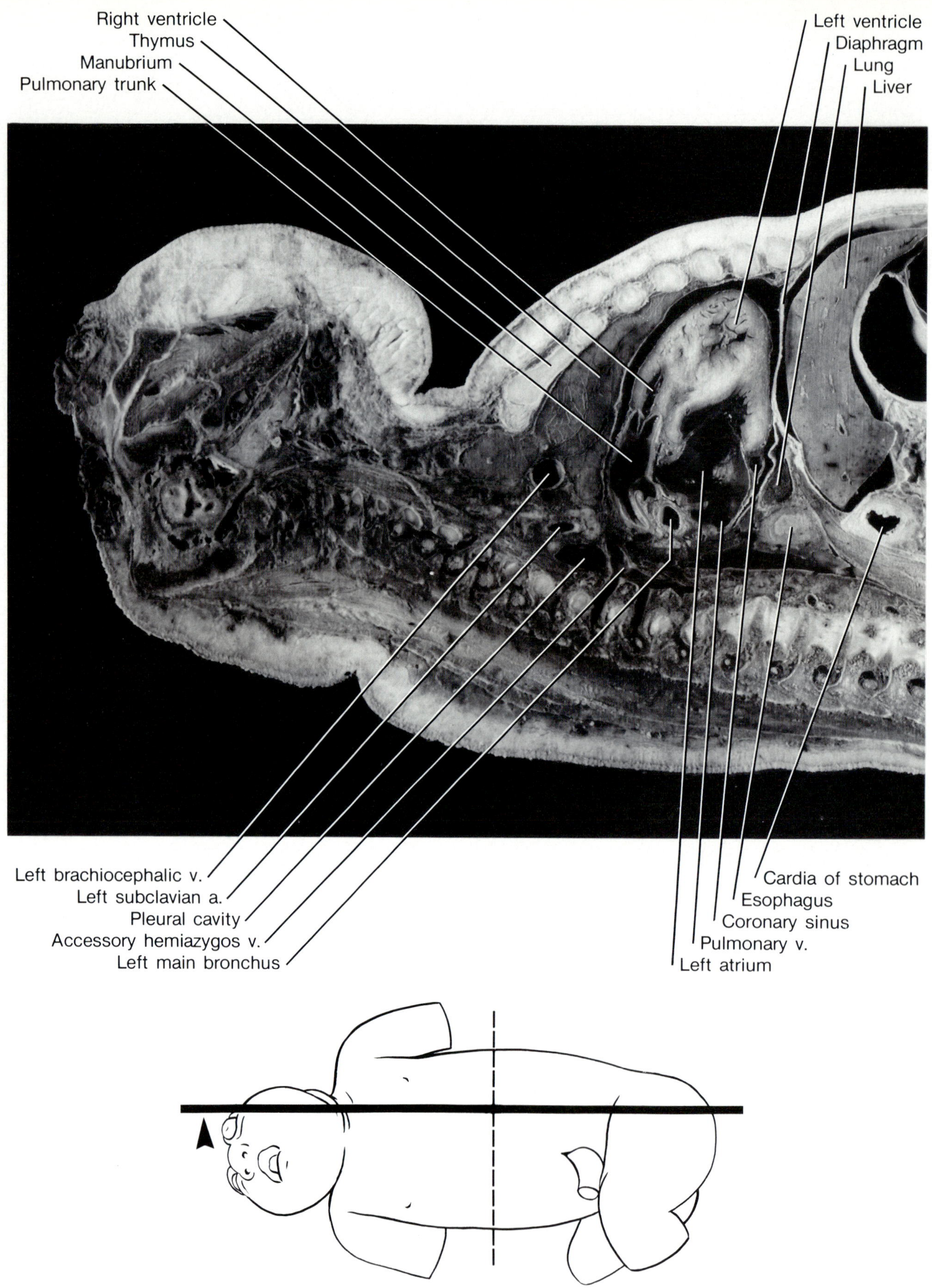

Figure 4.15

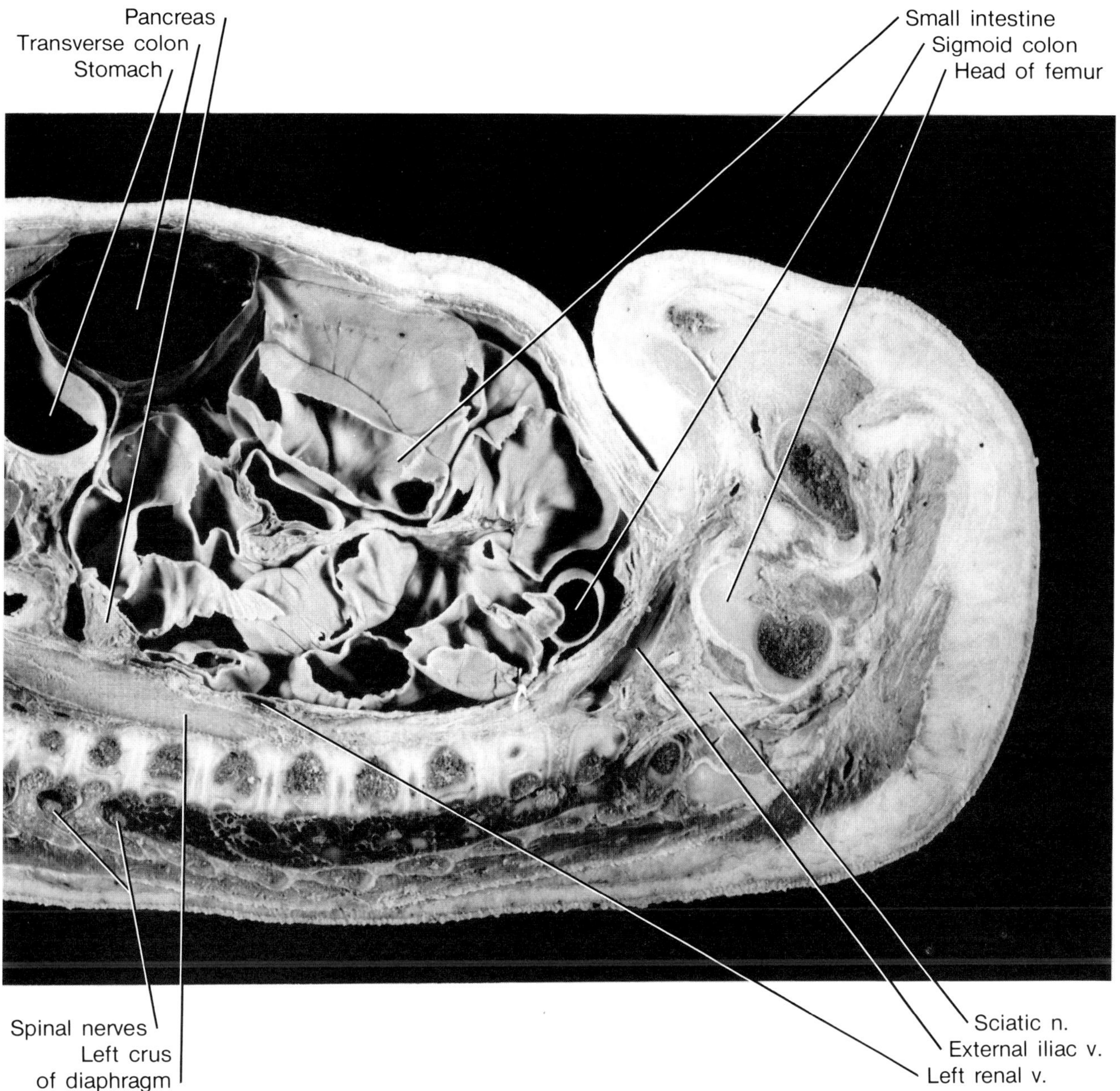

Pancreas
Transverse colon
Stomach
Small intestine
Sigmoid colon
Head of femur
Spinal nerves
Left crus
of diaphragm
Sciatic n.
External iliac v.
Left renal v.

Gluteus maximus m.
Head of femur
Acetabulum
Psoas m.
Spleen
Suprarenal gland
Left kidney
Left renal v.

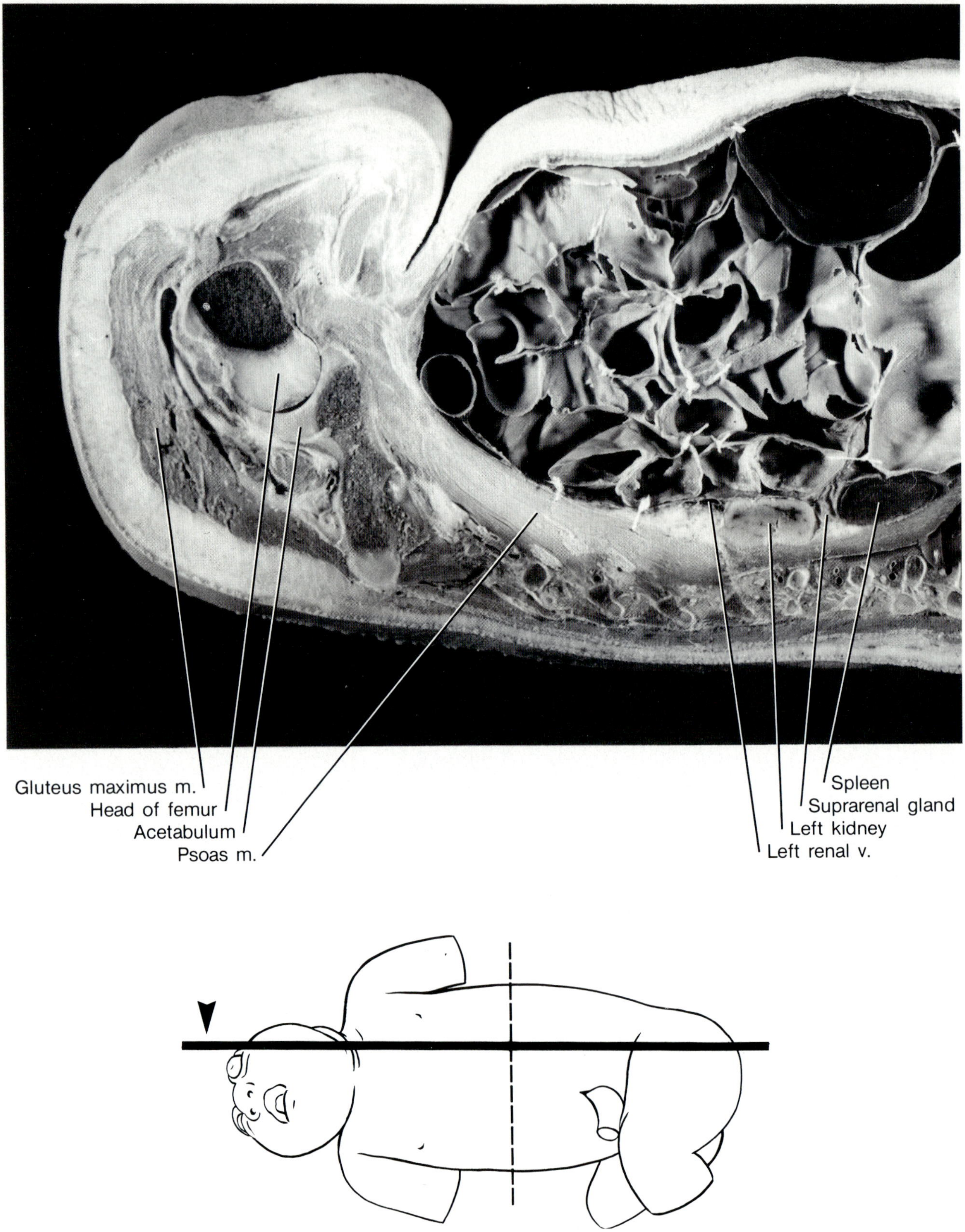

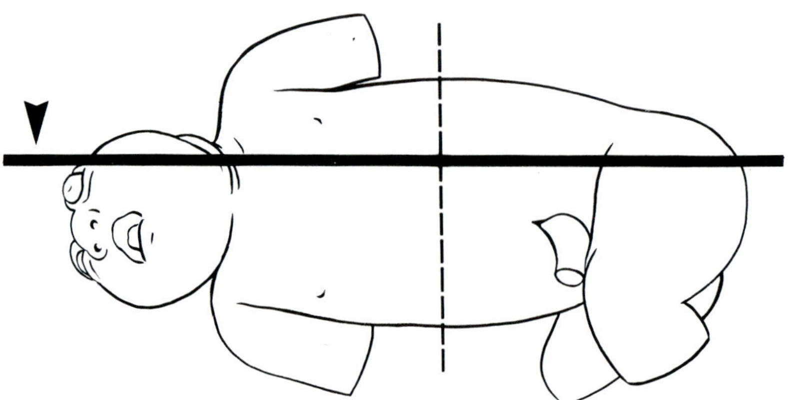

Figure 4.16

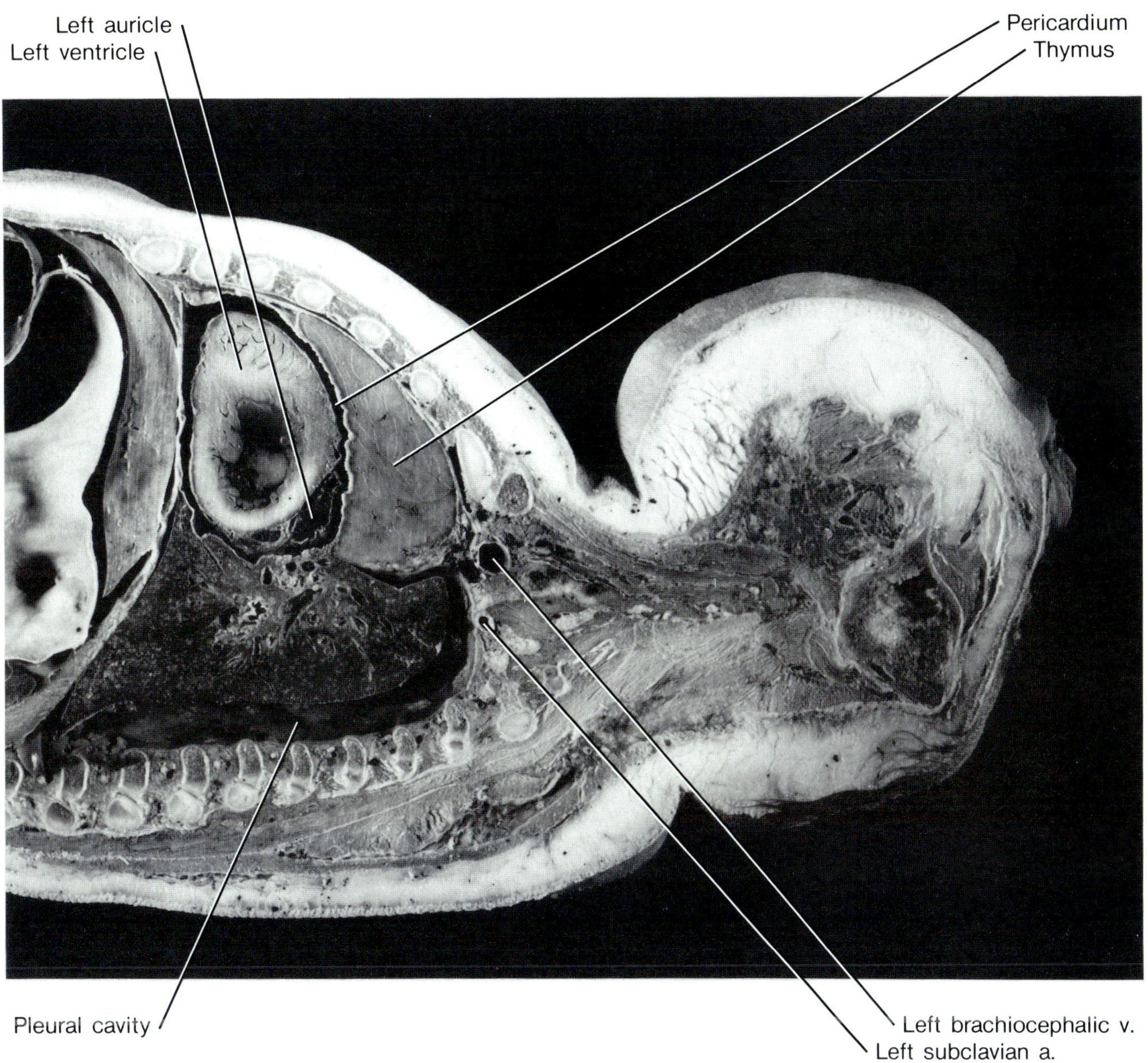

Left auricle
Left ventricle
Pericardium
Thymus
Pleural cavity
Left brachiocephalic v.
Left subclavian a.

Pericardial sac
Thymus
Clavicle
Left ventricle
Diaphragm
Left lobe of liver
Left brachiocephalic v.
Subclavian a.
Left lung
Pleural cavity

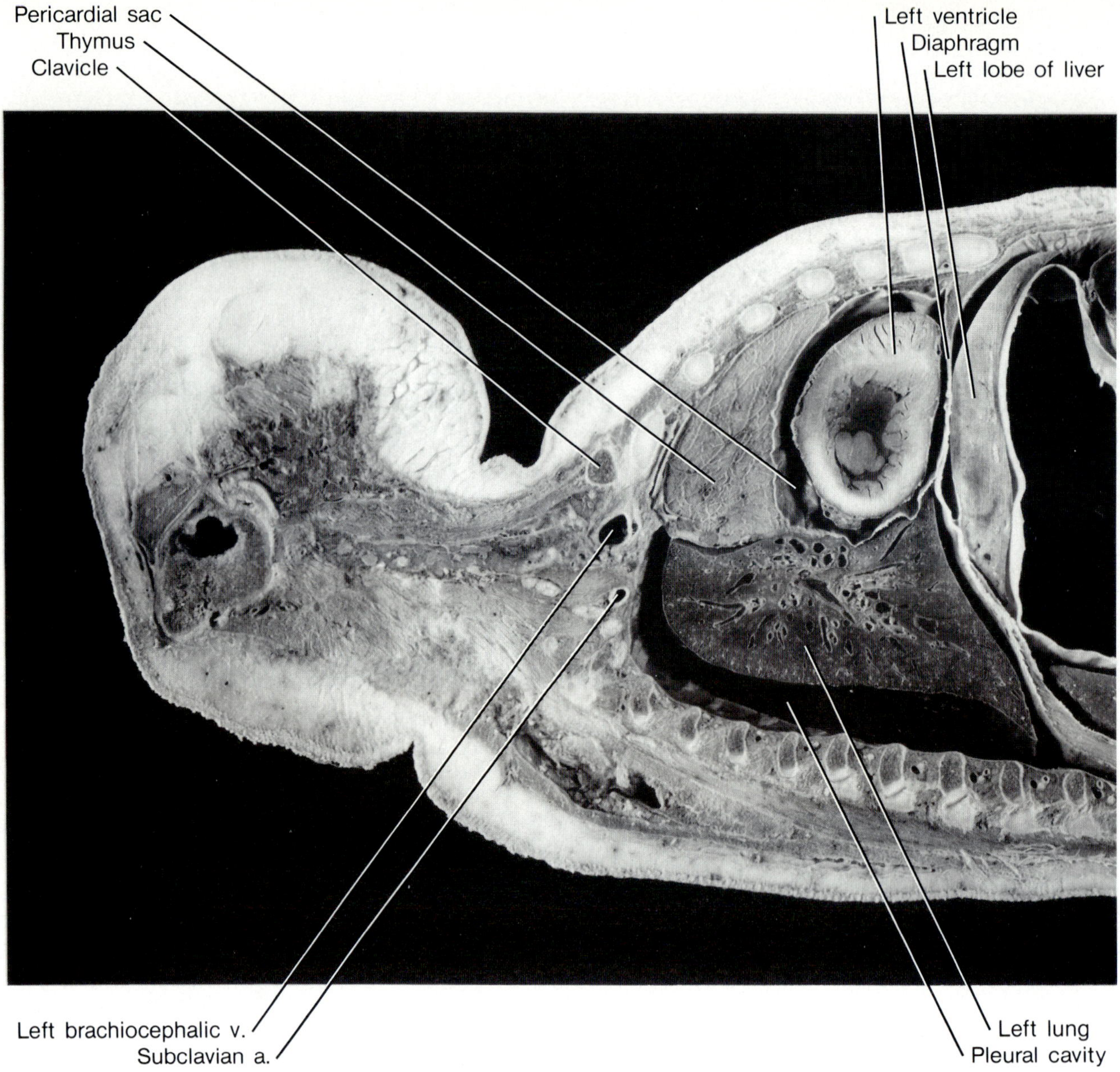

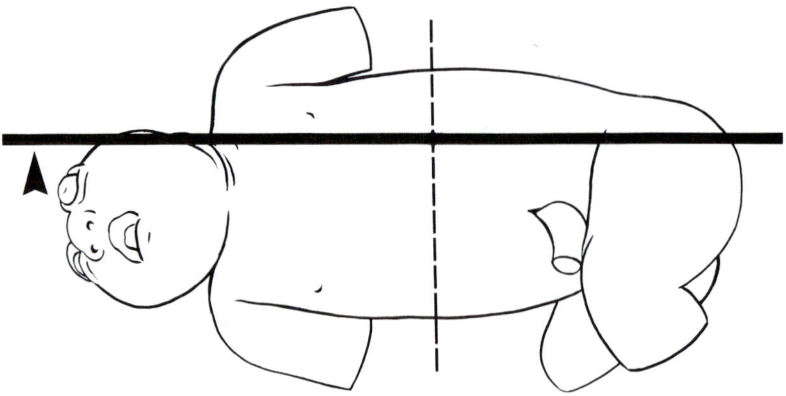

Figure 4.17

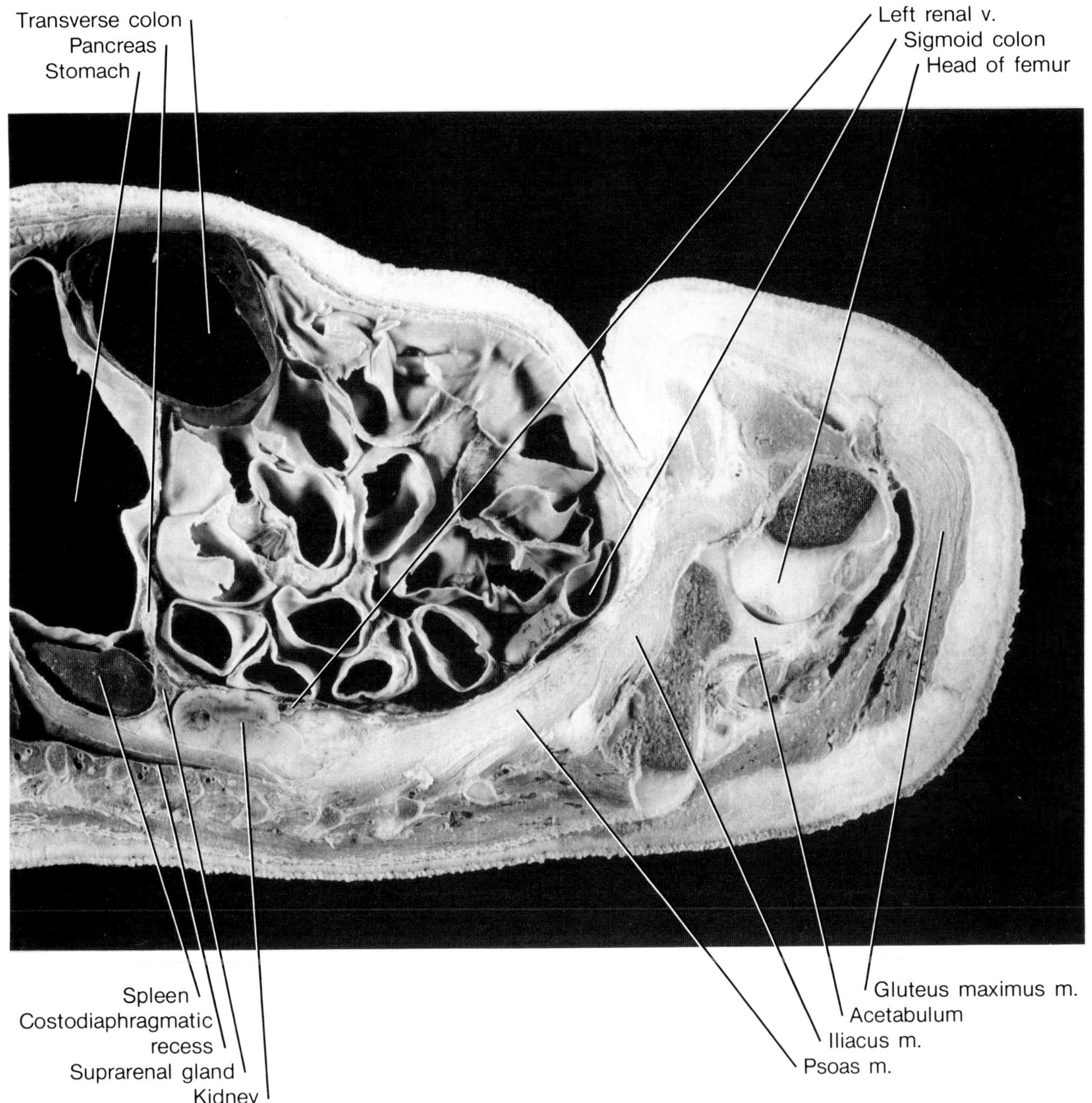

Transverse colon
Pancreas
Stomach
Left renal v.
Sigmoid colon
Head of femur
Spleen
Costodiaphragmatic recess
Suprarenal gland
Kidney
Gluteus maximus m.
Acetabulum
Iliacus m.
Psoas m.

Gluteus maximus m.
Pararenal fat
Splenic flexure
of colon
Kidney

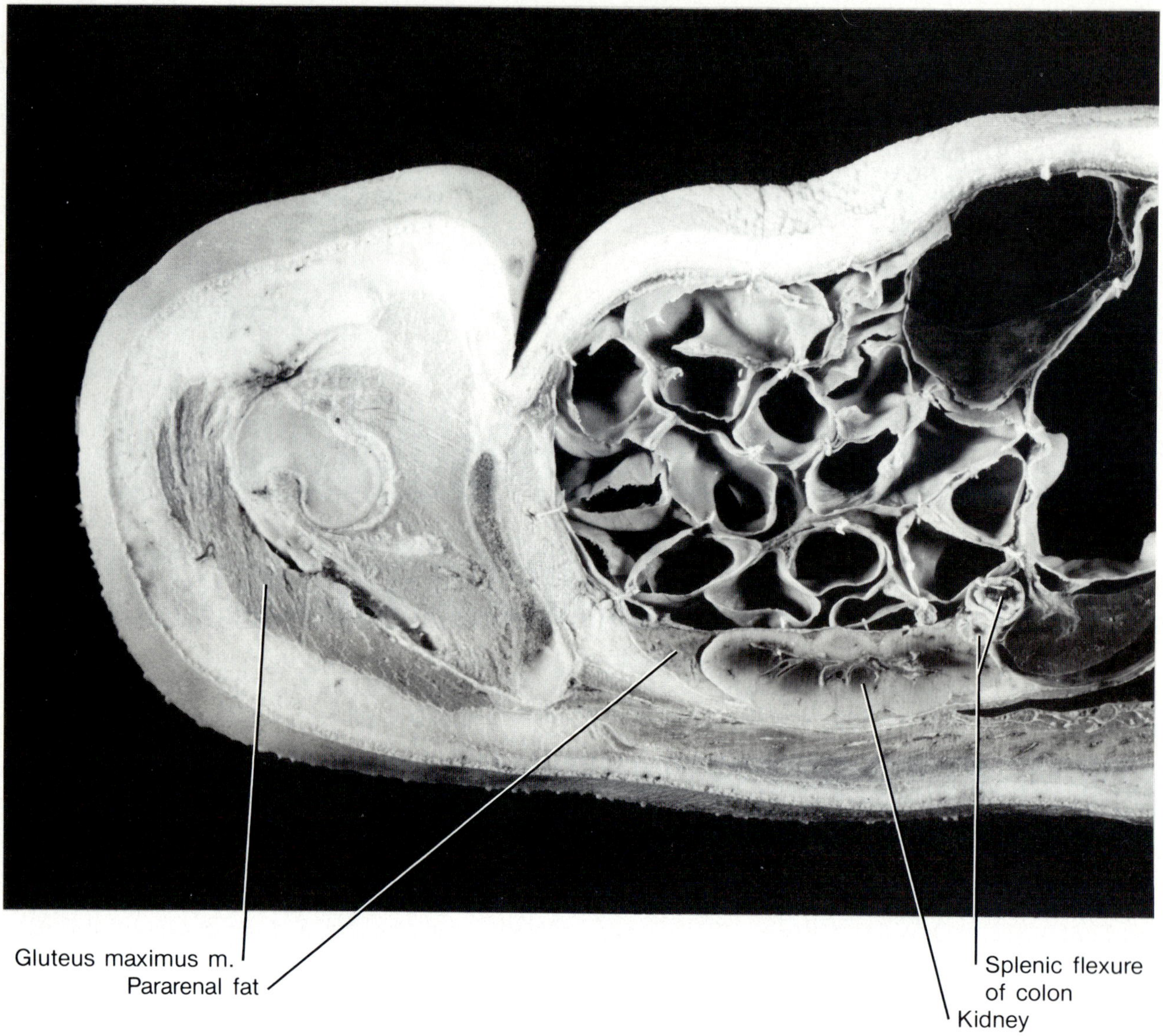

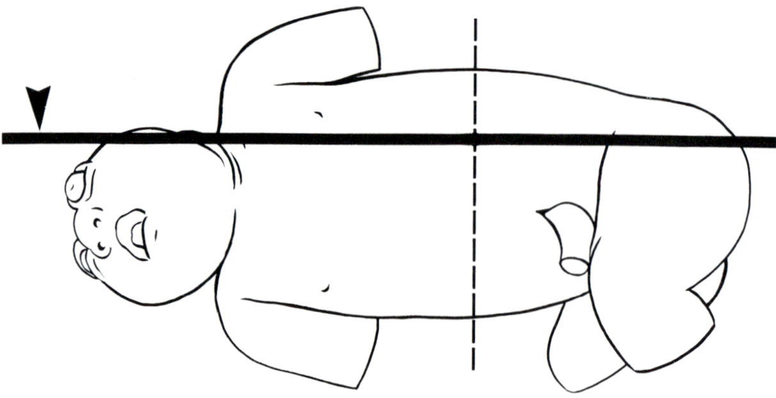

Figure 4.18

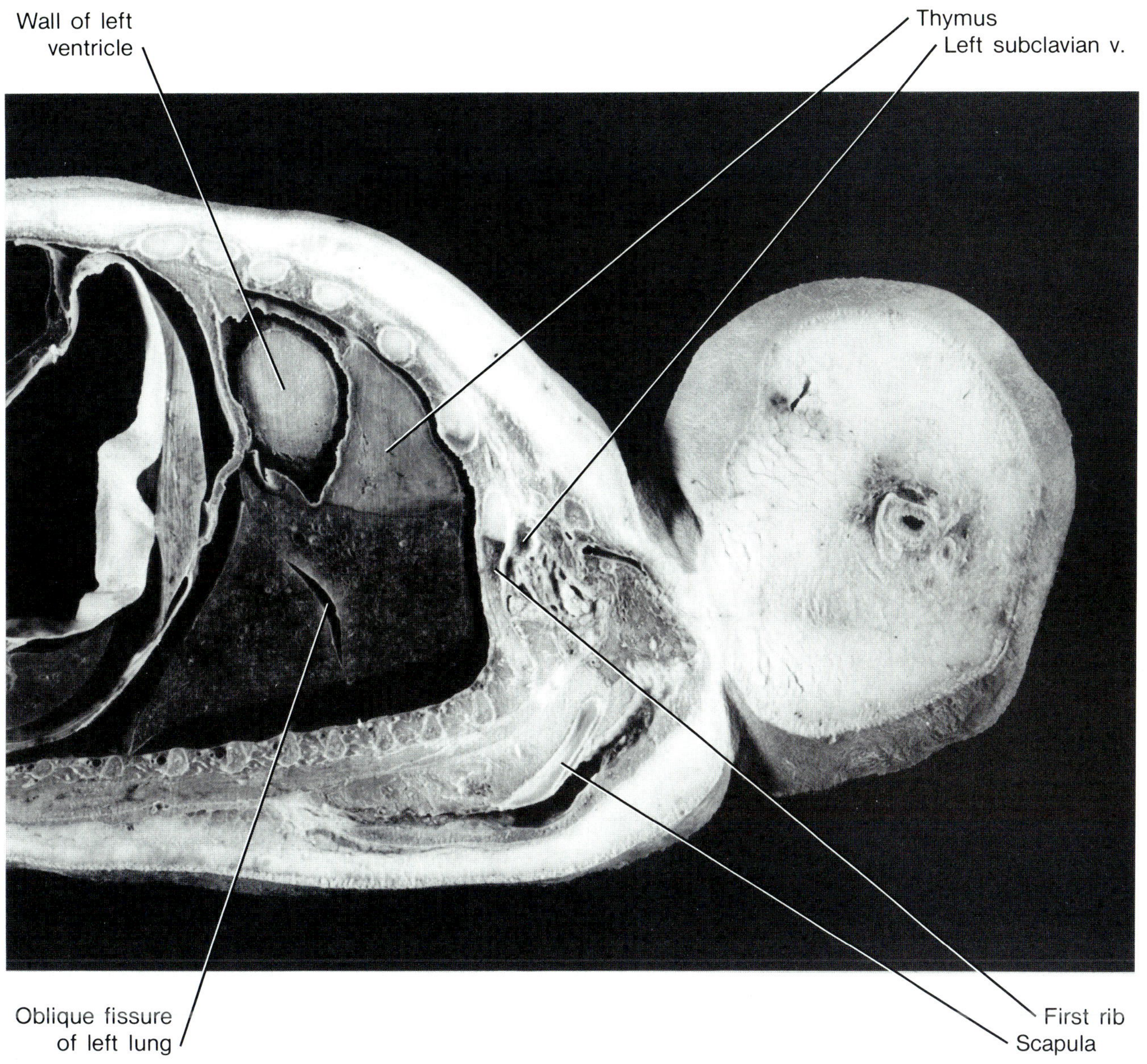

Wall of left
ventricle
Thymus
Left subclavian v.
Oblique fissure
of left lung
First rib
Scapula

Apex of heart
Thymus
First rib
Pericardial cavity
Liver
Stomach
Left subclavian a.
Scapula
Diaphragm
Oblique fissure of left lung

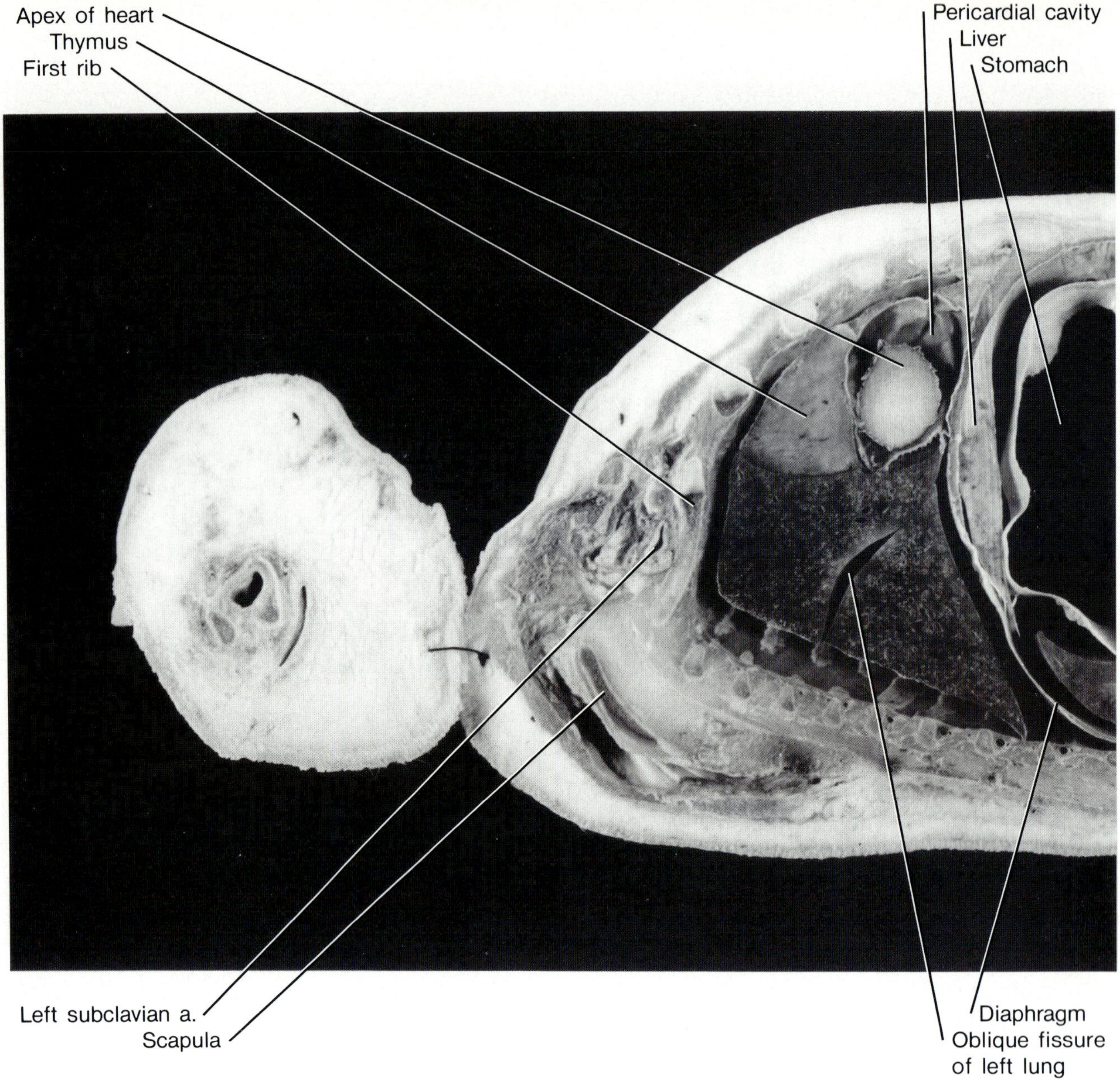

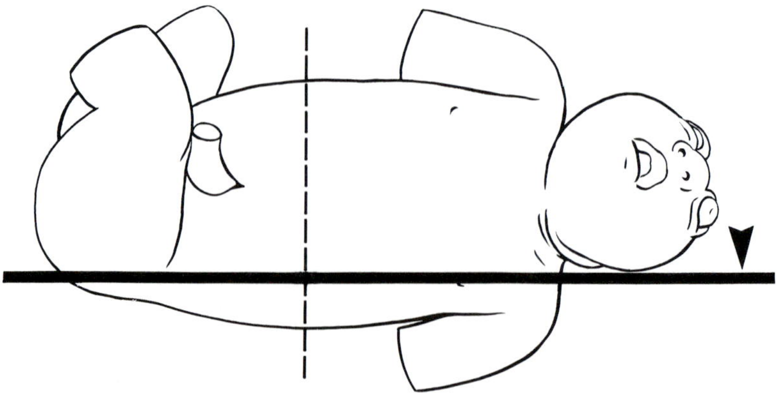

Figure 4.19

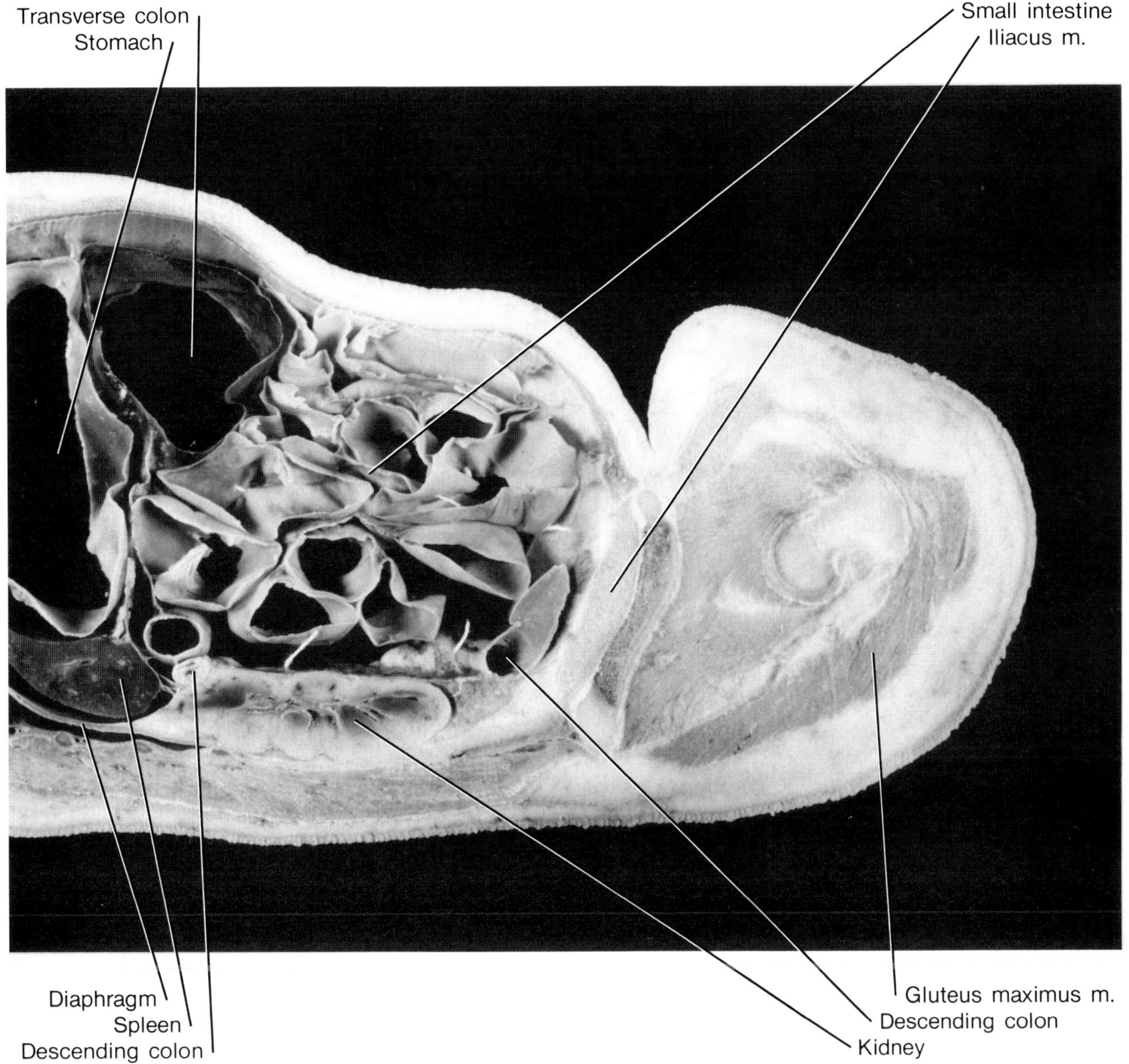

Transverse colon
Stomach
Small intestine
Iliacus m.
Diaphragm
Spleen
Descending colon
Gluteus maximus m.
Descending colon
Kidney

Anterior abdominal muscles
Transverse colon
Sigmoid colon
Kidney
Splenic flexure
Latissimus dorsi m.
Spleen
Diaphragm

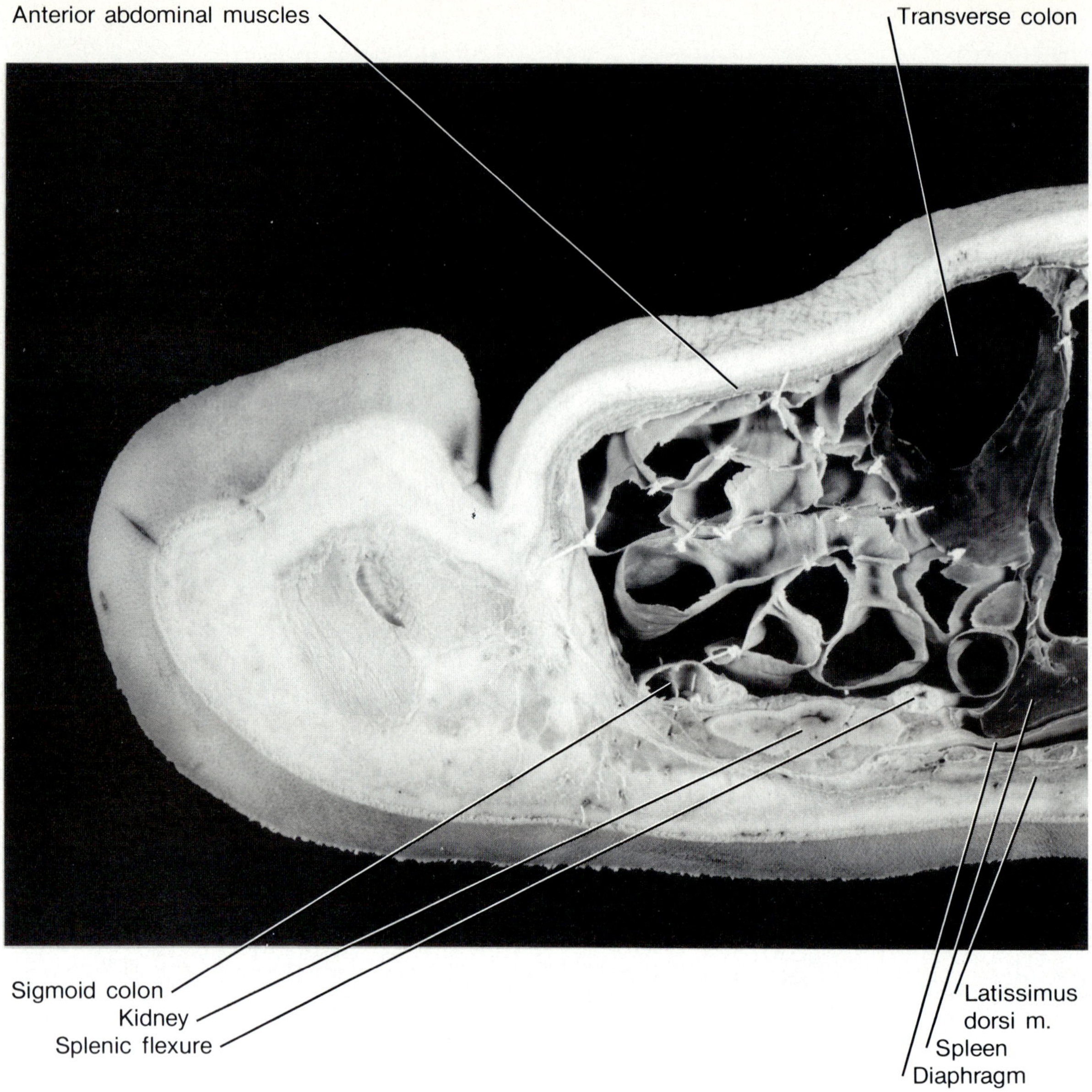

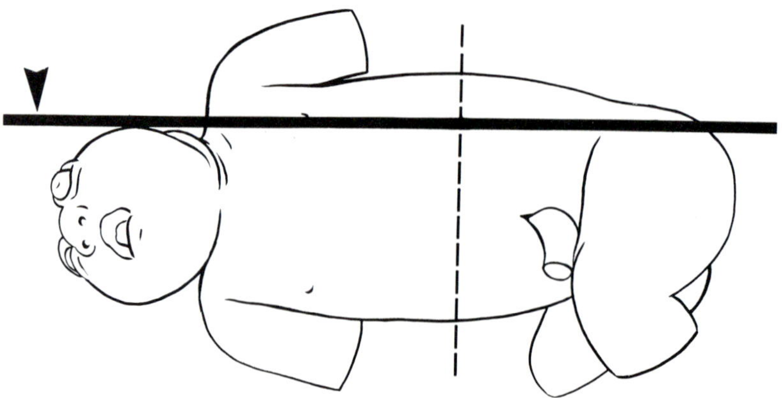

Figure 4.20

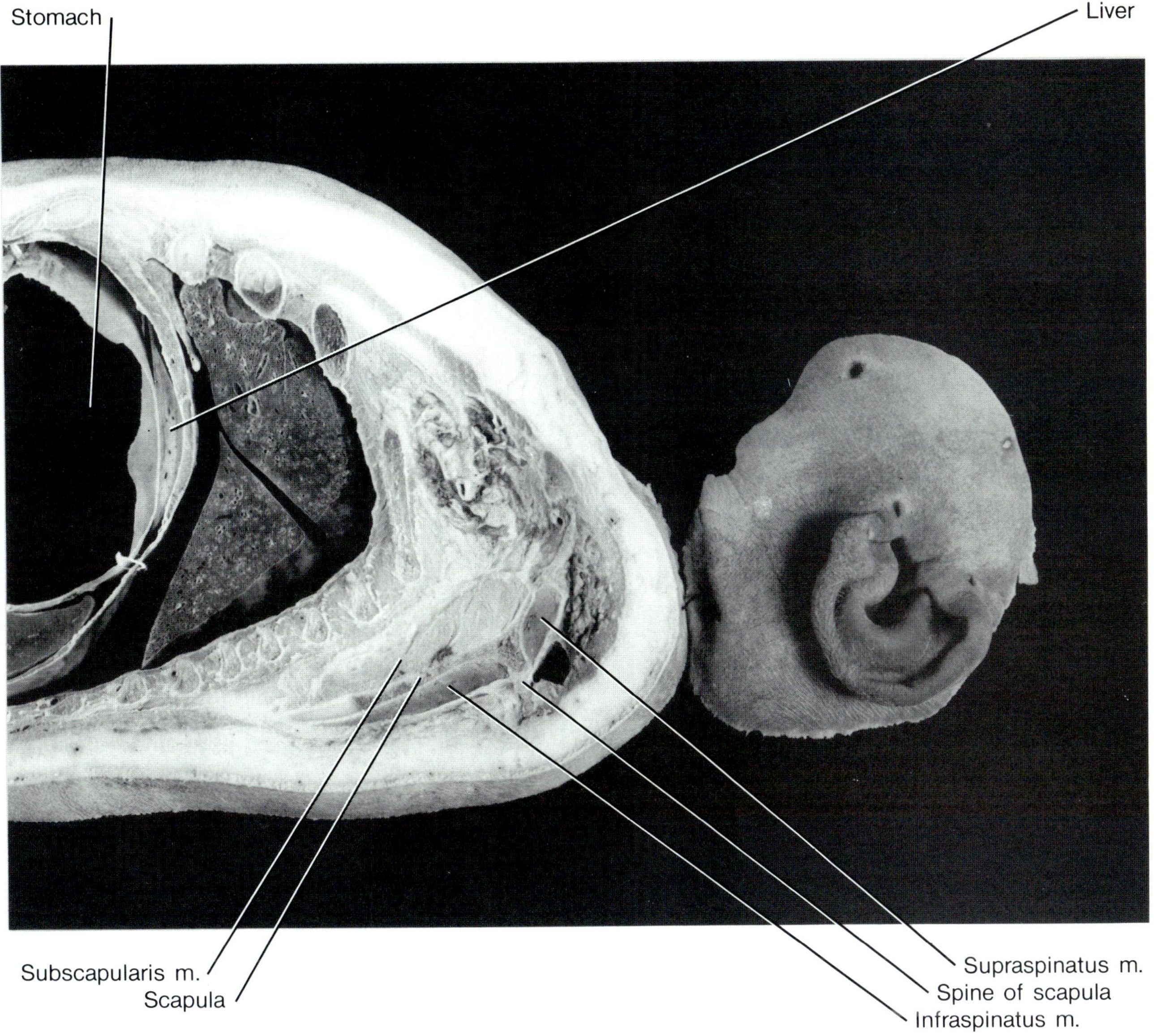

Stomach
Liver
Subscapularis m.
Scapula
Supraspinatus m.
Spine of scapula
Infraspinatus m.

Lung
Cords of brachial plexus
Clavicle
Diaphragm
Stomach
Transverse colon
Trapezius m.
Supraspinatus m.
Infraspinatus m.
Subscapularis m.
Spleen
Scapula

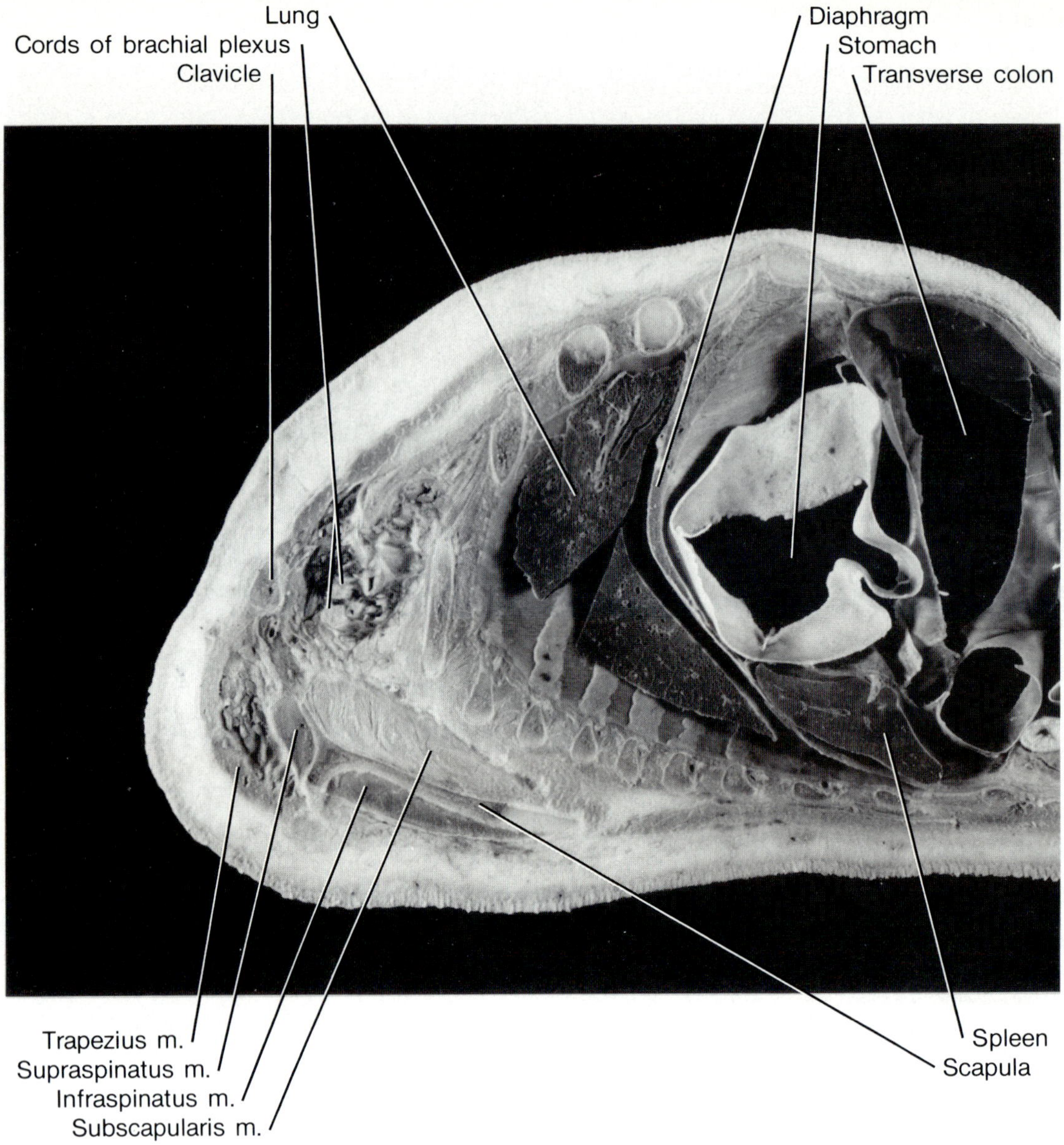

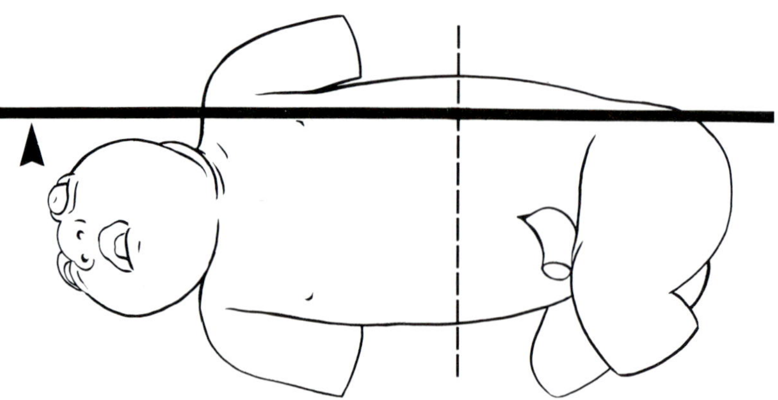

Figure 4.21

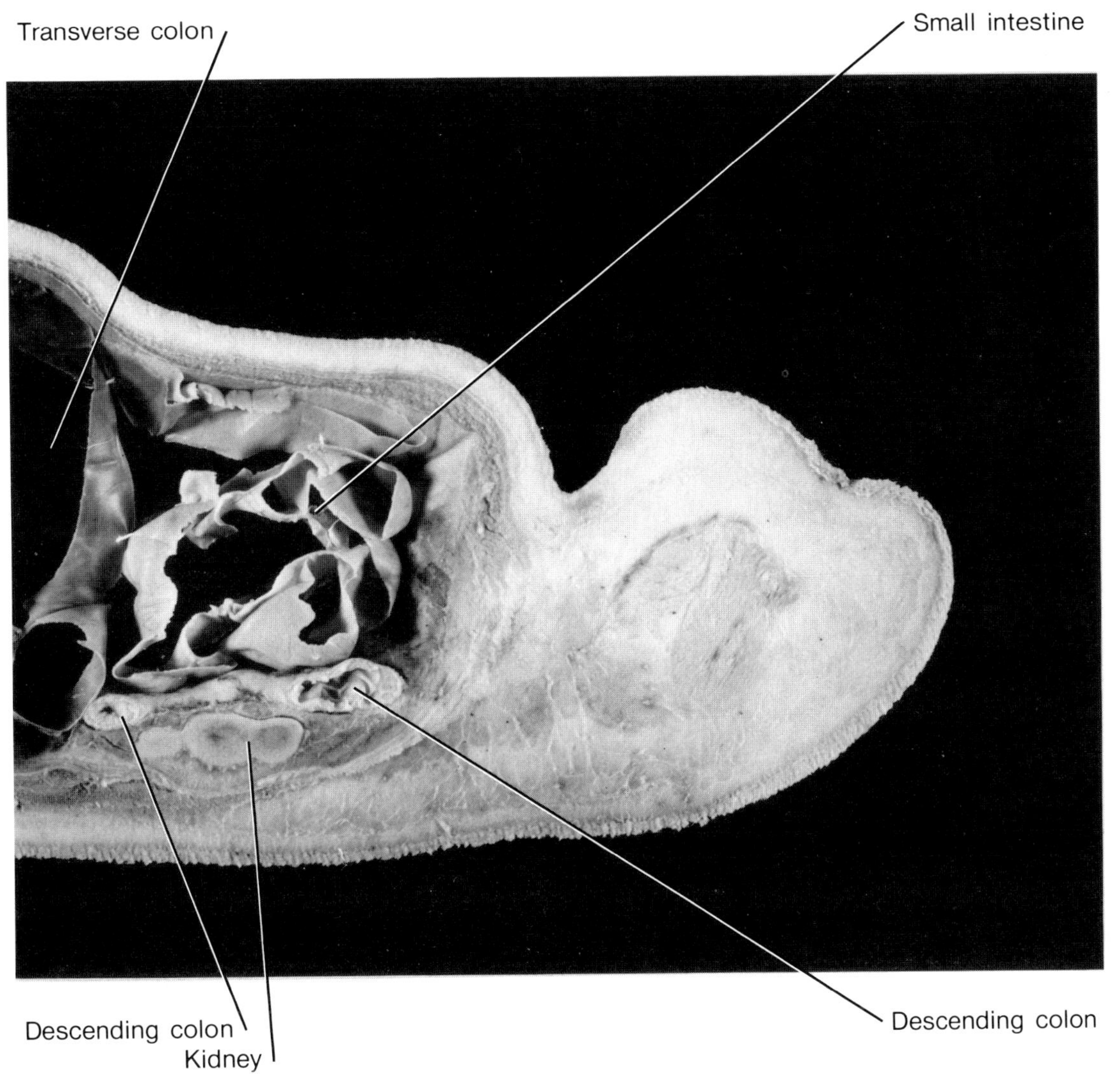
Transverse colon
Small intestine
Descending colon
Kidney
Descending colon

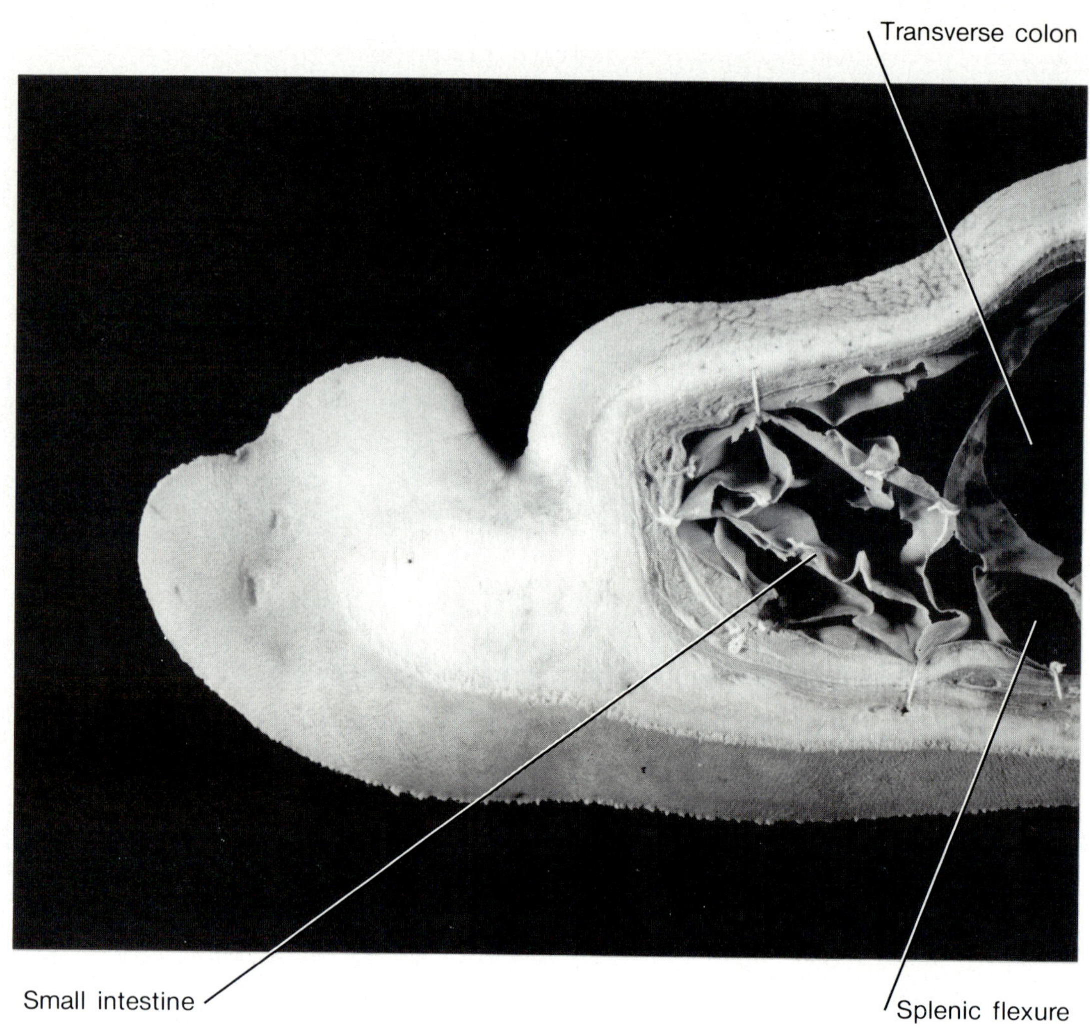

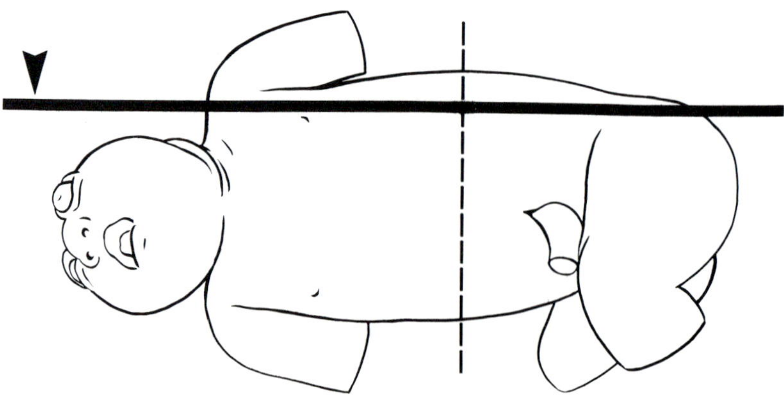

Figure 4.22

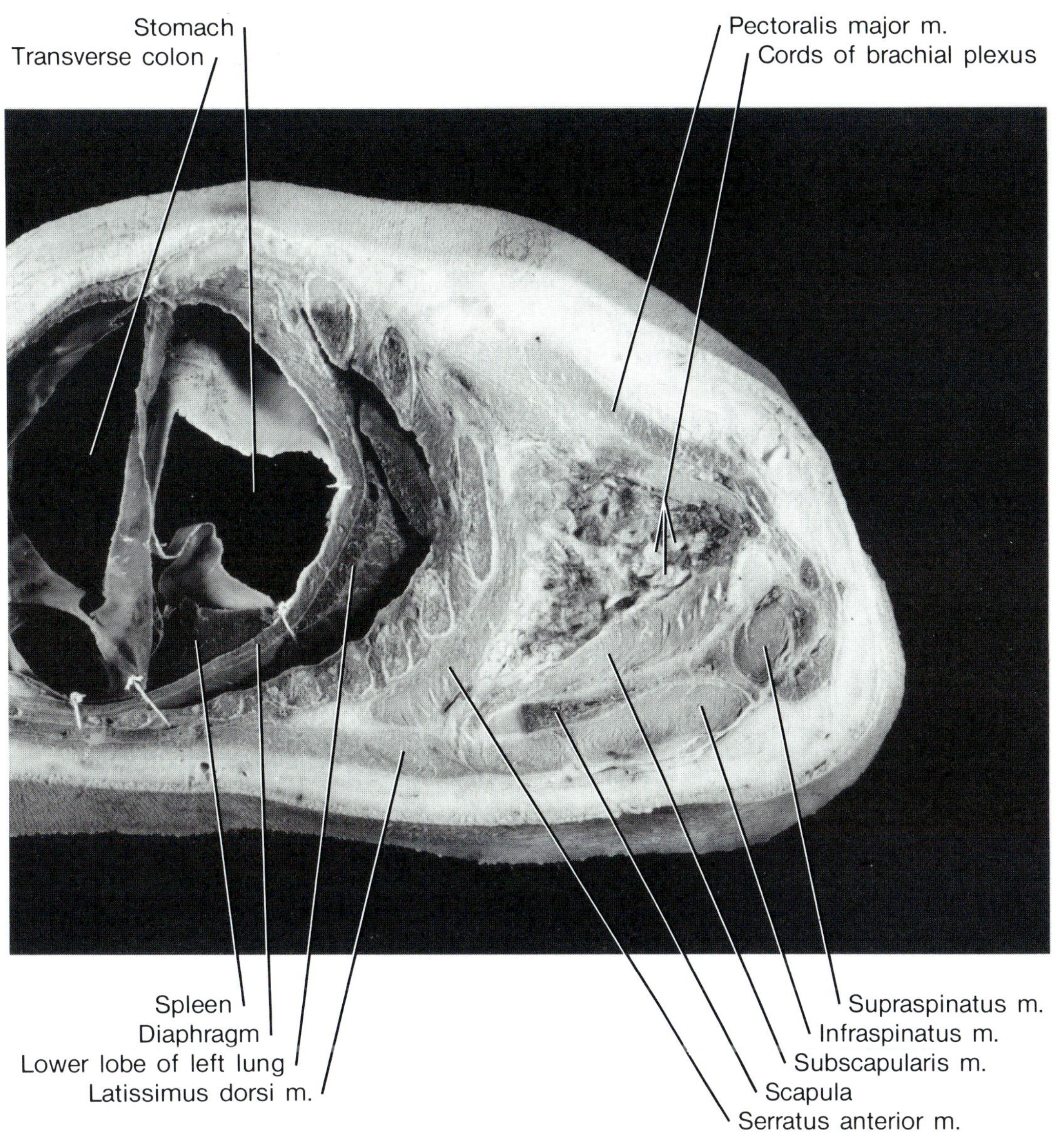

Stomach
Transverse colon
Pectoralis major m.
Cords of brachial plexus
Spleen
Diaphragm
Lower lobe of left lung
Latissimus dorsi m.
Supraspinatus m.
Infraspinatus m.
Subscapularis m.
Scapula
Serratus anterior m.

Subscapularis m.
Head of scapula
Clavicle
Second metacarpal
First metacarpal
Thenar eminence
Stomach
Supraspinatus m.
Infraspinatus m.
Scapula
Latissimus dorsi m.
Spleen
Diaphragm
Pleural cavity
Serratus anterior m.

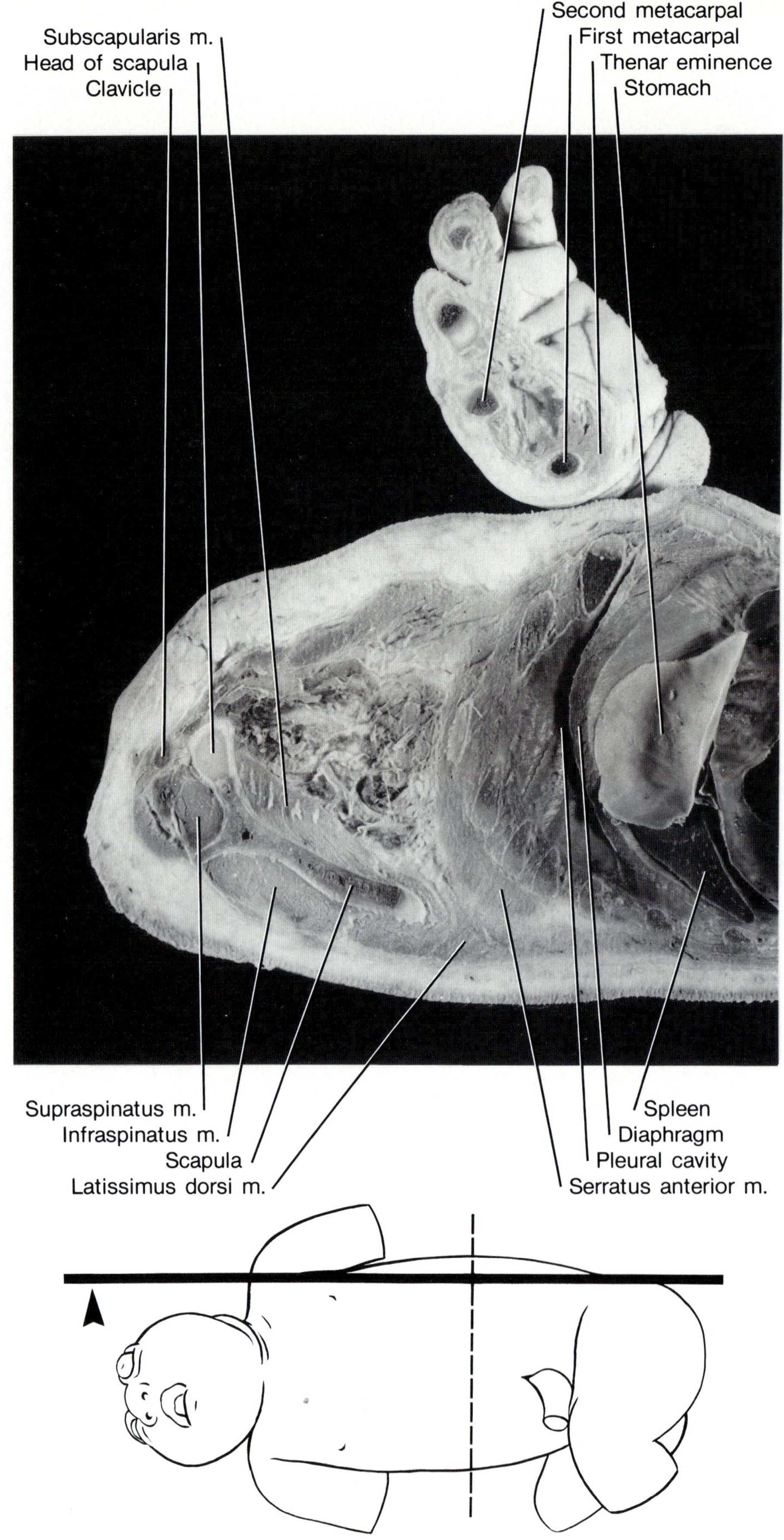

Figure 4.23

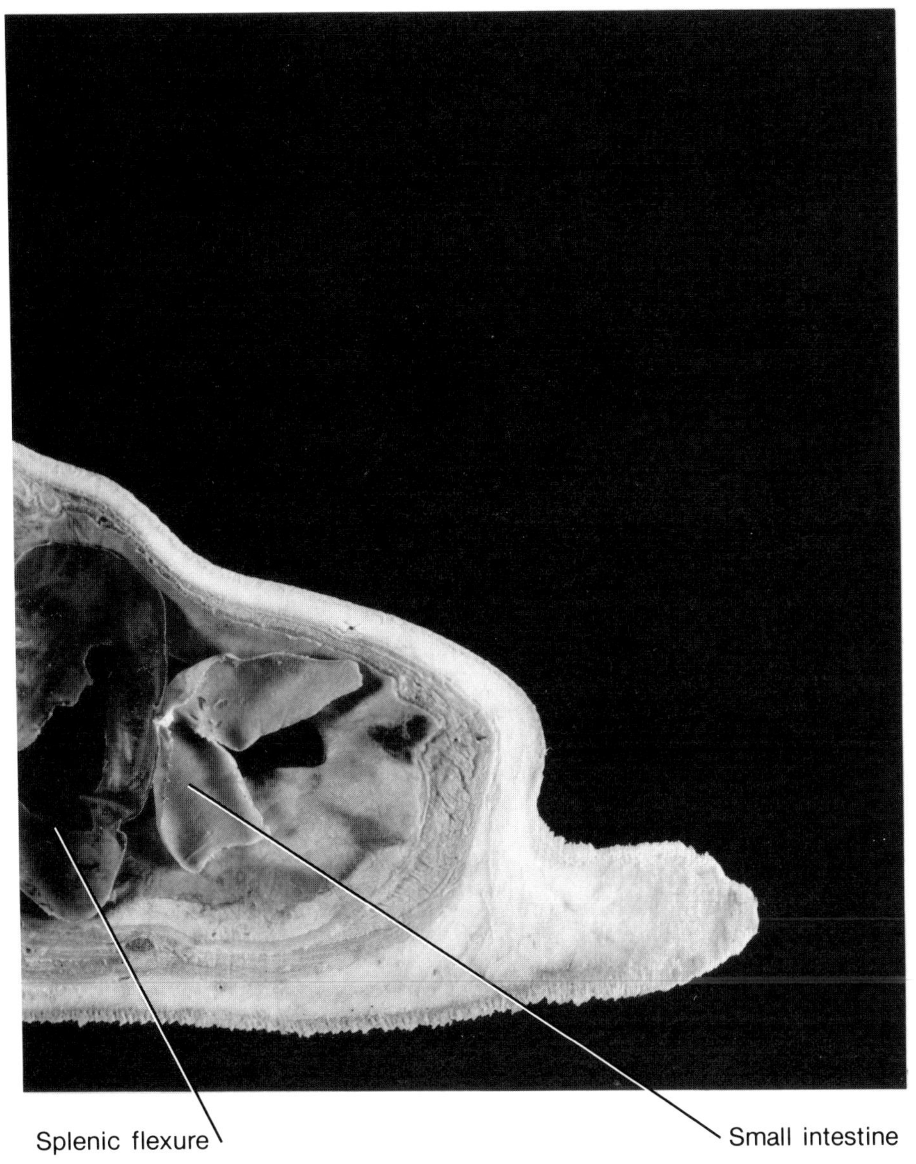

Splenic flexure
Small intestine

5

EXTREMITIES

Epiphyseal plate
Deltoid m.
Shaft of humerus
Brachialis m.
Biceps brachii m.
Head of humerus
Capsule of shoulder joint
Spine of scapula
Carpal bones
Epiphyseal plate
Shaft of radius
Triceps m.
Capitulum
Head of radius

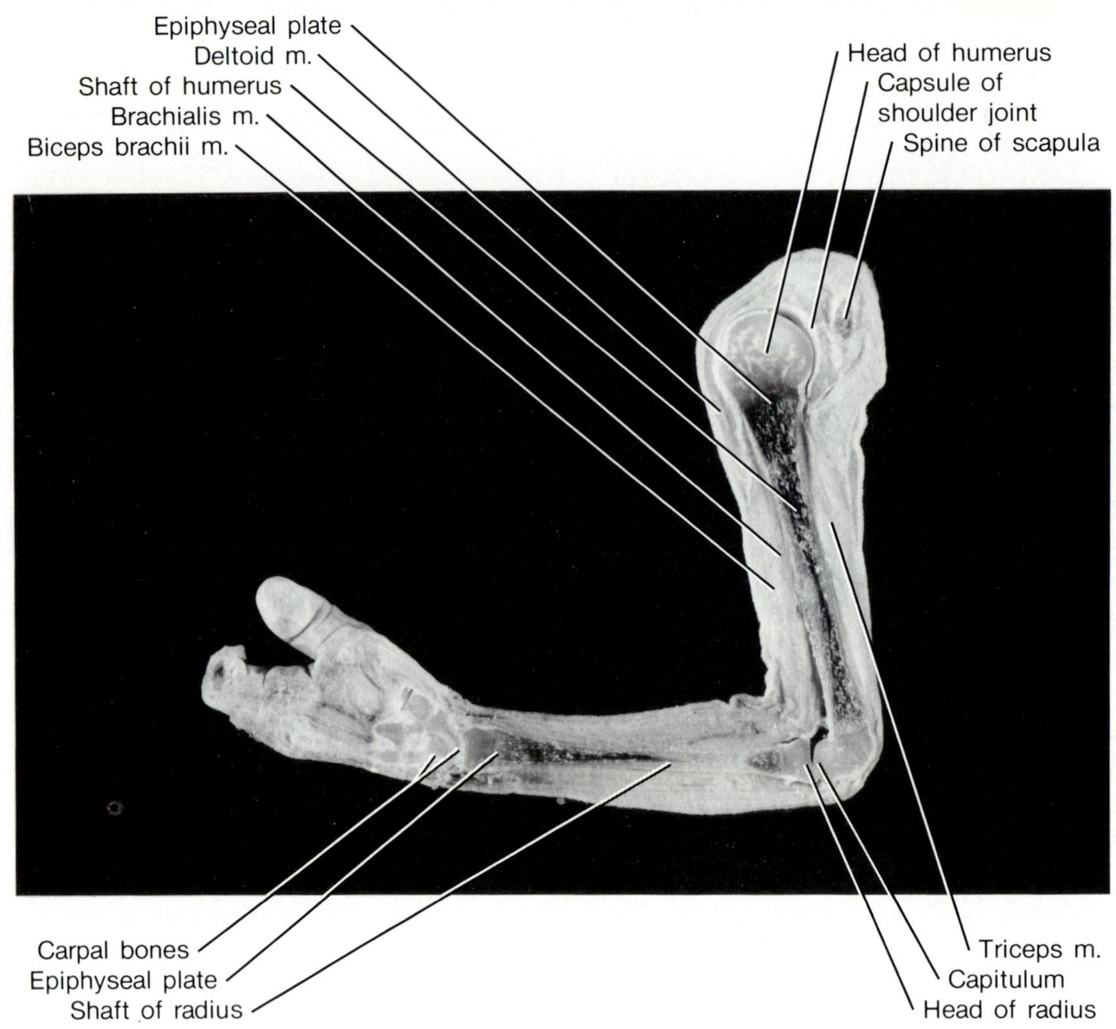

Figure 5.1

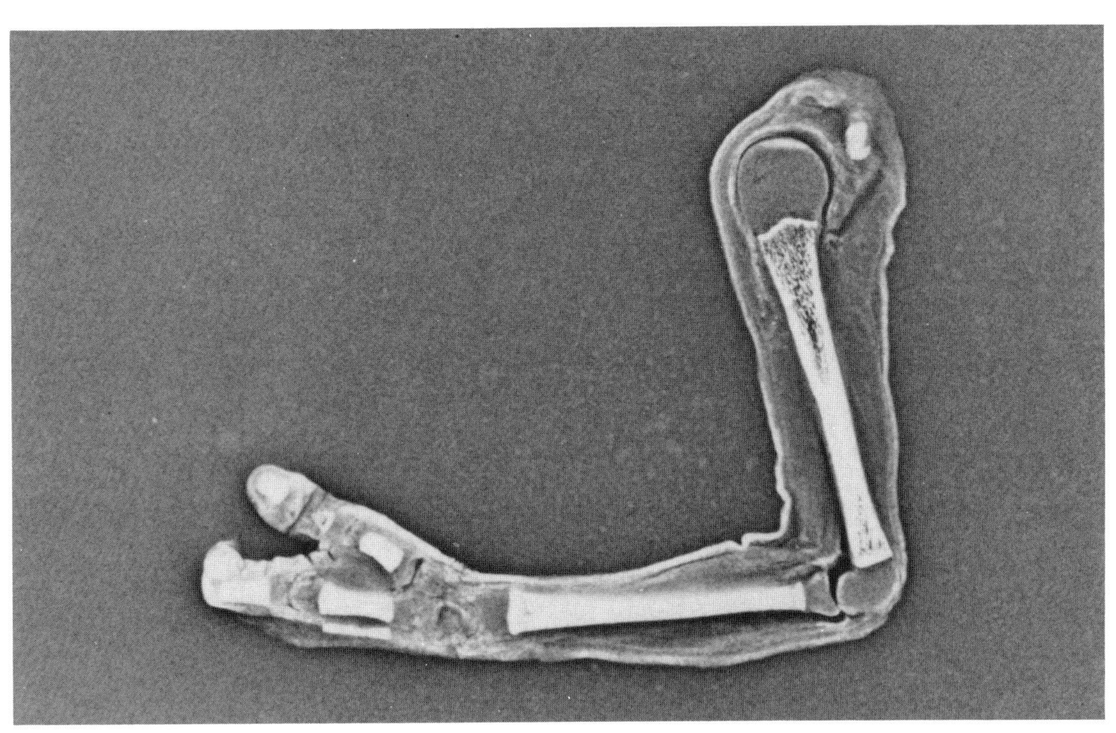

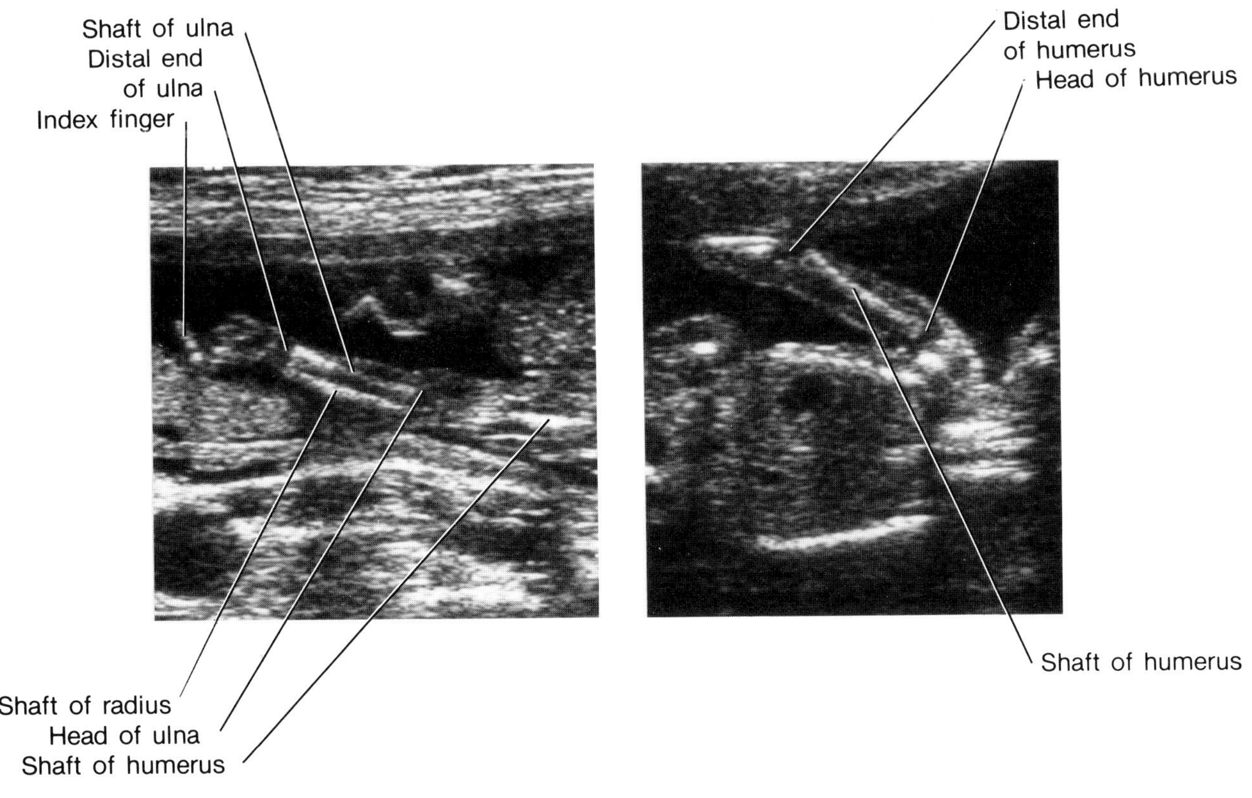
Shaft of ulna
Distal end
of ulna
Index finger
Distal end
of humerus
Head of humerus
Shaft of radius
Head of ulna
Shaft of humerus
Shaft of humerus

Shaft of femur
Extensor group
of muscles
Medial condyle of tibia
Flexor group of muscles
Popliteal vessels

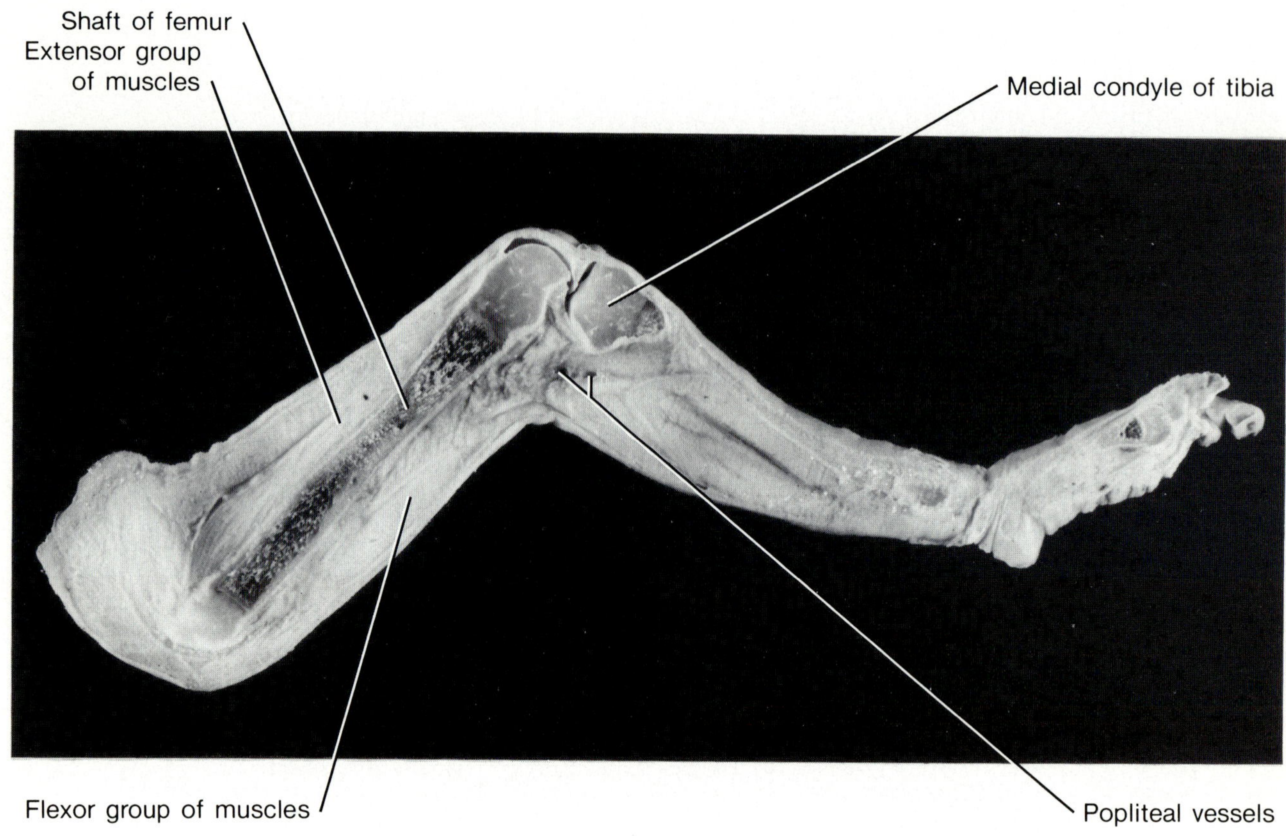

Figure 5.2

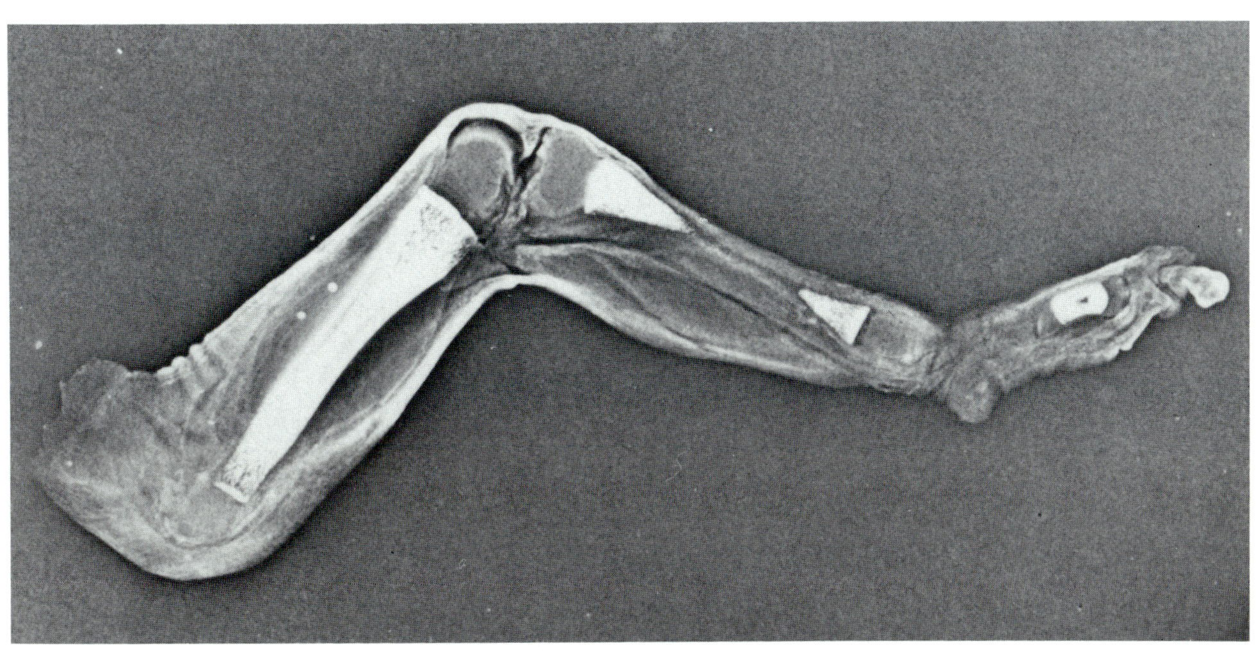

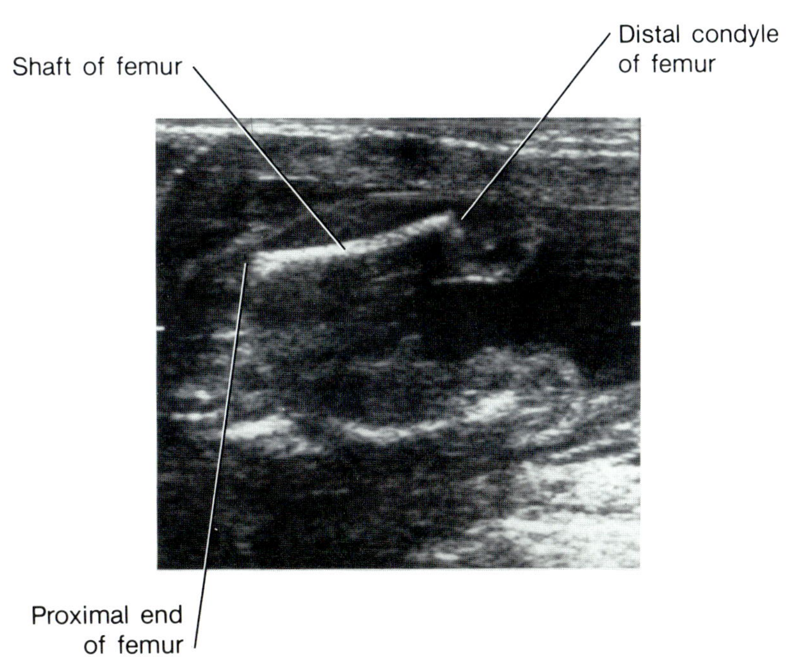

Shaft of femur

Distal condyle
of femur

Proximal end
of femur

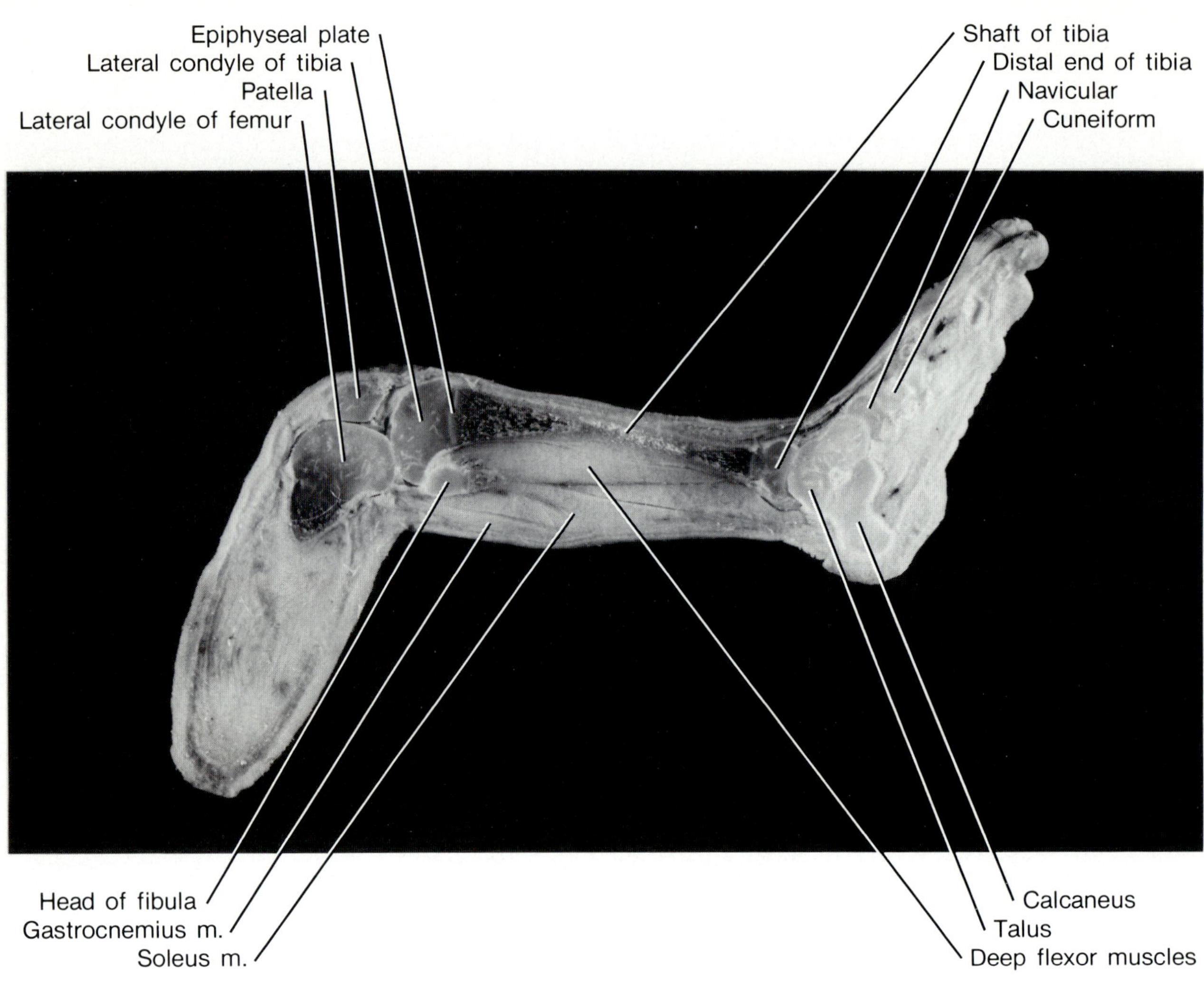

Figure 5.3

 FETAL SECTIONAL ANATOMY AND ULTRASONOGRAPHY

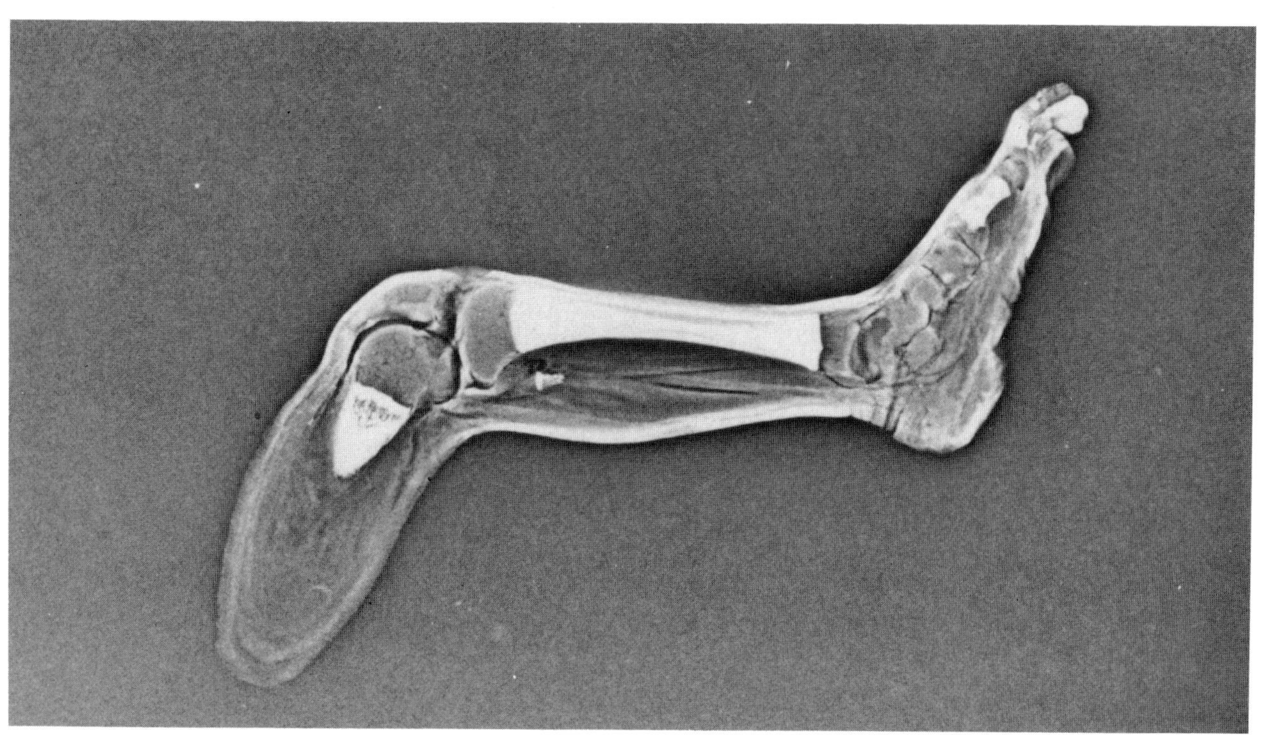

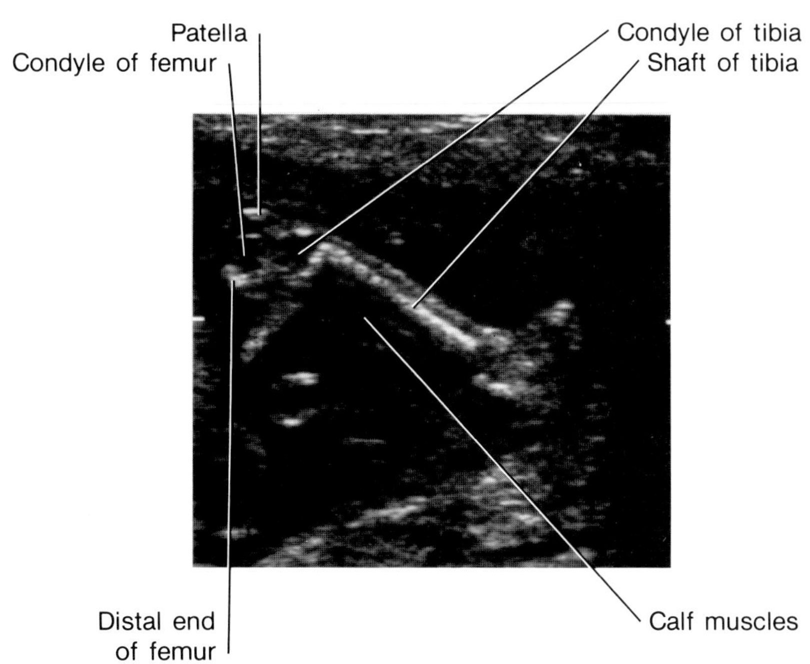

Patella
Condyle of femur
Condyle of tibia
Shaft of tibia
Distal end
of femur
Calf muscles

Lateral condyle
of tibia
Patella
Extensor group
of muscles
Talus
Lateral condyle
of femur
Head of fibula
Shaft of fibula
Cuboid
Calcaneus
Distal end of fibula

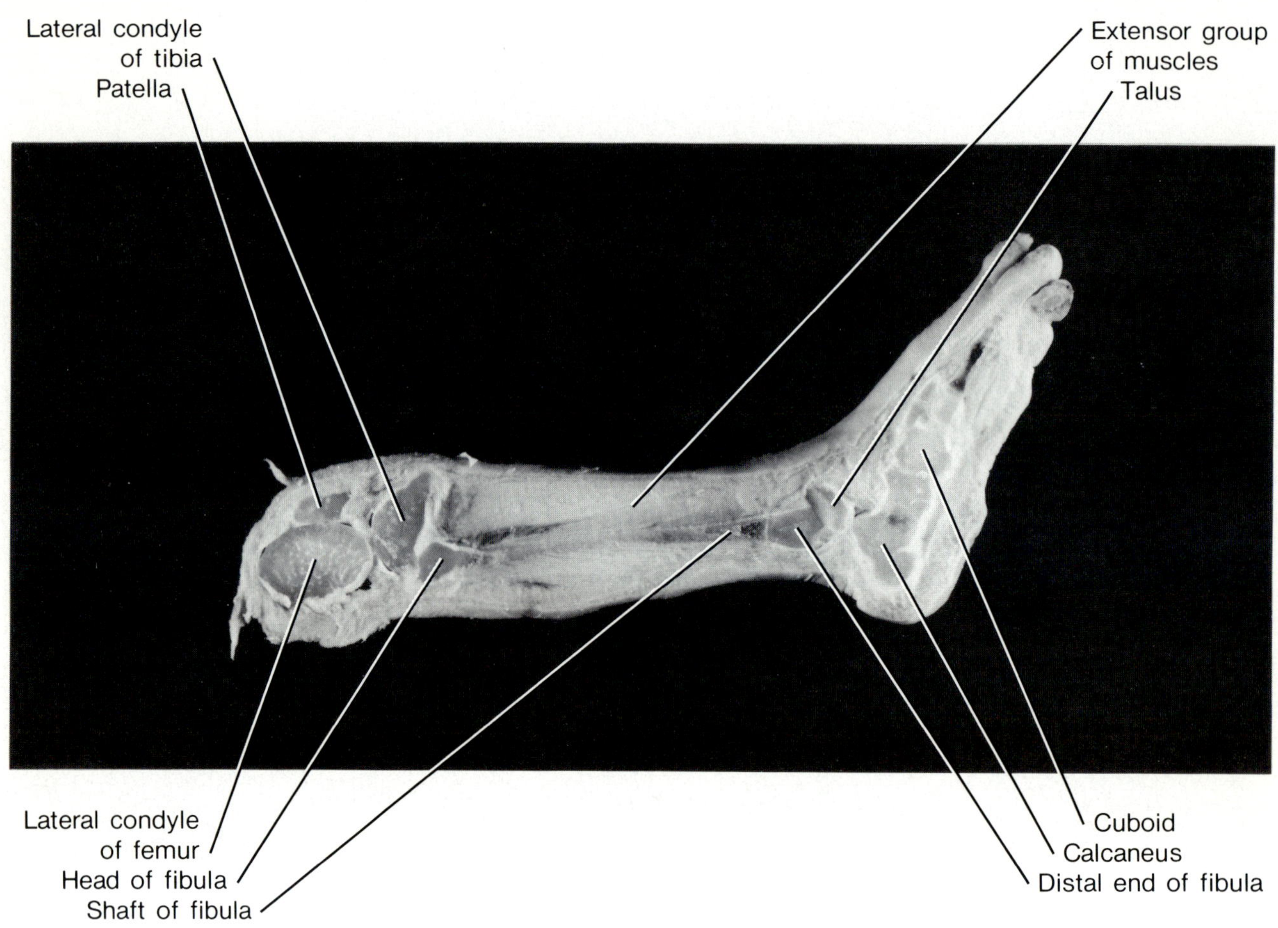

Figure 5.4

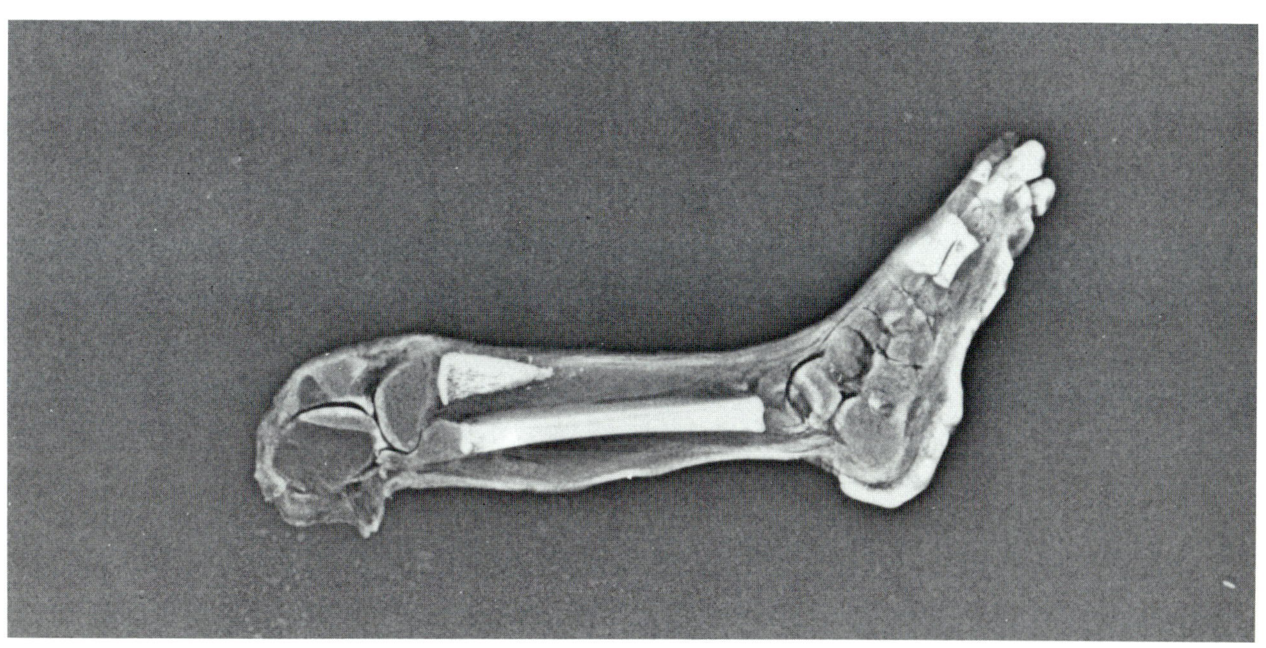

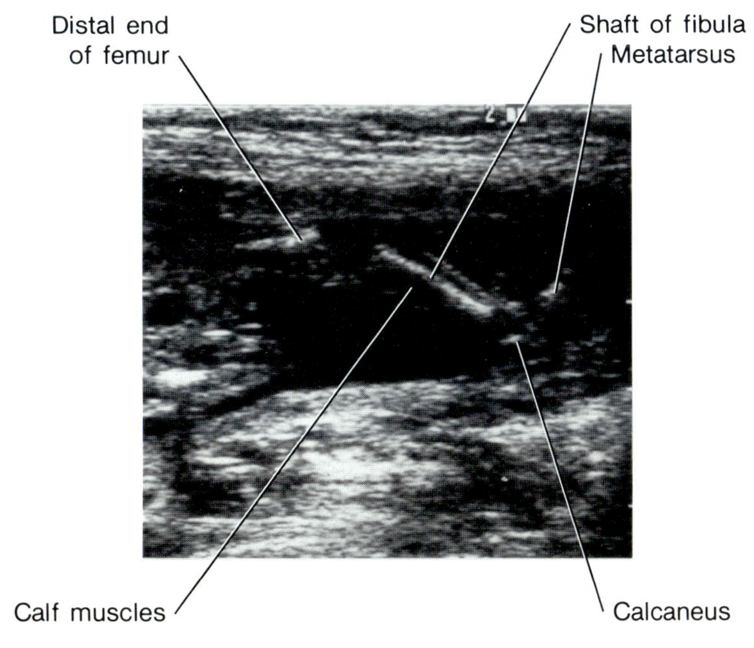

Distal end
of femur
Shaft of fibula
Metatarsus
Calf muscles
Calcaneus

INDEX

Page numbers in *italics* denote figures; those followed by "t" denote tables.